# Allergy Free

## An Alternative Medicine Definitive Guide

*by* KONRAD KAIL, N.D., *and* BOBBI LAWRENCE,
*with* BURTON GOLDBERG

ALTERNATIVEMEDICINE.COM BOOKS
TIBURON, CALIFORNIA

YEARY LIBRARY
LAREDO COMM. COLLEGE
LAREDO, TEXAS

AlternativeMedicine.com, Inc.
1640 Tiburon Blvd., Suite 2
Tiburon, CA 94920
www.alternativemedicine.com

Copyright © 2000 by AlternativeMedicine.com
All rights reserved.
No part of this book may be reproduced in any form without the expressed writ-
ten consent of the publisher, except by a reviewer, who may quote brief passages
in connection with a review.

Editor: John W. Anderson
Associate Editor: Ellen Cavalli
Art Director: Janine White
Production Manager: Gail Gongoll
Production Assistance: Victoria Swart

Manufactured in Canada.

10 9 8 7 6 5 4

REF.
RC
584
.K27
2000

Library of Congress Cataloging-in-Publication Data

Kail, Konrad.
    Allergy free: an alternative medicine definitive guide / by Konrad Kail
and Bobbi Lawrence, with Burton Goldberg.
            p.          cm.
    Includes bibliographical references and index.
    ISBN 1-887299-36-X (pbk.)
    1. Allergy—Alternative treatment. I. Lawrence, Bobbi. II. Goldberg, Burton,
1926- III. Title.

RC584.K27          2000
616.97'06—dc21                                          00-038575

                        CIP

OCT 1 0 2002

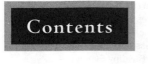

# Contents

# About the Authors

**Konrad Kail, N.D.**, is co-owner of Naturopathic Family Care, Inc., a naturopathic group practice in Phoenix, Arizona, that provides integrated—conventional as well as complementary and alternative (CAM)—medical services, emphasizing prevention and natural therapeutics. Dr. Kail was certified as a Physician's Assistant and received a B.S. in Medicine from Baylor College of Medicine in 1976 and a doctorate in Naturopathic Medicine (N.D.) from the National College of Naturopathic Medicine and Health Sciences in 1983. He is a Fellow of the American College of Naturopathic Family Medicine and Minor Surgery.

Dr. Kail is co-founder and serves on the Board of Directors of the Southwest College of Naturopathic Medicine and Health Sciences; past president and serves on the advisory board of the American Association of Naturopathic Physicians; and is a member of the Advisory Council to the National Center for Complementary and Alternative Medicine (NCCAM) at the National Institutes for Health. Dr. Kail is also president of the board of U.S. Complementary Health, Inc., a consulting and marketing corporation for his allergy research projects. He has appeared in the media and lectured nationally and internationally on allergies.

**Bobbi Lawrence** is a freelance writer based in Larkspur, California.

# Important Information

Burton Goldberg and the editors of *Alternative Medicine* are proud of the public and professional praise accorded AlternativeMedicine.com's (formerly Future Medicine Publishing) series of books. This latest book in the series continues the groundbreaking tradition of its predecessors.

Your health and that of your loved ones is important. Treat this book as an educational tool which will enable you to better understand, assess, and choose the best course of treatment when a health problem arises, and how to prevent health problems such as allergies from developing in the first place.

Remember that this book on allergies is different. This book is about alternative approaches to health—approaches generally not understood and, at this time, not endorsed by the medical establishment. We urge you to discuss the treatments described in this book with your doctor. If your doctor is open-minded, you may actually educate him or her. We have been gratified to learn that many of our readers have found their physicians open to the new ideas presented to them.

Use this book wisely. As many of the treatments described in this book are, by definition, alternative, they have not been investigated, approved, or endorsed by any government or regulatory agency. National, state, and local laws may vary regarding the use and application of many of the treatments discussed. Accordingly, this book should not be substituted for the advice and care of a physician or other licensed health-care professional. Pregnant women, in particular, are urged to consult a physician before commencing any therapy. Ultimately, you must take responsibility for your health and how you use the information in this book.

AlternativeMedicine.com and the authors have no financial interest in any of the products or services discussed in this book, with two exceptions. U.S. Complementary Health, Inc., is a consulting and product development company owned by Dr. Kail. The book also makes references in the text to AlternativeMedicine.com's other publications. All of the factual information in this book has been drawn from the scientific literature. To protect privacy, all patient names have been changed. Branded products and services discussed in the book are evaluated solely on the independent and direct experience of the health-care practitioners quoted. Reference to them does not imply an endorsement nor a superiority over other branded products and services which may provide similar or superior results.

One of the features of this book is that it is interactive, thanks to the following icons:

This means you can turn to the listed pages elsewhere in this book for more information.

Many times the text mentions a medical term that requires explanation. We don't want to interrupt the text, so instead we put the explanation in the margins under this icon.

This tells you where to contact a physician, group, or publication mentioned in the text. This is an editorial service to our readers. All items are based on recommendations from the clinical practice of physicians in this book. The publisher has no financial interest in any clinic, physician, or product discussed in this book.

This sign tells you there may be some risks, uncertainties, side effects, or special contraindications regarding a procedure or substance.

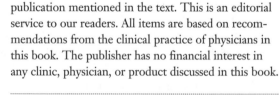

Here we refer you to our best-selling book, *Alternative Medicine: The Definitive Guide*, for more information on a particular topic.

Here we refer you to our book *Alternative Medicine Definitive Guide to Cancer* for more information on a particular topic.

Here we refer you to our book *Alternative Medicine Definitive Guide to Headaches* for more information on a particular topic.

This icon will alert you to an article published in our bimonthly magazine, *Alternative Medicine*, that is relevant to the topic under discussion.

Here we refer you to our book *The Enzyme Cure* for more information on enzymes and how they can be used to relieve health problems.

Here we refer you to our book *The Supplement Shopper* for more information on nutritional supplements for various health conditions.

# You Don't Have to Suffer with Allergies

**A**LLERGIES ARE NOT something you have to live with—alternative medicine has practical solutions for identifying and treating the underlying causes and can bring lasting relief to allergy sufferers. Many people have learned this the hard way, living with discomfort, sneezing, congestion, and pain for years before discovering that there is another option. Alternative medicine recognizes that allergies do not have one cause, but multiple factors that together overload your body systems. Looking at illness and health in this way makes for more effective treatment than the single-cause focus of conventional medicine. In this book, you will learn that once you identify the hidden factors that are combining to produce your allergies, you can treat each one and permanently eliminate your allergy symptoms. Patient success stories throughout the book provide practical details on how others were able to reverse their allergies.

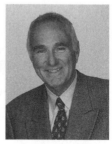

Today, an estimated 20% of Americans have allergies, making it one of the most prevalent chronic health problems. Conventional medicine offers antihistamines and other drug treatments that may temporarily relieve allergy symptoms, but also introduce serious side effects.

Alternative medicine physicians, on the other hand, focus on finding the root causes, rather than merely trying to alleviate symptoms. In this book, we show you how to prevent and reverse allergies using safe, noninvasive, and proven alternative therapies. Alternative medicine looks at the whole person, considering the individual's symptoms, health history, diet, and underlying imbalances. You can then use a combination of alternative treatments to heal these underlying causes leading to allergies, bringing lasting relief, not a simple masking of symptoms. This is the basic principle of alternative medicine and the reason why it succeeds where conventional medicine often fails in treatment of chronic disease.

You'll learn more about these treatment options:

■ Steps to prevent allergies from occurring in the first place, including advice to parents about breast-feeding and vaccinations for their children.

■ How to eliminate toxins from your home environment.

■ How to avoid foods that aggravate allergies and increase foods that support healing.

■ Strategies for supporting your digestive system, skin, and respiratory system— your frontline of defense against allergies.

■ Safe and effective allergy-stoppers—herbs, vitamins and minerals, essential fatty acids, and homeopathic remedies.

■ Physical therapies to improve allergy and asthma symptoms.

■ The role of stress in allergies and effective mind/body therapies to cope with stress.

**This book is here to tell you that you don't have to live with allergies, or with a continuing cycle of drugs and their side effects. By treating what is actually causing the condition, not only can allergies be reversed but your overall health will be improved.**

This book is here to tell you that you don't have to live with allergies, or with a continuing cycle of drugs and their side effects. By treating what is actually causing the condition, not only can allergies be reversed but your overall health will be improved. Start with the alternative therapies in this book to relieve your sneezing and congestion and eliminate your allergies for good. God bless.

—Burton Goldberg

# Visit our website at
# www.alternativemedicine.com

# 1

# Understanding Allergy and Sensitivity

I
F YOU FIND YOURSELF sneezing and coughing, with watery eyes and swollen sinuses each spring, you're probably aware that you have allergies. What might surprise you is that your child's ear infections or your spouse's digestive problems may stem from allergies, too. Recent research confirms that allergies manifest as various common ailments and disorders—from headaches to autism—that can occur any time of year, in just about anybody.

And just about everybody, it seems, has allergies. In industrialized nations, the number of people with allergies is rising at an alarming rate, and according to the American Academy of Allergy, Asthma & Immunology, more than 20% of the U.S. population—adults and children—has an allergic condition, making allergies the sixth-leading cause of chronic disease. Of those, more than 15 million have asthma[1] and 40 million experience chronic allergic rhinitis or its seasonal counterpart, hay fever, each year.[2] Studies have revealed that children from affluent backgrounds as well as those who have had fewer viral infections show a higher prevalence of allergic diseases, including asthma, atopic dermatitis, and allergic rhinitis.[3] The U.S. Department of Agriculture reports that 15% of the population has food allergies or sensitivities.[4] According to James Braly, M.D., medical director of Immuno Laboratories in Fort Lauderdale, Florida, food sensitivities and allergies can be the basis or a contributing factor in up to 80 medical conditions. Also pervasive are chemical sensitivities, in which some people expe-

## In This Chapter

- Allergy, Sensitivity, Intolerance: What's the Difference?
- Success Story: From Asthma to Tibet with Alternative Medicine
- Allergy 101: The Basics of Antibody–Antigen Reactions
- Types of Allergies and Allergic Conditions
- What Happens in a Non-Antibody–Mediated Event?

rience hives, headaches, muscle pains, and mental impairment, among other symptoms, when exposed to small amounts of everyday chemicals. According to a two-state study, 16% of the population reported "unusual sensitivity" to common chemicals, with another 2% to 6% diagnosed with multiple chemical sensitivity (MCS).[5] Multi-government studies reveal that Gulf War veterans experience MCS at a rate two to four times higher than undeployed personnel.[6]

Conventional medicine currently offers limited treatment options, generally medications, which provide only temporary relief of allergy symptoms. In some cases, the treatment may ultimately lead to new health problems. Alternative medicine practitioners, however, have found that by correcting the underlying causes of allergies, you can eliminate most allergy symptoms for good. Modifying your diet and restoring your allergy-defense functions may help you breathe, eat, and live normally again.

# Allergy, Sensitivity, Intolerance: What's the Difference?

Most people tend to think of any adverse reaction to an ordinarily innocuous substance as an allergy. Indeed, even the title of this book, *Allergy Free*, complies with this perspective. But if you've ever gone to a doctor expecting an allergy diagnosis, because eating bread always leads to a migraine, you know that the semantics of "allergy" is a tricky thing.

## Glossary of Terms

**Allergy:** Refers to the immune system's hypersensitivity upon re-exposure to a sensitizing agent, which results in the release of inflammatory chemicals and development of various symptoms. Although the presence of immunoglobulin E has traditionally been the marker of an allergy, the term *allergy* is correctly applied when diagnosing an adverse reaction involving elevation of specific antibodies due to antigen stimulus.

**Sensitivity:** Refers to adverse reactions in the body upon exposure to a sensitizing agent in the environment. It does not involve antibodies, although it may involve other immunological processes. Most food and chemical reactions are sensitivities. Also called "pseudo-allergy."

**Intolerance:** Refers to the absence of a particular chemical or physiological process needed to digest a food substance. The lack of the digestive enzyme lactase results in milk intolerance, or the inability to properly digest milk products. Gastrointestinal upset is often a sign of intolerance. Intolerance and sensitivity are used interchangeably or are simply referred to as "allergy"; however, intolerance is not a true allergy.

**Atopy:** Describes the inherited tendency to develop IgE-mediated immune responses. *Atopic* individuals have a higher risk for developing asthma, allergic rhinitis, and eczema.

## A Brief History of Allergy

The term *allergy* was first coined in 1906 by an Austrian pediatrician, Clemens von Pirquet, to describe the "altered reactivity" some of his patients had to substances ("allergens") that didn't affect most other people. The concept, however, goes back much further, and we can be fairly certain that an allergic reaction was what the Roman philosopher Lucretius had in mind when he stated over 2,000 years ago that "One man's meat is another man's poison."

The original meaning of allergy referred to any altered response to a substance, but by 1925 the majority of American allergists had accepted a narrower definition to describe an adverse immune system response, particularly one that could be scientifically demonstrated with the introduction of a substance, such as pollen, mold, animal dander, and dust, via a skin prick test. The reactions recorded by this testing method have become our classic allergic conditions: allergic rhinitis and hay fever, asthma, eczema, hives, and the life-threatening cascade of symptoms leading to anaphylactic shock. In the 1960s, scientists discovered that the skin prick test was actually measuring the presence of an antibody (SEE QUICK DEFINITION) called immunoglobulin E (IgE) in the immune system. The definition of allergy became even more specific: an adverse response that could be detected by the presence of IgE; in clinical jargon, "IgE-mediated."

For more on the **skin prick test**, see Chapter 3: Allergy/Sensitivity Testing, pp. 70-105.

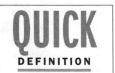

# QUICK
## DEFINITION

An **antibody** is a protein molecule made from amino acids by white blood cells in the circulation and set in motion by the immune system against a specific foreign protein, or antigen. An antibody is also referred to as an immunoglobulin and may be found in body fluids (the blood, lymph, saliva, gastrointestinal and urinary tracts), usually within three days after the first encounter with an antigen. The antibody binds tightly with the antigen in order to remove it from the system or destroy it. This is when the inflammatory chemicals (histamine and others) are released into the tissues causing irritating symptoms. The resulting antigen–antibody complexes are then excreted in the urine.

As mainstream medicine took a progressively more restrictive approach to allergy diagnosis, several physicians, including Theron Randolph, M.D., began investigating largely overlooked sources of adverse reactions, particularly food and chemical agents. They found that IgE was not involved in all types of adverse reactions, especially those that occurred hours or days after exposure to a food or environmental substance. Conventional medicine frowned upon what they construed as an aberration of allergy research, and food manufacturers, some of whom were funding allergy research, were wary of their products being implicated in allergies.[7] However, despite discouragement from mainstream medicine and special interest groups, respected physicians such as Dr. Randolph continued to research and validate the existence of "hidden" or "latent" food and environmental reactions, calling them "sensitiv-ities" and "intolerances" to distinguish them from antibody-antigen allergies.

These doctors taught that sensitivity reactions to commonly eaten foods could cause a range of symptoms in susceptible individuals, including headaches, eczema, fatigue, arthritis, depression, and various gastrointestinal disorders. Their research further revealed that chemicals in the environment could have profoundly negative effects on the body. In 1962, Dr. Randolph pub-lished the first textbook in the nascent field of environmental medicine (SEE QUICK DEFINITION), *Human Ecology and Susceptibility to the Chemical Environment.*[8]

Since then, may other physicians have followed in Dr. Randolph's footsteps, educating the public that the widespread use of insecticides, herbicides, formaldehyde, plastics, food additives, petroleum products, and other chemicals can—and does—lead to sensitivity. Among the most debilitating is a multiple chemical sensitivity called *environmental illness*, of which fatigue, memory loss, and an inability to concentrate are major symptoms.

**QUICK**

**DEFINITION**

**Environmental medicine** explores the role of dietary and environ-mental allergens in health and ill-ness. Dust, molds, chemicals, cer-tain foods, and many other sub-stances can cause adverse reac-tions, which can be linked to dis-orders such as chronic fatigue, asthma, arthritis, headaches, depression, gastrointestinal prob-lems, and environmental illness. Environmental medicine physi-cians identify and treat patients' sensitivities and allergies as a means to resolve their health con-dition. Environmental medicine also addresses "sick building syn-drome," which is when the physi-cal environment of a building—its construction materials, furnish-ings, paints, lighting, and ventila-tion—directly contributes to the ill health of those living or working in it.

Since medical terminology must be precise in order to facilitate the proper diagnosis and treatment of health conditions, we will abide by the distinctions between allergy and sensitivity/intolerance throughout this book. Allergy will refer to an antibody-antigen reaction. Sensitivity and intolerance will refer to non-antibody-mediated events. However, since both types of reactions are caused by many of the same underlying factors, alternative medicine prac-titioners often use the same therapies and strategies to eliminate allergy as well as sensitivity. This book will help you on your way to being *reaction* free.

# Success Story: From Asthma to Tibet with Alternative Medicine

Marianne, a popular 36-year-old jazz guitarist, began to notice that she was often short of breath. Since she'd had breast cancer, she was worried that the shortness of breath was related to her cancer. She consulted New York City–based Leo Galland, M.D., F.A.C.P., F.A.C.N, author of *The Four Pillars of Healing*, who diagnosed her with asthma. "Actually, [the diagnosis] was pretty obvious" says Dr. Galland, who noted that Marianne had a childhood history of allergies. "She was wheezing. I did some pulmonary [lung] function tests and she just had regular asthma."

Since Marianne's job required that she often work in smoke-filled clubs, which exacerbated her condition, Dr. Galland decided that the best course of action would be to build up her respiratory barrier functions with supplements. "Asthma can be treated with selenium, magnesium, and vitamin C," all immune system stimulants, he states. "Antioxidants [SEE QUICK DEFINITION] such as vitamin E are helpful as is quercetin, a bioflavonoid that is an anti-inflammatory."

For more information on **how to allergy-proof your home**, see Chapter 5, Environmental Control, pp. 128-157. For more on **building up your respiratory barrier function**, see Chapter 10: Supporting the Respiratory System, pp. 260-277.

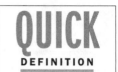

# QUICK
### DEFINITION

An **antioxidant** (meaning "against oxidation") is a natural biochemical substance that protects living cells against damage from harmful free radicals. Antioxidants work against the process of oxidation—the robbing of electrons from substances. If unblocked or left uncontrolled, oxidation can lead to cellular aging, degeneration, arthritis, heart disease, cancer, and other illnesses. Antioxidants in the body react readily with oxygen breakdown products and free radicals, and neutralize them before they can damage the body. Antioxidant nutrients include vitamins A, C, and E, beta carotene, selenium, coenzyme Q10, pycnogenol (grape seed extract), N-acetyl cysteine, L-glutathione, superoxide dismutase, and bioflavonoids. When antioxidants are taken in combination, the effect is stronger than when they are used individually.

Specifically, Dr. Galland prescribed a multivitamin for Marianne that included vitamin B6 (25 mg), magnesium chloride (300 mg), selenium (200 mcg), vitamin C (1,200 mg), and vitamin E (400 IU). She also took quercetin (900 mg, twice a day on an empty stomach) and essential fatty acids in the form of evening primrose oil (six capsules daily) and flaxseed oil (one tablespoon daily).

Dr. Galland recommended that Marianne allergy-proof her home by ridding it of dust and mold, using air purifiers, and eliminating as many potential allergens as possible. This step was particularly important because Marianne often encountered irritants such as cigarette smoke at the nightclubs. Minimizing her exposure to allergens at home helped control her asthma symptoms.

Within three months of adopting these measures, Marianne noticed an improvement in her breathing. After five years on the regime, she has remained mostly free from asthma, except for an occasional episode due to her work environment. "Before treatment, she was seriously inhibited by shortness of breath. Now, she has become very active physically," says Dr. Galland. "In fact, she has even studied karate and gone hiking in Tibet."

# Allergy 101: The Basics of Antibody-Antigen Reactions

An allergy is an adverse immune system reaction—sometimes mild, sometimes severe—to a substance that other people find harmless. Quite often, an allergen (a substance provoking allergy symptoms) is a protein that the body judges to be foreign and dangerous and thus attacks it. The adverse reaction that follows is called an allergic response. Common manifestations of this allergic response include fatigue, headaches, sneezing, watery eyes, and stuffy sinuses following exposure to an allergen. Allergic reactions fall into two categories, immediate and delayed. Food allergy symptoms tend to be delayed, manifesting two to 72 hours after eating the offending food. True food allergies occur in up to 5% of children under the age of three and in 1.5% of the general population, amounting to a total of four million Americans.[9]

## Biological Cycles Affect Allergic Reactions

Scientists believe that every physiological function follows a natural rhythm. Sleep/wake patterns, body temperature, and hormone release fluctuate on a daily basis; heart rates follow a much shorter cycle measured in seconds; menstrual periods repeat approximately every 28 days. These biological cycles also affect the severity of allergic reactions.

Several studies have shown that the magnitude of asthma attacks oscillates daily, with symptoms worsening during late night and early morning. Studies on both healthy and asthmatic subjects have found that lung function is at its peak (called "peak expiratory flow") at approximately 4 p.m. and at its lowest at 4 a.m. Asthmatics, however, suffer from significantly diminished lung function compared to healthy people in the early morning hours.[10] This reduction in expiratory flow often causes an asthma attack. According to one study, 74% of 8,000 asthmatic subjects claimed to have at least one bout of nocturnal asthma per week.[11] The menstrual cycle also affects lung function. In a recent study on 14 women diagnosed with mild to moderate asthma, all experienced a 20% decrease in peak expiratory flow in the days preceding menstruation.[12] Low levels of the hormone estradiol are associated with decreased lung function and higher risks for asthma attacks.

The severity of allergic rhinitis symptoms follows daily (circadian) rhythms. In one study, 70% of sufferers experienced a greater intensi-

# Top Triggers of Allergic Reactions

**INHALANTS**

- Plant Pollen (ragweed, timothy grass, etc.)
- Animal Dander (cat, dog, other furry pets)
- Cockroach Casings
- House Dust Mite Casings
- Mold Spores
- Tobacco Smoke
- Vehicle Exhaust
- Chemical Products (paint and cleaning solution fumes, etc.)

**INGESTANTS**

- Foods[14]

  *In Children:* Milk, Egg, Peanuts, Wheat, Soy, Tree Nuts

  *In Adults:* Peanuts, Tree Nuts, Fish, Shellfish

- Medications

  Antibiotics (penicillin, amoxicillin, etc.)

  Non-steroidal anti-inflammatory drugs (aspirin, etc.)

**CONTACTANTS**

- Plants (poison ivy, oak, sumac)
- Jewelry (nickel, copper, chromates, etc.)
- Latex Gloves
- Beauty Products (hair dyes, cosmetics, etc.)

**INJECTANTS**

- Insect Stings/Bites
- Some Medications

ty in respiratory problems upon awakening in the morning; symptoms dramatically abated by nighttime, only to return in the morning.[13]

**Common Triggers of Allergic Reactions**—Almost any agent can trigger allergic reactions. However, substances you inhale or eat are the main allergens. The most common source of environmental allergies is the pollen of plants, particularly trees, weeds, and grasses, and molds. The most common culprits in food allergies are yeast, wheat, corn, milk and other dairy products, eggs, soy, shellfish, peanuts, chocolate, and food dyes and additives.

**Common Symptoms of a Typical Allergic Reaction**—True allergy is manifested by numerous symptoms. The most common are breathing congestion, inflamed, bloodshot, or scratchy eyes, watery eyes, sneezing, coughing, itching, nosebleeds, puffy face, flushing of the cheeks, dark circles under the eyes, runny nose, swelling, hives, vomiting, stomachache, and intestinal irritation or swelling.

**Common Health Problems Partly Caused by Allergens**—Among the most frequently associated allergic conditions are allergic rhinitis and its seasonal counterpart hay fever, arthritis, asthma, bed-wetting, chronic runny nose, diarrhea, ear infections, eczema, fatigue, headache, irritability, concentration problems, hyperactivity, and attention deficit disorder.

# Common Allergy and Sensitivity Symptoms

Any symptom or physical sign can be caused by allergy or sensitivity reactions, because the symptoms are related to the tissues in which inflammatory chemicals are released. Symptoms may manifest immediately after exposure to a sensitizing agent or hours or days later. (Chapter 3: Allergy/Sensitivity Testing describes how alternative medicine physicians can detect the causes of both immediate and delayed symptoms.)

## HEAD

Dark circles under eyes (allergic shiners), swelling and wrinkles under eyes (Dennie's sign), cluster headaches, vascular headaches, migraines, faintness, dizziness, feelings of fullness in the head, excessive drowsiness or sleepiness soon after eating, insomnia, frequent awakenings during the night, early morning awakenings with inability to return to sleep

## SINUSES

Blurred vision, watery eyes, earache, ear drainage, fullness in ears, fluid in middle ear, hearing loss, itching ears, recurrent ear infections, tinnitus (buzzing, roaring, ringing, popping of the ears), excessive nasal mucus, postnasal drip, runny nose, stuffy nose, canker sores, chronic cough, gagging, hoarseness, itching of the roof of the mouth, sore throat, recurrent sinusitis

## HEART AND LUNGS

Palpitations, irregular heartbeat (arrhythmias), increased heart rate, rapid heart rate (tachycardia), congestion of the chest, asthma, exercise-induced asthma, anaphylaxis

## GASTROINTESTINAL SYSTEM

Candidiasis, mucus in stools, undigested food in stools, inflammatory bowel diseases (ulcerative colitis, Crohn's disease), celiac disease, colitis, anal itching, symptoms of gallbladder disease, nausea, vomiting, diarrhea, constipation, bloating after meals, belching, gas, abdominal pains or cramps, extreme thirst, coated tongue

## SKIN

Hives, rashes, eczema, contact dermatitis, pallor, dry skin, dandruff, brittle hair and nails

## DISEASES AND ILLNESSES

Adult-onset diabetes, chronic fatigue syndrome, lupus, rheumatoid arthritis, urinary tract disorder symptoms (urgency, frequency)

## BEHAVIORAL AND PSYCHOLOGICAL

Abnormal food cravings/binge eating, aggressive behavior, alcoholism/addiction, anorexia/bulemia, anxiety, autism, confusion, crying jags, depression, excessive daydreaming, hyperactivity, inability to concentrate, indifference, irritability, learning disabilities, mental dullness, mental lethargy, mental nervosa, panic attacks, restlessness, schizophrenia, slurred speech, stuttering

## OTHER SYMPTOMS

Autoimmune weakness, fatigue, muscle aches, swelling of hands and feet, obesity, rapid daily weight fluctuations (2-10 pounds), vaginal itching/discharge
*In Children:*
Colic, epilepsy, failure to thrive in infants, growing pains

## What Happens in an Allergic Response

The body has three main immune defense mechanisms—called "barrier functions"—that, when healthy, prevent foreign and potentially harmful substances from entering the bloodstream. The mucous membrane barrier, consisting of the respiratory system including the throat, nasal passages, and lungs, protects us from inhaled substances (pollen, animal dander). The skin barrier keeps us safe from contactant (poison ivy, jewelry) or injected (insect bites) antigens. And the gut barrier, including the stomach and intestines, wards off ingested antigens, primarily those found in food. The adrenal and thyroid glands are primary adjuncts to the barrier defense system, since they provide the hormones and energy essential for the proper operation of the entire immune system. When any or all of the barrier functions are broken down, due to poor diet, enzyme deficiency, bacteria overgrowth, and other factors, foreign molecules are able to pass through the barriers and enter the bloodstream.

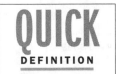

**DEFINITION**

The **immune system** guards the body against foreign, disease-producing substances. Its "workers" are various white blood cells including one trillion lymphocytes and 100 million trillion antibodies produced and secreted by the lymphocytes. Lymphocytes are found in high numbers in the lymph nodes, bone marrow, spleen, and thymus gland.

Upon its first exposure to a specific foreign molecule in the bloodstream (a process called *sensitization*), the immune system (SEE QUICK DEFINITION) determines whether the substance may be harmful to the body. If it does find the molecule to be potentially dangerous (antigen), it records the antigen's identification information (cellular memory) and begins production of a type of protein called an antibody, which is specifically designed to deactivate the antigen. When the body is exposed again to the antigen, the immune system identifies the antigen and mobilizes the release of the pre-selected antibody, setting in motion a complex series of events involving many biochemicals. These chemicals then produce the inflammation and other typi-

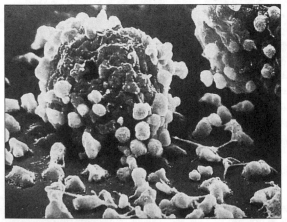

**Mast cell "degranulating" (releasing histamine granules) upon exposure to an allergen.**

cal symptoms of an allergy response. (See "Inflammatory Chemicals: A Lot More Than Histamine," p. 24.)

The antibody most commonly involved in the allergic response to pollens and other aeroallergens is IgE, one of five immunoglobulins, or specially designed antibody proteins, involved in the immune system's defense response to foreign substances. The main types of immunoglobulins, grouped according to their concentration in the blood, are: IgG (80%), IgA (10%-15%), IgM (5%-10%), IgD (less than 0.1%), and IgE (less than 0.01%). Mast cells, which produce the allergic response and are found throughout the body's tissues, next come into play; they tend to be concentrated in the skin, nose, and lung linings, gastrointestinal tract, and reproductive organs. When the IgE antibody senses an allergen, it triggers the mast cells to release histamine and 28 other chemicals and the allergic response flares into action. The IgE molecules also attach themselves, like a key fitting a lock, to the allergens. Both IgG and IgM antibodies neutralize bacteria, viruses, and toxins so they can be destroyed by other white blood cells. IgA antibodies, which are especially important in the gut, protect mucous membranes and neutralize antigens before they enter the bloodstream to trigger an allergic response. The immune function of IgD is not presently known.

## Early and Late Stages of Allergic Reactions

The allergic response consists of an early- and late-phase reaction. During the early stage, allergens attach to antibody receptors located on mast cells, triggering the release of chemical mediators into the blood vessels, nerves, and glands. Sneezing, runny nose, and nasal congestion are symptoms. During the late phase, the cellular mediators in the tissues stimulate secondary immune responses within the cells that result in further, more systemic symptoms like fatigue and joint pains. These pains are the result of antibody complexes being deposited into the tissues. At this point in the allergic reaction, you may treat the symptoms, by controlling the chemical responses (the reaction). However, if you don't treat the heart of the problem—the cause of your allergy or sensitivity—you risk developing serious health problems and diseases.

### Immediate vs. Delayed Allergic Reactions

The most common allergic reactions occur immediately after exposure to a certain substance (peanuts, pollen, bee venom, or cats, for example). These reactions are typically caused by IgE antibodies, resulting in a runny nose, watery eyes, itching, and skin rashes; more severe reactions include constriction of the bronchial tubes and difficulty breathing. Delayed allergies are another type of allergic reaction, which can manifest symptoms up to 72 hours after exposure to a trig-

# Inflammatory Chemicals:
# A Lot More Than Histamine

**Histamine:** This substance causes the blood vessels to widen, enabling more fluid to pass into body tissues, resulting in swelling; it also triggers the smooth involuntary muscles in the lungs, blood vessels, heart, stomach, intestines, and bladder to contract. Histamine gives us runny noses, red itchy eyes, hot, tender, or swollen body parts, flushing, and the other symptoms associated with allergic reactions. In general, the allergic response, in the form of an inflammation, swelling, or tenderness, is the body's attempt to heal itself from the effect of the allergen. These responses are normal ways the body takes care of itself, albeit in the process they can make us feel miserable. However, if they continue unchecked for too long, your health will suffer.

**Heparin:** Increases blood flow to the site of inflammation and swelling.

**Platelet-Activating Factor:** Causes blood platelets to group together so that they release chemicals to change the diameter of blood vessels, affecting blood pressure.

**Serotonin:** A brain chemical known as a neurotransmitter, found in the mucous membrane cells of the gastrointestinal tract, and involved in the allergic response to foods.

**Lymphokines:** Produced by white blood cells (lymphocytes) and involved in communications among cells.

**Leukotrienes:** Found in cell membranes and involved in making the lung muscles contract and the lungs to retain more air, as in the bronchial spasm of asthma.

**Prostaglandins:** Hormone-like substances that help dilate blood vessels, affect smooth muscle contraction, increase pain in affected areas, and heat up inflamed tissues.

**Thromboxanes:** These chemicals contract blood vessels and bronchial tubes.

**Bradykinin:** Supports the cascade of inflammatory symptoms set in motion by the mast cells.

**Interleukins:** Antibodies involved in the activity of lymphocytes.

**Interferons:** Produced by lymphocytes to regulate the speed of immune responses.

gering substance. These symptoms often appear as illnesses or disorders seemingly unrelated to allergy, such as lethargy, attention deficit disorder, fatigue, hyperactivity, itchy skin, mood swings, insomnia, and joint inflammation. Many of these reactions are caused by IgG immunoglobulins. Up to 80 different medical conditions—from arthritis, asthma, and autism to insomnia and diabetes—have been clinically associated with IgG food allergy reactions.

# Types of Allergies and Allergic Conditions

Almost anything a susceptible person ingests, inhales, or touches can trigger allergies—foods, food additives, drugs, insects, plants, dust, molds, metals, fabrics, household cleaners, and industrial vapors, among others—but there are only four types of antibody-mediated reactions to allergens. These types, which may be immediate or delayed, are defined according to the presence of certain antibodies and immune system cells.

### Type I: Immediate Hypersensitivity (IgE-Mediated)

The presence of the antibody immunoglobulin E (IgE) in the body distinguishes Type I allergies from the other three reaction types. This reaction occurs within minutes after exposure to the allergen. Reactive airway disease, hay fever, most skin allergies, and anaphylaxis are Type I or "classic" allergic conditions. Because symptoms are readily visible, these allergies are also classified as "active" allergies.

In the case of an allergy to goldenrod pollen, for instance, a typical reaction would be as follows: the allergic individual breathes in the goldenrod allergen and the immune system signals a type of lymphocyte called B cells (SEE QUICK DEFINITION) to begin production of IgE antibodies specifically designed to target the goldenrod protein molecules. These IgE antibodies then attach themselves to the surface structures of mast cells, located in the respiratory and gastrointestinal tracts, and of eosinophils, similar cells found in the bloodstream.

Upon a subsequent exposure to goldenrod, the pollen binds to the waiting IgE antibody receptors. This triggers the mast cells and eosinophils to release a group of chemicals, of which histamine is the most well known. The symptoms caused by these

> ## Common Allergic Conditions
>
> - Allergic Rhinitis (Hay Fever)
> - Anaphylaxis (Anaphylactic Shock)
> - Reactive Airway Disease/Asthma
> - Atopic Dermatitis (Eczema)
> - Urticaria (Hives)
> - Allergic Contact Dermatitis
> - Otitis Media (Ear Infections)
> - Rhinosinusitis

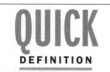

**QUICK DEFINITION**

A **lymphocyte** is a specialized form of white blood cell, representing 25%-33% of the total count, whose numbers increase during infection. Lymphocytes are produced in the bone marrow and come in two basic forms: T cells, which mature in the thymus gland (located behind the breastbone and just above the heart) and are sensitized to attack and kill invading pathogens (this is known as cell-mediated immunity); and B cells, which mature in the bone marrow and produce antibodies to neutralize specific invaders.

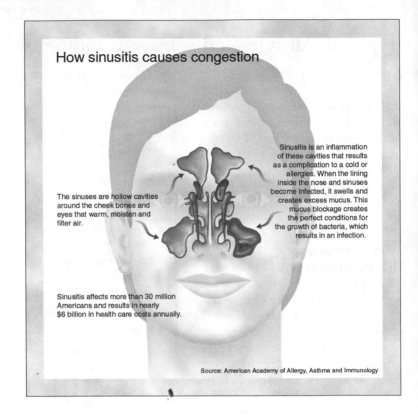

**How sinusitis causes congestion**

The sinuses are hollow cavities around the cheek bones and eyes that warm, moisten and filter air.

Sinusitis is an inflammation of these cavities that results as a complication to a cold or allergies. When the lining inside the nose and sinuses become infected, it swells and creates excess mucus. This mucus blockage creates the perfect conditions for the growth of bacteria, which results in an infection.

Sinusitis affects more than 30 million Americans and results in nearly $6 billion in health care costs annually.

Source: American Academy of Allergy, Asthma and Immunology

chemicals (called mediators) depend on the tissues in which inflammatory chemicals are released. Some common manifestations include mucus membrane inflammation, swelling, itching, redness, pain, watery eyes and nose, contraction of smooth muscles in the bronchial tract, and capillary permeability. The response itself is the body's attempt to eliminate the pollen from its system, and unless the body is desensitized, these symptoms will occur every time exposure to goldenrod occurs. Symptoms in a classic reaction appear immediately to two hours within contact, and their manifestations depend upon which area of the body the allergen affects.

Type I allergies are usually associated with airborne and inhalant allergens such as pollen, mold, dust mites, and animal dander. The most common foods that bring on this reaction are milk, eggs, corn, chocolate, strawberries, tree nuts, and peanuts (a legume).[15] However, food allergies may be undiagnosed due to false negatives to skin and other IgE–measurement tests.

**Allergic Rhinitis/Hay Fever**—Allergic rhinitis is a general term that indicates an inflammation of the nasal mucous membranes. The release of histamine and other inflammatory substances during an allergic reaction produce the other symptoms associated with this condition: sneezing, a runny nose, ear and throat congestion, swollen sinuses, postnasal drip, and red, watery, itchy eyes.

An estimated 40 million Americans suffer from hay fever (seasonal allergic rhinitis) and its year-round counterpart, perennial rhinitis, with women and people living in the southern United States being slightly more susceptible to it than others. Allergic rhinitis accounts for more than 8 million physician office visits each year;[16] total direct medical costs amount to $4.5 billion per year.[17] There is a significant correlation between allergic rhinitis and asthma. Approximately 38% of patients with allergic rhinitis also suffer from asthma, higher than the 3% to 5% prevalence in the general population.[18] Allergic rhinitis often coincides with chronic ear infections (otitis media), and half of children over three years of age with chronic ear infections also suffer from allergic rhinitis.[19] Allergic rhinitis can also lead to rhinosinusitis, or sinus infection, which affects 14% of the U.S. population annually.[20]

Some well-known rhinitis allergens are mold spores and the pollens from an estimated 65 types of trees as well as those from weeds, flowers, and grasses. Ragweed pollen alone triggers approximately 75% of allergic rhinitis cases.[21] These substances are carried by the wind, generally between February and October, and are inhaled through the nose and mouth. Contrary to popular belief, most vividly colored flowers are not sources of allergic reactions, since their pollen is too heavy for airborne pollination.

As we now spend up to 90% of our time indoors, often in energy-efficient buildings that recirculate the same stale air, indoor air irritants such as dust mites, mold spores, cockroach casings, animal dander, smoke, and chemicals are likely triggering more cases of allergic rhinitis than do outdoor sources. Conventional doctors treat allergic rhinitis with one or a combination of antihistamines, decongestants, allergy shots, cromolyn sodium, and topical nasal steroids.

**Reactive Airway Disease/Asthma**—You might be sleeping, jogging, even reading this book when you suddenly start wheezing and coughing. You struggle to breathe, your chest tightens, and anxiety floods your body. You're experiencing an asthma attack. (See

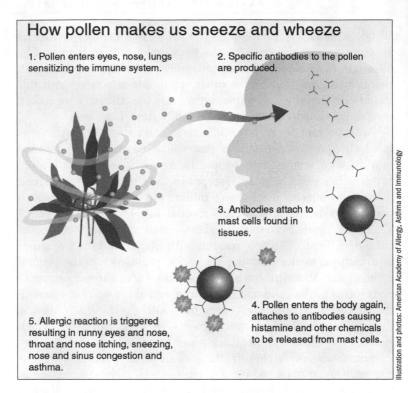

# How pollen makes us sneeze and wheeze

1. Pollen enters eyes, nose, lungs sensitizing the immune system.

2. Specific antibodies to the pollen are produced.

3. Antibodies attach to mast cells found in tissues.

5. Allergic reaction is triggered resulting in runny eyes and nose, throat and nose itching, sneezing, nose and sinus congestion and asthma.

4. Pollen enters the body again, attaches to antibodies causing histamine and other chemicals to be released from mast cells.

Illustration and photos: American Academy of Allergy, Asthma and Immunology

**EDITOR'S NOTE**

Most consumer medical literature and many doctors do not make the distinction between reactive airway disease and asthma, because the symptoms of both conditions are identical. Thus, many of the statistics in this book refer to the symptomatic definition of asthma. When seeking treatment, however, it's crucial that you understand the differences between these two respiratory conditions; reactive airway disease is reversible but asthma is not.

"Reactive Airway Disease and Asthma," p. 31, for clarification on the use of the term *asthma* throughout this book.)

During an asthma attack, IgE antibodies activate histamine and other chemicals, which trigger the bronchioles (bronchial tubes) to become inflamed and flooded with mucus. The bronchial lining's smooth muscles contract, narrowing the bronchial passages and obstructing the airways. Symptoms can range from minor difficulties in breathing to severe wheezing and coughing accompanied by mucus excretion.

More than 15 million Americans have asthma, a 33% increase from 1990 and 66% increase from 1980.[22] In 1997, more than 5,400 people died from severe asthma attacks,[23] more than double the asthma death rate in 1980.[24] Occupational asthma, which develops in adults due to substances they are exposed to at work, accounts for 15.4% of all cases of asthma in United States.[25] Five million children under the age of 18 suffer from asthma,[26] making it the leading cause of hospitalization and school absenteeism for children.[27] Asthma is more prevalent among African-American children than in other groups (26%), and is more likely to culminate in death.[28] Asthma takes a high toll on health-care finances as well, with total related medical costs at an estimated $14.5 billion per year.[29] Asthma patients tend to also suffer from allergic rhinitis. A recent study showed allergic rhinitis occurred in 99% of asthmatic adults and 93% of asthmatic adolescents; the same study reports that severe rhinitis is associated with an exacerbation of asthma.[30]

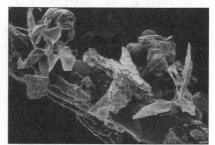

**Animal dander**

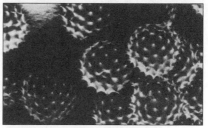

**Ragweed pollen**

Common food allergens that trigger asthma attacks include cow's milk, eggs, fish, tree nuts, peanuts, seeds, soy, wheat, corn, citrus fruits, chocolate, some spices, and various food additives and colorings, especially sulfites. Aspirin and acetaminophen also can prompt asthma. Some other triggers are animal dander, dust mites, mold, chlorine, car exhaust fumes, tobacco smoke, smoke

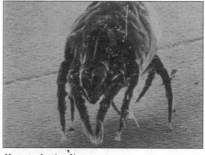

**House dust mite**

from a wood-burning stove or fireplace, latex, cleaning chemicals, newsprint and fabric dyes, and formaldehyde-containing sprays, polishes, building materials, fabrics, and personal hygiene products.

Conventional drug treatment for asthma focuses on controlling or preventing symptoms. Common prescription medications include oral and inhaled corticosteroids (cortisone), epinephrine (adrenaline) shots, including home kits for emergencies; theophylline (methylxanthine), a mild-to-moderate bronchodilator; cromolyn sodium, a preventive anti-inflammatory; and the newer adrenaline mimics called beta agonists (such as albuterol), usually prescribed in bronchodilator form.

## Why asthma makes it hard to breathe

Air enters the respiratory system from the nose and mouth and travels through the bronchial tubes.

In an asthmatic person, the muscles of the bronchial tubes tighten and thicken, and the air passages become inflamed and mucus-filled, making it difficult for air to move.

In a non-asthmatic person, the muscles around the bronchial tubes are relaxed and the tissue thin, allowing for easy airflow.

Inflamed bronchial tube of an asthmatic

Normal bronchial tube

American Academy of Allergy, Asthma and Immunology

**Atopic Dermatitis (Eczema)**—Eczema often begins in infancy after the baby is weaned from breast milk and is characterized by an inflammation of the skin, usually associated with blisters, red bumps, swelling, oozing, scaling, crusting, and itching. In infants two to 18 months, it appears as weeping, crusty red spots on the face, scalp, and extremities. In older children and adults, it may be more localized and chronic. Eczema often subsides by age three or four, but may reoccur in adolescence or adulthood as a skin condition or other allergy.

Eczema most frequently occurs in families with a history of allergies. Between 10% and 15% of the U.S. population has experienced eczema during childhood, half during the first year of life.[31] Eczema often precedes other allergic conditions, with more than half of patients ultimately developing asthma[32] and approximately 75% developing allergic rhinitis.[33]

Eczema-triggering allergens include cow's milk, eggs, peanuts, fish, wheat, soybean, dust mites, fabrics, plastics, smoke, chemicals such as fluoride, and items containing orris root (face powder, creams, cosmetics, perfume, scented soap or shampoo, shaving cream, teething rings, and toothpaste). Conventional treatment is usually with a topical cortisone cream and may include antihistamines.

**Urticaria (Hives)—**Up to 20% of the U.S. population has experienced an outbreak of hives.[34] Known technically as *urticaria*, hives are characterized by eruptions of red, raised, swollen welts that can appear on any part of the body but tend to cluster on the arms, legs, and trunk. They resemble mosquito bites and vary in size. Extremely itchy, they spread when scratched and can last from hours to days.

Common triggers are drugs, such as penicillin, aspirin, sulfur, anticonvulsive drugs, and phenobarbital. Other common allergens include strawberries, shellfish, peanuts, soy, beef, citrus, tomatoes, milk, eggs, and various chemicals found in laundry soaps, fabric softeners, and cosmetics. Insect stings, pollens, molds, dust, and animal dander may also spark hives, and sometimes sunlight or cold weather will heighten the reaction. Hives are conventionally treated with cortisone creams, antihistamines, and other anti-inflammatory drugs.

## Reactive Airway Disease and Asthma

In common parlance, the term *asthma* describes a condition marked by constriction of the airways, which causes wheezing and difficulty in breathing. For the purposes of this book, however, it's important to differentiate between reversible and irreversible forms of this respiratory problem, specifically, between reactive airway disease and asthma.

If you experience bronchial spasm and constriction only upon exposure to an allergen, for example, to food or pollen, you have reactive airway disease (RAD). This condition is likely due to defaults in barrier functions (e.g., intestines or respiratory system) and if treated early enough with alternative therapies, it can be cured. Chronic episodes of RAD, however, put a high-pressure load on your lungs, ultimately damaging the lung tissue. This damage leads to asthma, a chronic, degenerative, and irreversible disease. In asthmatic patients, bronchial constrictions are no longer solely triggered by allergens, but also by exercise, strong emotions, and other events. Asthma can kill. Managing asthma is more difficult and requires a long-term strategy, often incorporating conventional drugs.

**Anaphylaxis (Anaphylactic Shock)—**The severest form of IgE-mediated allergy is anaphylaxis, also called anaphylactic shock. In an anaphylactic reaction, the IgE antibodies respond to the invasion of an allergy by signaling a massive release of chemical mediators. This rush of histamine and other chemicals causes the blood vessels throughout the body to dilate, leading to a rapid drop in blood pressure and pulse. Air pathways constrict and breathing becomes difficult. Symptoms, which appear immediately but may take up to two hours to fully manifest, include heart palpitations, hives, headache, nausea and vomiting, sneezing and coughing, stomach cramps, swelling of the lips and joints, and diarrhea. The body is ready to shut down. Anaphylaxis requires immediate medical assistance in the form of an adrenaline (epinephrine) injection to reverse the symptoms. Oxygen, steroids, and antihistamines may also be used.

Alternative remedies can alleviate and reverse many allergic conditions, but anaphylaxis is not one of them. Anaphylaxis can be deadly if not treated immediately. Patients who are susceptible to anaphylactic reactions to food, insect stings, and other allergens should keep an epinephrine kit on hand. Be sure that caretakers of children or elderly patients prone to anaphylaxis can identify the signs of anaphylactic shock. Also, teach them how to administer emergency epinephrine shots.

Food-induced anaphylaxis is the leading cause of anaphylaxis in children.[35] The foods most frequently eliciting this response are seafood, peanuts, tree nuts, eggs, and milk.[36] Pharmaceuticals such as penicillin (made from a mold) and aspirin as well as insect stings also are common triggers of anaphylaxis. Each year, approximately 100 people in the U.S. die from food-related anaphylaxis and 40 die from anaphylactic shock triggered by insect stings.[37] People who have had an episode of anaphylaxis often keep an emergency medical kit containing epinephrine handy.

### Type II: Cytotoxic Allergies

This is an immediate allergic reaction triggered by food allergens or the transfusion of incompatible blood types as well as some drugs. Symptoms may include anemia (called immune hemolytic anemia), jaundice, or even kidney failure in the case of blood transfusions.

Preceding the Type II allergic response, antigens bind to blood or tissue cell membranes. Their invasion prompts the B cells to produce IgG or IgM antibodies, which seek out and attach to the antigens. The antibodies inject toxic protein enzymes (cytotoxin) into the antigen cells, killing them. However, cytotoxic reactions have one drawback. If antigens have invaded blood or tissue cells, the antibodies will also inject cytotoxin into the infected cells, producing cell damage or death. If too many red blood cells are destroyed during the reaction, immune hemolytic anemia can set in. It's estimated that cytotoxic reactions sparked by foods may damage body cells 75% of the time.[38] Intestinal cells bear the brunt of cytotoxic reactions because food antigens and immunoglobulins often meet in the intestines.

### Type III: Arthus Allergies

This reaction, also known as serum sickness, is typically triggered by food and to a lesser degree, insect stings and pharmaceutical drugs. The reaction occurs several hours to up to ten days after exposure. Here, as in type II, the antibody IgG binds to an invading protein molecule (virus, venom, or undigested food resulting from leaky gut syndrome, or defaults in the gut barrier function), but in this case the process forms a circulating immune complex (CIC). In a healthy person, immune cells called phagocytes neutralize the CICs, but in someone with weakened immunity, the CICs tend to accumulate in the bloodstream. If too many CICs accumulate, the kidneys cannot excrete enough of them via the urine and they are deposited in soft tissues, causing inflammation and damaging the healthy tissue, leading to such diseases as arthritis. Resulting symptoms include hives, joint pain, headaches, gastrointestinal disturbances, and fatigue. It is estimated that 80% of food allergies are Type III reactions.[39]

### Type IV: T Cell–Mediated Allergies

Type IV symptoms typically appear two to three days after exposure.

Allergic contact dermatitis, as well as autoimmune diseases such as allergic colitis (inflammation of the colon), Crohn's disease (regional ileitis, or inflammation of the ileum in the small intestine), and graft-transplant rejections are the main manifestations of Type IV allergies. Common triggers include poison ivy and other plants as well as pharmaceutical drugs.

In a Type IV reaction, T cells, not antibodies, are activated to directly attack an antigen. When someone brushes against poison ivy, for instance, the urushiol (oily toxin in the leaves) does not immediately cause a reaction in the person's tissues. Upon a subse-

## Allergic Addiction Syndrome

With food allergies, there is a strange paradox: often a person becomes addicted to a food that produces an allergic response. This is called allergic addiction syndrome. When a person stops eating an allergy-producing food to which their body is "addicted," such as coffee or chocolate, there is a three-day period in which they experience unpleasant withdrawal symptoms, such as fatigue and anxiety; eating more of this addictive substance can actually improve the situation by suppressing these withdrawal symptoms. This becomes an unhealthy cycle of addiction, craving, and fulfillment that eventually leads to more serious health problems. Allergy experts call this suppression of symptoms by an allergenic food *masking*, because it masks or disguises the true allergic symptoms. See Chapter 6: Therapeutic Diets, to learn more about allergic addiction syndrome.

For more information on **leaky gut syndrome**, see Chapter 2: Causes of Allergy and Sensitivity, pp. 38-69, and Chapter 7: Healing Leaky Gut Syndrome, pp. 184-211.

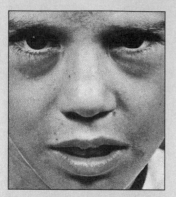

## Common Physical Signs of Food Allergy

- Dark circles under eyes ("allergic shiners")
- Puffiness under eyes
- Horizontal creases in the lower lip
- Horizontal crease across the nose
- Chronic swollen glands
- Chronic noncyclic fluid retention

quent exposure, however, the immune system determines that the urushiol may be an antigen and proceeds to mobilize helper and natural killer T cells. When the body is exposed to the poison ivy again, the activated T cells travel from the bloodstream to the affected skin area, congregate, initiate the release of inflammatory chemicals, and neutralize the allergen. It takes approximately one day for the T cells to amass in sufficient numbers to fight the allergen; for that reason the allergic symptoms are delayed, primarily manifesting as allergic contact dermatitis one to three days after exposure to the allergen.

**Allergic Contact Dermatitis**—This term applies to an inflammation with redness, itching, scales, and blisters produced by allergenic substances that touch the skin. Typical examples would be poison ivy, oak, or sumac, in which oil from the leaves (urushiol) comes in contact with the skin, causing burning or itching. The skin starts to swell, a rash spreads, and blisters—which may ooze—form. According to the American Association of Dermatology, 10-50 million Americans suffer from rashes from poison ivy, oak, or sumac each year. Of the approximately 3,000 known contact allergens, nickel, mercury, chromates, plastic products, rubber products, hair dyes, cosmetics, and latex are among the most common.[40] Bananas, pineapple, papaya, kiwi, and avocado, all of which belong to the same plant family as latex, may also spark an allergic rash.[41]

Not all cases of contact dermatitis are allergic reactions. If you touch bleach or another noxious chemical, for example, it's normal to get a rash ("irritant" contact dermatitis). If you experience a skin reaction after touching typically innocuous substances such as jewelry or latex gloves, then you have allergic contact dermatitis. Typically, the allergic reaction starts 24 hours to up to six days after contact and may last a week or longer; irritant contact dermatitis develops within two days after exposure and disappears within 96 hours, depending on the toxicity of the substance and duration of exposure. Conventional physicians usually advise dermatitis sufferers to wash any clothing that has come in contact with an allergenic substance. They may also recommend antihistamines or corticosteroid creams.

# What Happens in a Non-Antibody-Mediated Event?

As discussed earlier, sensitivities are distinguished from allergy in that no antibodies respond to the allergen invasion. Additionally, sensitivities can come and go spontaneously and may be more related to the individual's ability to metabolize and detoxify substances than to any other factor. Allergy, on the other hand, is permanent in that your body will always make antibodies when challenged with the allergen, but the response is dictated by the amount of antibodies present at the time of exposure.

Conventional medicine has been slow to recognize that both foods and chemicals can trigger adverse responses in the body. Part of the problem is that conventional skin tests do not identify sensitivities. Additionally, the symptoms may change after each exposure to a sensitizing agent—smelling an offending chemical gives you a headache one time and makes you nauseous the next. Hence, numerous mainstream doctors, unable to determine a cause for their patients' symptoms, refer them to psychiatrists for psychological counseling. However, recent research in the field of environmental medicine confirms that the body can respond negatively—without the mediation of antibodies—to specific food and chemical stimuli.

## Food Sensitivity

Most adverse reactions to foods are sensitivities, not true allergies. The U.S. Department of Agriculture reports that 15% of the total population suffers from both immunologic and nonimmunologic reactions to foods. Of that, 1.5% experiences true, antibody-mediated allergy; the remaining 13.5% suffer from food sensitivities. However, some environmental medicine doctors believe that up to 50% of the U.S. population is sensitive to foods. Symptoms of food sensitivities can be immediate or delayed and often manifest as gastrointestinal problems, such as belching, bloating, gas, and diarrhea, headaches, lack of mental clarity, and fatigue. Additives in foods, such as monosodium glutamate (MSG), tartrazine (FD&C Yellow Dye #5), aspartame (found in NutraSweet™ and Equal™), and sulfites have been shown to trigger adverse

To learn about **tests that detect food and chemical sensitivities**, see Chapter 3: Allergy/Sensitivity Testing, pp. 70-105.

reactions, including headaches and hyperactivity in children.

Several physiological responses can cause pseudo-allergic reactions to food. Excessive intake of histamine-containing foods (exogenous histamine), such as sausage, sauerkraut, tuna, wine, preserves, spinach, and tomato, can mimic the body's natural histamine response, causing inflammation. Eating too many animal products, which contain fats called arachidonic acid, can boost production of pro-inflammatory prostaglandins, which also provoke symptoms similar to allergic reactions. Other foods also facilitate the release of a chemical called platelet-activating factor into the bloodstream. This chemical causes the cells (platelets) that are responsible for blood-clotting to clump together. (Platelet-activating factor is also released during a true allergic reaction.) The activation of platelets results in the release of serotonin, a neurotransmitter or brain chemical. Serotonin can contract smooth muscles and stimulate mucus secretion—other signs of pseudo-allergic as well as true allergic reactions.

Additionally, some people suffer from food intolerances caused by enzyme deficiency. The most common case of this intolerance is due to a deficiency of lactase, the enzyme that breaks down milk sugars. It is important to recognize that this is an intolerance, not sensitivity, since there is no sensitization mechanism (a leaky gut). Some intolerances of this nature are temporary, due to pancreatic disturbance such as viral illness, while other cases are permanent, due to genetic lactase deficiency.

## Chemical Sensitivity

Chemical sensitivity is a modern phenomenon. It has been directly linked by the work of environmental medicine pioneer Theron Randolph, M.D., to the increasing prevalence of chemicals and toxins in our environment— pesticides in foods, heavy metals in water, vehicle exhaust in the air, and numerous synthetic chemicals in personal hygiene products, cleaning supplies, and building materials. Chemically sensitive people experience adverse reactions from minute, seemingly harmless amounts of chemical agents. Many symptoms of chemical sensitivity are cerebral in nature—an inability to concentrate or think clearly, depression, or debilitating fatigue—which is why chemical sensitivity is so often misdiagnosed as a psychological problem rather than a reaction to the environment.[42] Chemicals that are unable to be eliminated by normal detoxification means are deposited in body fat, including the brain, which has a very high fat content. Chemically sensitive people have been shown to have slow or sluggish liver detoxification processes.

A recent report established that the physiological reactions of allergy and chemical sensitivity are similar. As discussed above, in an allergic reaction, an allergen protein binds to the IgE antibody on mast cells, which leads to the release of inflammatory mediators. In a chemical reaction, low molecular–weight chemicals bind to chemoreceptors (which detect taste and smell) on sensory nerve C-fibers (primary components of the nerves that conduct impulses from a sense organ to the spinal cord and brain). This in turn leads to the release of inflammatory chemicals.[43] The report also acknowledges the spreading phenomenon of chemical sensitivity.

For more on the **link between sensitivity and liver detoxification**, see Chapter 8: Intestinal Detoxification, pp. 212-235.

**Multiple Chemical Sensitivity**—Multiple chemical sensitivity (MCS), also known as environmental illness, is an extreme variation of chemical sensitivity, in which patients have a prolonged, heightened, and often incapacitating reaction to a number of common substances found in their environment. While the prevalence of MCS in the U.S. is pegged at anywhere from 2% to 6%, it's difficult to substantiate these numbers because MCS is not generally diagnosed as such. Therefore, it is often mislabeled and may underlie numerous other illnesses. For example, in a 1994 study of patients with chronic fatigue syndrome (CFS) and fibromyalgia, up to 67% also had multiple chemical sensitivities but none had ever received the diagnosis.[44]

A distinguishing feature of MCS is its "spreading" effect. After the sensitizing event or chronic low-level exposure to one or more chemicals, an individual becomes sensitive to an increasing number of substances. This may include chemicals that had never triggered reactions before the sensitization, such as glue, perfumes, air fresheners, or gasoline. It may also spread to include foods, drugs, alcohol, caffeine, or even airborne allergens. "Switching" is another phenomenon associated with MCS, in which one symptom is replaced by another. For instance, whereas the smell of paint used to make you dizzy, it now gives you headaches.

For more on **sick building syndrome and multiple chemical sensitivity**, see Chapter 5: Environmental Control, pp. 128-157.

Many MCS patients can identify the chemical event that caused the onset of their disease. In one survey of 6,800 chemically sensitive persons, 80% claimed that they knew exactly "when, where, with what, and how they were made ill." Of those individuals, 60% cited pesticide exposure as the major trigger.[45] Formaldehyde and "sick" (airtight) buildings are also named as the most frequently initiating causes by many MCS patients.

# CHAPTER

# 2

# Causes of Allergy and Sensitivity

**D**O YOU BREAK INTO HIVES whenever you eat strawberries? Suffer an asthma attack when you pet a cat? Do you likewise believe that strawberries or cats cause your allergies? If so, you are mistaken. Strawberries, cats, and many other agents do indeed spark allergic reactions, but they are not the reasons you suffer from this condition. The underlying causes of allergy and sensitivity are dietary and lifestyle factors that break down your immune system and barrier defenses. Specifically, genetic susceptibility, some child-rearing practices, barrier function default, and toxic overload are in varying degrees responsible for the development and continuation of allergy and sensitivity.

## In This Chapter

## Allergy Susceptibility May Be in Your Genes

Recently, the Human Genome Project has garnered much media attention, as participating research groups around the world announce that they're close to finding biotechnology's holy grail—the map of the human gene code. The findings of this project may determine once and for all the roles genes play in the development of disease. For example, is there an allergy gene, that is, a gene that causes allergies?

For several years, scientists have been conducting studies with this question in mind. Their research suggests that there are genetic factors that predispose people to allergy and asthma (a condition called atopy), but that no specific gene ultimately causes the onset of allergic conditions. Studies have found that up-regulation (abnormal increase in function) of a gene that controls the production and activity of specific immune cells (interleukin 4 and T-helper cells) are implicated in the onset of allergy and asthma.[1] The researchers clarify that the presence of this gene doesn't necessarily mean certain individuals will develop allergy. Rather, changes in the function of this gene appear to promote susceptibility to allergy. Scientists have narrowed down chromosomal locations that are likely to contain "susceptibility genes" for asthma and allergy, although the exact genome locus has not been determined.[2] Further research has found that variations in a gene called NOS1, which synthesizes the nitric oxide gas we exhale during breathing, are common in patients with asthma.[3]

Hence, it seems likely that some people are genetically predisposed to developing allergy and asthma. But not everyone with susceptibility gene or genes will suffer from allergies. Something has to provoke or deregulate the gene to increase atopy risk. Additionally, even people without susceptibility genes can develop allergy and sensitivity. Other factors, which are described below, contribute to the onset of allergy and sensitivity in both genetically predisposed and non-predisposed individuals.

# Early Childhood Practices Lead to Allergy and Sensitivity

Children should be the healthiest age group. They haven't been exposed to years of toxins, stress, and poor eating habits. And on the whole, they are well-nourished, well-loved, and cared for. So why then do children bear the brunt of allergy and asthma? Ironically, their parents' and doctors' best intentions can set the stage for allergic disorders. Breast-feeding mistakes and immunizations are among the leading contributors of early childhood allergies. Early introduction of solid foods is also implicated.

## Prenatal Exposure and Breast-feeding by Allergic Mothers
Research shows that up to 34% of infants borne to women who have allergies will develop allergies as well.[4] This is not due to genetic inheritance of allergy for, as we've discussed above, there is no

research supporting the existence of an allergy-causing gene. But the allergic mothers do pass something to their progeny—antigens and their associated antibodies. James Braly, M.D., medical director of Immuno Laboratories, in Fort Lauderdale, Florida, explains one way this can happen. "One of the immune mechanisms that mediate allergies, an antibody called IgG, transfers through the placenta from the mother's blood into the fetal blood supply," he says. "This causes the fetus to passively develop allergies to the same foods that the mother is allergic to." Mother's milk, which generally reduces the risk of allergy in children, can also transfer allergens and antibodies to infants.[5]

In one study, for instance, a one-month-old breast-fed infant who suffered from chronic allergy-related intestinal problems experienced a full recovery of symptoms when his mother eliminated cow's milk products, egg, and pork—all commonly allergenic foods—from her diet.[6] Food allergies aren't the only conditions "inherited" in utero. Pollen contact in utero can sensitize the developing baby to these aeroallergens, leading to allergic rhinitis and other allergies upon birth.[7] In one study, infants whose mothers were exposed during pregnancy to high amounts of the common aeroallergens birch pollen and house dust mites were more likely than other infants to develop allergies to these substances within one month of birth. These infants also experienced higher allergic asthma rates by one year of age.[8]

The transfer of allergen and antibody, however, doesn't fully explain why breast-fed infants become hypersensitive. As it does in all cases of allergy, barrier function default (see "Barrier Function Default: The Root of Allergy and Sensitivity," p. 44) often contributes to infantile allergy development. In fact, the one-month-old infant mentioned above suffered from intestinal permeability, or intestinal barrier function default. It's likely that maternal exposure to factors that cause barrier function default can also damage the barrier functions of developing fetuses. In such cases, it doesn't matter if the mother is allergic or not.

To learn **how to prevent childhood allergies**, see Chapter 4: Prevention of Sensitization, pp. 106-127.

## Vaccinations Impair the Immune System

During the past century, vaccinations (SEE QUICK DEFINITION) have become regarded almost as a rite of passage for American children. Beginning as early as a few weeks after birth, the vast majority of children are inoculated against numerous illnesses, including measles, mumps, whooping cough, polio, and tetanus. Most schools actually require immunizations as part of its admissions process. At the same time, childhood cases of allergy and asthma have skyrocketed.

According to many alternative medicine and Anthroposophic (SEE QUICK DEFINITION) practitioners, this correlation is no coincidence.

Recent evidence indicates that routine childhood vaccinations contribute to the emergence of chronic allergic problems such as eczema, ear infections, and asthma. While this contention is controversial, a growing number of scientists and physicians maintain that most standard vaccinations impair a child's developing immune system, setting the stage for hypersensitive reactions to foods and other common substances. In fact, childhood illnesses such as measles, mumps, and whooping cough may actually reduce the risk of allergy.

The immune system has two different aspects: the humoral (B cell) immune system, whereby antibodies are produced to recognize and neutralize antigens in the body, and the cell-mediated (T cell) immune system, which involves white blood cells and immune cells called macrophages that "eat" antigens. They also help drive the antigens out of the body, by causing skin rashes and discharges of pus and mucus from the throat and lungs. Both are typical signs of a beneficial acute inflammatory illness of childhood. (Polio and tetanus, in contrast, do not belong to this group of beneficial illnesses.)

The two poles of the immune system have a reciprocal relationship. When the humoral pole is over-stimulated (for example, from allergies), the cell-mediated pole tends to be relatively inactive. Vaccines do not stimulate the cell-mediated pole, so their contents never get discharged. On the other hand, an acute inflammatory childhood illness—measles, mumps, rubella, chicken pox, scarlatina, or whooping cough—develops the cell-mediated immune system. The difference here is crucial, because it is the cell-mediated response that protects the child from future illness and provides the deeper immunity.

Physicians who practice Anthroposophic medicine generally believe that having acute but limited inflammatory diseases as a child helps protect one as an adult against more serious, long-term, chronic illnesses. On the other hand, not having these childhood illnesses because of multiple

## QUICK DEFINITION

A **vaccine** is a preparation containing a weakened (attenuated) or "killed" solution of a specific bacteria, virus, or germ believed to produce a disease. Some vaccines are live viruses, which are more dangerous. After it is injected into the body, the immune system wages a protective response, developing antibodies to the disease-organism's foreign proteins. The theory is that the antibodies "remember" how to respond and neutralize the vaccine antigen in the future, thereby bestowing immunity to the illness.

**Anthroposophic medicine** is an extension of conventional Western medicine developed by Austrian scientist Rudolf Steiner in the 1920s, in conjunction with other European physicians. It is based on a spiritual model of the human being and its medicines are extensions of homeopathic remedies. In the United States, there are about 60 practitioners, all M.D.s or D.O.s, plus many hundreds of nurses and adjunctive therapists, but in German-speaking countries, there are thousands of practitioners plus several hospitals in Germany and Switzerland devoted exclusively to this medical approach.

# Do Vaccines Delay Children's Development?

The nation is seemingly in the midst of an autism epidemic: the California Department of Developmental Services found a 273% increase of autism between 1987 and 1998. Maryland has reported a 513% increase in autism between 1993 and 1998 and several dozen other states have reported similar findings. Hearings in the House Government Reform Committee were held in August 1999 and April 2000 to investigate the possible causes. Testimony given before the committee included those from parents of New Jersey's Brick Township where one in 149 children suffers from autism, a much higher incidence than national statistics. These parents contend that their children developed autistic symptoms after receiving common childhood vaccinations.

Unfortunately, there has been very little scientific study into the possible connection between autism and vaccines. It is suspected that autism might be connected to the MMR (measles-mumps-rubella) vaccine. One report published by Dr. Vijendra Singh, Department of Pharmacology, University of Michigan, found a higher incidence of MMR antibody in autistic children than normal children.[9]

The National Vaccine Information Center in Vienna, Virginia, has also noted a strong association of the MMR with autistic features (as well as DPT vaccine with infantile spasms). The Encephalitis Support Group in Sinnington, England, reports that, according to parents who have contacted the organization, children who became autistic after the MMR vaccine started showing early symptoms of autism about 30 days after vaccination. They also report that the DPT vaccine (given at two, four, and six months) has triggered autistic symptoms.

The common denominator for both the DPT and MMR vaccines is their potential to interrupt myelinization (formation of fatty wrappings or insulation of nerves) in developing infants. The MMR vaccination may also be the proverbial straw that breaks the camel's back. In this case, the "camel" is the infant's immune system.

Some research suggests that autism may develop in utero when the fetus is only 16-24 weeks old. Perhaps, the mother had the flu during the early months of her pregnancy or was exposed to a pathogen; such an event could compromise her fetus' immune and central nervous systems during the critical stage of development. Some mothers of children with autism have high blood levels of rubella. This may be due to the mother's own childhood reaction to vaccination. Her high blood levels then have an impact on the fetus.

For whatever reason, the infant enters the world with an immune system unable to handle certain stresses, such as vaccinations given at birth or subsequent months in the first year of life. Many children, in fact, don't respond well. In Europe and Asia, doctors wait until the infant is much older before vaccinating; in Japan, the DPT vaccine is not given until the child is two years old, while in the United States. it is given when the infant is one month old.

vaccinations can lead to a greater incidence of adult health problems. The same is true when childhood illnesses are routinely suppressed with antibiotics rather than helping the cell-mediated immune system to work out the illness in a rash or mucous discharge.

Recent research confirms this view. In early 1997, a team of British physicians writing in *Science* made this provocative statement: "Childhood infections may paradoxically protect against asthma." The British physicians noted that the incidence of asthma has doubled in Western countries since 1977. In the United States, it is responsible for 33% of all pediatric emergency-room visits. Yet this growing incidence of asthma seems to be related more to the suppression or absence of respiratory infections than to the commonly perceived cause of air pollution. Highly polluted European cities where the use of antibiotics and immunizations is less than in the U.S. have lower asthma rates than comparable U.S. cities. Conversely, in Tucson, Arizona, despite the dry heat and lack of irritants (such as dust mites) in the air, the rate of asthma is the same as elsewhere in the country.

The *Science* research suggests that diseases such as tuberculosis and whooping cough may permanently alter a child's immune system such that they confer a lifetime protection against asthma. Certainly they were not saying that children should have tuberculosis, but they noted that the humoral immune system needs to be tempered by the cell-mediated response, and this best happens during an infectious childhood disease.

When a child undergoes an intense but short-term lung infection, for example, this provides the necessary exercise of the cell-mediated immune system. If this does not happen, the humoral system is left unbridled and subject to overreaction (allergies) to otherwise harmless substances such as pollen and dust particles. Eventually, this may lead to asthma.

Let's follow this idea in the case of measles. When a child gets a measles rash, the body excretes the virus through the skin, usually within about four days after rash onset. If the child does not get a measles rash, some of the measles virus remains un-neutralized in the body where it can act as a chronic irritant to the immune system and contribute to degenerative disease later.

The fever and rash of measles enable the body to burn up the virus; having a measles vaccine is like planting a seed of future infection in the body and tricking the body not to reject it. This is because a vaccine results in only a partial immunity—the humoral system is triggered while the cell-

For more information on **vaccinations**, see Chapter 4: Prevention of Sensitization, pp. 106-127.

## Does Sanitation Encourage Allergies?

The rise in allergy and asthma has coincided with many changes in the Western world—use of chemicals, widespread immunizations, and consumption of more processed foods—leading many researchers to conclude that these factors are responsible for the increased prevalence of allergic disorders. Two recent studies also suggest that sanitization is also partly to blame for the rapid jump in allergy.

In one paper published in the *British Medical Journal*, Italian scientists reported that respiratory allergy (allergic rhinitis and asthma) occurred less frequently in people heavily exposed to orofecal and foodborne pathogens, such as *Helicobacter pylori*. Of the 680 test subjects, 245 had been exposed to at least two infections. In this group, only one (0.4%) had asthma while only 16 (7%) had allergic rhinitis—significantly lower rates compared to the other participants.[11]

In another study, published in the *American Journal of Respiratory and Critical Care Medicine*, 1,199 rural youth in Canada between the ages of 12 and 19 years old were surveyed for prevalence of asthma. Half of the subject had been raised on a farm and exposed to various aeroallergens, such as animal dander, bacteria, fungi, and dust, while the rest had not been raised in a farming environment. The researchers found that adolescents who were raised on farms had far fewer incidences of asthma than the others.[12] (Additionally, farm children reported that they were more likely to grow up with a pet, but that pets were not allowed in the bedroom, attesting to the efficacy of environmental control.)

The researchers in both of these studies speculated that viral infections enable children to better respond to potential allergens. Excessive sanitation and low exposure to viruses and other pathogens appears to make children more susceptible to developing allergies.

mediated system (which offers long-term protection) remains dormant or can even be inhibited by the vaccine.

It is significant to note that in a recent study, adults who received the pertussis (whooping cough) vaccine were not at risk for developing allergies.[10] This is because both poles of the immune system usually function properly by adulthood.

# Barrier Function Default: The Root of Allergy and Sensitivity

Barrier function is an important concept in understanding and treating allergy/sensitivity. Barrier functions are those things that keep the patient from becoming sensitized (experiencing a negative body response) to substances. There are three major barriers and some supporting organs to consider.

The barrier function for food sensitivity or intolerance is digestion. If the patient can digest and metabolize normally, they do not become sensitized to foods. Inadequate digestion for any reason (infection, inflammation, malabsorption) may result in digestive barrier default, and particles that are too large are absorbed into the bloodstream. If that occurs, sensitization becomes a random event. That is, the patient may or may not become sensitized to any food or chemical constituent or metabolite of that food. Clearly, those substances highest in the patient's food chain (the things they eat the most) are the most suspect. Remember that due to digestion and delayed (rather than immediate) hypersensitivity responses, it is very difficult to correlate food symptoms to exposure. Allergy testing must consider IgG as well as IgE antibodies to foods.

The second, most difficult, barrier to assess and control is for inhaled substances (dust, pollens, dander, molds, etc.) That barrier is the mucus that covers the membranes of the sinuses and respiratory passages. If there is too much mucus, the passages can't drain and infection results. The purpose of the mucus is to trap any irritants and particulates so that they do not come in contact with the membranes and can be removed (blowing the nose, sneezing, or coughing). If the nose, sinuses, or respiratory passages have areas without mucus, however, a pollen that comes in direct contact with the membrane may irritate it enough so that the pollen is absorbed into the bloodstream and sensitization occurs. Adequate fluid intake, humidification of the air, nasal application of isotonic saline drops, and use of mucilaginous plant substances (slippery elm, plantain, marshmallow root) are protective measures for the mucous membranes.

The third barrier is the skin. Any break in the skin (cut, scrape, burn, rash, or other skin defect) compromises the barrier. Sensitization may occur with any substance that comes in contact with that area of the skin. Cosmetics, eyeglasses, jewelry, perfumes, deodorants, sunscreen, as well as skin organisms are all commonly sensitized.

Organs that support the barrier functions are the adrenal, thyroid, and endocrine glands, and the pancreas, which regulates blood sugar. Numerous factors can lead to functional defaults in all three barriers and their support organs. These causes are discussed below.

For more on **testing**, see Chapter 3: Allergy/Sensitivity Testing, pp. 70-105.

## Digestive Dysfunction and Leaky Gut Syndrome

The digestive tract is an elaborate system that involves organs from the mouth to the colon (see "A Primer on Digestion," p. 47). One of the system's components, the small intestine, performs an essential barrier function in keeping the body free from allergy. The intestine's membrane acts as a wall separating undigested food and the bloodstream; this function allows the digestive tract organs to properly break down food into smaller, usable molecules, which then are sent through the bloodstream to nourish the body's tissues. Some amount of wall permeability is common. In people with a normal, intact gut, up to 2% of undigested protein molecules can pass through the mucous membranes.

But when there is an inflammation in the gastrointestinal mucosa, the intestinal wall becomes excessively permeable—a condition called leaky gut syndrome. If bits of food have not been properly broken down due to imbalances in the digestive tract, food molecules (macromolecules), which are usually too large to pass through the intestinal barrier, slip through the gaps in the gut wall and enter the bloodstream. When this happens, the immune system treats these foreign substances as antigens, setting off an allergic response in which antibodies are secreted in the bloodstream to couple with and immobilize the macromolecules.

> ## The Body's Barrier Functions
>
> ■ Intestinal Wall/Digestion
> ■ Skin
> ■ Mucous Membranes
>    (Respiratory System)

This antigen and antibody combination is known as a circulating immune complex (CIC). In a healthy person, CICs are neutralized, but in someone with an immune system compromised by other factors, such as childhood vaccinations, poor diet, or stress, they tend to accumulate in the blood where they burden the detoxification pathways or initiate an allergic reaction. If too many CICs accumulate, the kidneys and liver cannot get rid of enough of them via the urine or stool. The CICs then settle in soft tissues, causing inflammation and bringing further stress to the immune system, leading to more allergies.

There are many instigators of leaky gut–induced allergies. Some factors, such as parasites, directly inflame the mucosal barrier, leading to excessive permeability. Others, such as enzyme deficiency, disrupt the pH balance in the digestive tract, preventing the proper breakdown of large food molecules. The early introduction of solid foods, internal dysbiosis, and alcohol ingestion can do both. The common causes of both leaky gut and digestive dysfunction are described below.

## A Primer on Digestion

Digestion begins in the mouth with digestive enzymes secreted by the salivary glands. These enzymes include amylase, lipase, and some protease. Also at work in the mouth are the enzymes (plant enzymes) present in foods being eaten.

Salivary enzymes combined with the plant enzymes continue digestion in the upper (cardiac) portion of the stomach. Amylase will digest up to 60% of carbohydrates, protease up to 30% of protein, and lipase up to 10% of fat, before HCl (hydrochloric or stomach acid) and pepsin (a stomach enzyme) begin to work in the stomach.

After about an hour, stomach cells secrete enough HCl to further acidify the

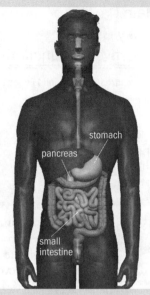

predigested food to a low pH. This acidic pH temporarily deactivates the plant enzymes and the predigested food passes to the lower portion of the stomach, where cells in the stomach lining secrete more pepsin; it is here that pepsin continues the digestion of protein. Adequate HCl is required to activate pepsin from its inactive form and to maintain the stomach pH below 3.0, the optimum level for pepsin to work.

In the next stage of digestion, the partially digested food and deactivated plant enzymes pass into the upper part of the small intestine (the duodenum). Here, digestion continues with the help of bile, pancreatic enzymes, and an alkalizing substance (bicarbonate) that reactivates the food enzymes by reducing acidity. Then digestion proceeds to the jejunum (the next section of the small intestine), where disaccharidases (sugar-digesting enzymes) are secreted. From the small intestine, the majority of nutrients from digested food are absorbed into the blood.

**Early Introduction of Solid Foods**—Although fetuses undergo the vast majority of their physiological development in the womb, it isn't until after birth that all organ systems become fully formed and independently functional. Immunity, as we discussed above, is one of these systems. So too are intestinal barrier function and the digestive system.

A recent study postulates that the high occurrence of food allergy in young infants is likely the result of immature intestinal barrier function.[13] A healthy balance of intestinal bacteria (called microflora) is needed to build strong gut and digestive function. However, research has found that

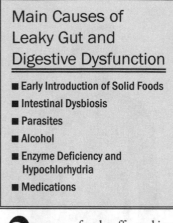

## Main Causes of Leaky Gut and Digestive Dysfunction

■ Early Introduction of Solid Foods

■ Intestinal Dysbiosis

■ Parasites

■ Alcohol

■ Enzyme Deficiency and Hypochlorhydria

■ Medications

For information about **introducing solid foods to infants**, see Chapter 4: Prevention of Sensitization, pp. 106-127.

microbial colonization of the intestine doesn't begin until just after birth, and numerous variables at birth—such as degree of hygiene, mode of delivery, administration of antibiotics and other medications, and use of incubators—can impair this process.[14]

In addition, any of the formulas and processed solid foods fed to young infants, such as cow's milk, cereal (wheat) products, corn, eggs, and meat, contain difficult-to-digest proteins. Infants' developing digestive tracts are not able to properly break down these foodstuffs, and immature gut walls cannot contain the partially undigested protein molecules. Thus, these macromolecules leak through the gut wall into the bloodstream, resulting in sensitization. Several studies prove that early introduction of solid food causes allergies. For example, in a 10-year study involving 1,265 children in New Zealand, children who were introduced to four or more types of solid foods before the age of four months were 2.9 times more likely to develop recurrent eczema than children not exposed to early solid feeding.[15]

**Intestinal Dysbiosis—**As we briefly discussed above, intestinal strength and integrity depend on proper colonization of microflora, or bacteria. There are more than 400 species of bacteria living in the human body and the majority of these bacteria reside in the gastrointestinal tract. Under conditions of intestinal health, "friendly" bacteria (such as *Lactobacillus acidophilus* and *Bifidobacterium bifidum*) predominate and contribute to digestion and the overall health of the body. But, increasingly, the shift observed today is towards a predominance of pathogenic bacteria, a condition called intestinal dysbiosis. Of particular concern in the development of allergy/sensitivity is the overgrowth of *Candida albicans* (SEE QUICK DEFINITION), which is called candidiasis. *Candida* and other unfriendly or pathogenic bacteria that dominate the intestines impair digestion, the absorption of nutrients, and the normal elimination cycle. They also contribute to the erosion of the intestinal membrane and the infiltration of inappropriate substances into the bloodstream.

*Candida* overgrowth can also trigger allergic reactions on its own by stimulating a non-cellular part of the immune system known as the complement pathway. This is a technical term referring to a series of 28 proteins that are activated in a chain reaction when the immune system senses that an antigen is present. The complement system's legitimate job is to amplify inflammation, because the body's goal is to clean itself, to flush out of the tissues the circulating immune complexes. The complement system summons additional white blood cells to the contaminated tissues to start cleansing them of the inappropriately deposited *Candida* antigens. When the inflammatory response gets out of control, however, then the disease process shifts and localized healthy tissues get damaged by the excessive white blood cell activity. White blood cells release powerful peroxides (such as hydrogen peroxide) that oxidize invaders as well as healthy tissues. When this continues long enough, delayed hypersensitivity reactions, such as reactive airway disease and arthritis, are initiated.

The liver is also involved in this short-lived, natural inflammatory response. Under normal conditions, the liver traps about 99% of the bacteria that has escaped form the intestines. *Candida* overgrowth and other pathogenic bacteria activate the Kupffer cells, immune cells residing in the liver, which cause a release of interleukin 2. Interleukin 2 is a lymphokine, a chemical that calls in other white blood cells to the area to clean up the "gut garbage," a process that increases inflammation. If the liver is overburdened or compromised by poor diet, excessive toxins, or other factors, it becomes less efficient at processing circulating immune complexes. (See "Toxic Overload Impairs All Barrier Functions," p. 56, for more details on how overburdened detoxification organs cause allergies.)

**Parasites**—Parasites (SEE QUICK DEFINITION) are often-overlooked contributors to a leaky gut. Parasites tend to reside in the intestines, where they can cause extensive damage. Rarely, they also migrate to the blood, lymph, heart, liver, gallbladder, pancreas, spleen, eyes, and brain. While in place, they can produce numerous symptoms in addition to

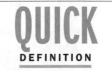

**DEFINITION**

**Candida albicans** is a yeast-like fungus found widely in nature, in the soil, on vegetables and fruits, and in the human body. It is frequently present in small quantities in the intestines and in a woman's vagina. When its numbers are few, *Candida* is generally not harmful to the human body. A *Candida* overgrowth, a condition called candidiasis, can become pathogenic and cause toxic reactions throughout the body. The toxic reactions are from absorption of candidatoxin, which is produced by the yeast and absorbed through the membranes. These reactions can lead to a wide range of symptoms, including depression, fatigue, weight gain, anxiety, rashes, headaches, and muscle cramping.

A **parasite** is any organism that lives off another organism (called a host), and draws nourishment from it. Specifically, parasites are the protozoa (single-cell organisms), arthropods (insects), and worms that infect the body and cause serious damage to tissues and organs. Common forms of the protozoan parasites are *Giardia lamblia*, which causes giardiasis; *Entamoeba histolytica*, which causes dysentery; and *Cryptosporidium*, which causes diarrhea, in people with immunologic diseases such as AIDS. The most common arthropod parasites are lice, mites, ticks, and fleas. Worm parasites include pinworms, roundworms, tapeworms, whipworms, hookworms, and filaria (threadlike worms that inhabit the blood and tissues).

# Causes of Candidiasis

Medications and foods are largely responsible for the development of candidiasis. Antibiotic drugs, frequently prescribed for even the smallest of infections, severely alter the intestinal flora by killing off bacteria, including beneficial microorganisms. As the bacterial communities repopulate after prolonged use of antibiotics, the colonic environment favors the growth of disease-causing organisms such as Candida in lieu of the healthier bacteria. Additionally, conventionally produced meats contain large amounts of antibiotics used to make the animals grow larger and more rapidly. When we eat these antibiotic-tainted meats, the effects on the microflora are the same as ingesting the antibiotics firsthand.

The Standard American Diet (SAD), high in sugar, refined carbohydrates, and chemically laden foods, also stimulates the growth of unfriendly bacteria. Simple sugars, in particular, are a favorite Candida food. Many of these foods are deleterious to pH balance of the stomach and intestines, decreasing the amount of intestinal secretions that aid in the proper breakdown of foods, and further promoting the overgrowth of pathogenic microorganisms. Birth control pills, steroid medications, antacids, and anti-ulcer drugs also disrupt the pH in the intestines by making them more alkaline. Candida and other pathogenic bacteria flourish in alkaline environments.

allergies: constipation, diarrhea, gas, bloating, irritable bowel syndrome, joint and muscle aches, anemia, skin problems, sleep disturbances, chronic fatigue, and gradual immune dysfunction. Parasites release toxins that damage tissues, resulting in pain and inflammation, particularly in the gastrointestinal tract; over time, they can depress, even exhaust, the immune system.

People assume they are vulnerable to parasites only if they travel in tropical areas, but this is a dangerous misconception, says parasite specialist Ann Louise Gittleman, M.S., author of *Guess What Came to Dinner*. Anyone can get them from merely staying at home. *Giardia lamblia*, for instance, is the major cause of diarrhea in day care centers; and *Cryptosporidium* and *Giardia* are found in many municipal water supplies.[16]

Undiagnosed parasitic infections may account for a great deal of otherwise unexplained allergic conditions, according to Leo Galland, M.D., of New York City. "I have seen hundreds of patients with chronic illnesses involving allergies, food intolerances, fatigue, or toxic feelings, who have parasitic infections. Frequently, they also complain of inflammatory skin disorders, joint pain, or arthritis. I always look for parasites when faced with those conditions and about one-third of the time, I will find them." Dr. Galland goes on to say that eliminating the parasites produces significant improvement in those patients an estimated 80%-85% of the time.

**Medications**—Certain drugs such as antacids, anti-ulcer and steroid medications, and oral contraceptives, are alkalizing. When they enter the stomach, they can impair hydrochloric acid's ability to break down food molecules, enabling macromolecules to escape through the leaky gut (which these drugs also indirectly cause by stimulating *Candida* overgrowth).

**Hypochlorhydria and Enzyme Deficiency**—Hypochlorhydria and enzyme deficiencies are major causes of the digestive dysfunction that leads to allergies and sensitivities. Hypochlorhydria is hydrochloric acid (HCl) deficiency. As we age, HCl levels decline; however, other factors, such as excess fat and sugar in the diet, overeating, bacterial (*Helicobacter pylori*) infections, weakened adrenal function, and stress also can lead to HCl depletion. Adequate HCl is absolutely essential for proper digestion. HCl is necessary to activate the stomach enzyme pepsin, which is needed for digestion.

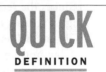

Enzymes (SEE QUICK DEFINITION) are required for the proper digestion of fats, carbohydrates, and proteins. If the pH in the stomach is higher than 3, digestive enzymes will not be activated. Furthermore, if your stomach contents are not at a pH of 3 or less, the pH downstream in the duodenum (where the pancreas enzymes are secreted into the gut) will also be abnormal. Although the enzymes will be released into the gut as normal, they will not be activated due to the overly alkaline pH. Thus, food will not be adequately digested. If we do not have an adequate supply of enzymes, we will not only be malnourished but, according to enzyme-therapy pioneer Howard F. Loomis, Jr., D.C., of Madison, Wisconsin, large undigested protein molecules may seep into our bloodstream through a leaky gut. Allergic sensitization is the result.

> **DEFINITION**
>
> **Enzymes** are specialized proteins fundamental to all living processes in the body, necessary for every chemical reaction and the normal activity of our organs, tissues, fluids, and cells. Enzymes are essential for the production of energy required to run cellular functions. There are hundreds of thousands of these "Nature's workers." Enzymes enable the body to digest and assimilate food. There are special enzymes for digesting proteins, carbohydrates, fats, and plant fibers. Specifically, protease digests proteins, amylase digests carbohydrates, lipase digests fats, cellulase digests fiber, and disaccharidase digests sugars. Enzymes also assist in clearing the body of toxins and cellular debris.

We can also derive enzymes from external sources, such as food and supplements. Enzymes are present in raw foods and contribute a small amount to digestion, but studies have shown that food enzymes like bromelain (pineapple) and papain (papaya) are far less effective than pancreatic enzymes in digesting food and correcting malabsorption.

When pancreatic enzymes, necessary for digestion, are in short supply due to malnourishment or toxic overload (see "Toxic Overload Impairs All Barrier Functions," p. 56), the body will search elsewhere for replacement enzymes to do the job. White blood cells called leukocytes, top players in the body's immune defense, are rich sources of similar enzymes. They readily relinquish their enzymes to perform the priority process of digestion, leaving the immune system unable to decipher allergens and antigens.[17] In his book *The Complete Guide to Food Allergy and Intolerance*, Jonathan Brostoff, M.D., reports that in one study, 90% of people with chemical sensitivities and food intolerance were enzyme-deficient. He further notes that hyperactive children appear to have a deficiency of the enzyme phenolsulphotransferase-P (PST-P), a detoxification enzyme that can be deactivated by some food colorings.[18]

**Alcohol—**The health risks of excessive consumption of alcohol are well-known, but even moderate alcohol consumption can increase your chances of developing allergies. According to Dr. Braly, alcohol reduces the secretion of hydrochloric acid in the stomach. When the digestive tract is rendered more alkaline due to alcohol consumption, not only will enzymes not be activated and food not properly digested, but unfriendly intestinal flora such as *Candida* will flourish. Alcohol also inhibits the efficiency of an enzyme called delta-6-desaturase, which is necessary in the production of anti-inflammatory prostaglandins (hormone-like fats that can cause or block inflammation), protection against autoimmune disease, inhibition of inflammation in the intestinal wall, and maintenance of skin barrier function.[19]

## Skin Barrier Default

Most of us don't view the skin as an organ, but it happens to be the largest and one of the heaviest, albeit simplest, organs of the body. Skin performs many important functions for the body—regulating heat loss through perspiration, assisting the detoxification process, and helping produce and store vitamin D, which is crucial for calcium absorption. A major component of the immune system, the skin is also able to identify potentially dangerous substances from beneficial ones, and deters such external elements, such as viruses, toxins, and chemicals, from entering the body. This barrier function is crucial in preventing allergies and sensitivities.

When the skin is irritated, either by dry conditions, sunburn, cuts and abrasions, acne, and chemicals, it is no longer able to "remember" which substances are bad and which are good. Consequently, it may randomly allow some antigens to literally get under your skin and enter your bloodstream, while blockading beneficial substances from entering the body. The immune system, however, is still able to identify invading antigens and begins the allergic response.

People become most sensitized to what touches damaged skin most frequently. Clothing, fabric chemicals and dyes, laundry products, cosmetics, perfume, aftershave lotions, creams, sunscreens, and even topical medicines can trigger allergic reactions, such as eczema and allergic contact dermatitis. Perspiration mixed with any of the above substances increases the likelihood of sensitization, since sweat promotes absorption.

Properly nourished, the skin can resist these irritations and quickly rebuild its protective layers, keeping the barrier—and its cellular immune memory—intact. However, deficiencies in water and essential fatty acids, ultraviolet radiation, hormonal irregularities, and stress, can impair the skin's repair process, leading the way to allergy and sensitivity.

**Essential Fatty Acids and the Skin**—The stratum corneum (see "The Skinny on Skin," p. 54) is the most important skin structure in terms of barrier function. This layer of skin is made up of skin cells and three types of fats—ceramides, cholesterol, and essential fatty acids. These fats provide the water barrier function of the skin. If there is an imbalance in these fats, holes open between stratum corneum cells, resulting in water loss and increased risk of sensitization. The body usually makes enough ceramides and cholesterol to replenish the skin barrier function. However, the body cannot manufacture essential fatty acids (EFAs), so they must be derived from the diet. There are two primary groups of EFAs, omega-6 and omega-3.

For more about **essential fatty acids and the skin**, see Chapter 9: Supporting the Skin, pp. 236-259.

An omega-6 EFA called linoleic acid (LA) is required in the skin barrier. Linoleic acid is found in the oils of safflower, sunflower, corn, soy, and sesame. The body converts linoleic acid into the more usable EFA, gamma-linolenic acid (GLA). GLA is found naturally in evening primrose oil, black currant oil, and borage oil. Dietary deficiency of LA (and by extension, of GLA) has been shown to cause epidermal water loss (manifesting as dry, scaly skin), reduced production of anti-inflammatory prostaglandins, and skin allergies such as eczema. Many people cannot metabolize LA into GLA because the enzyme that does that, delta-6-desaturase, is often inactive. Many factors—aging, stress, vitamin B6 deficiency, zinc or magnesium deficiency, and sunlight—block this enzyme. Among the results of this metabolic problem are increased risks of skin allergies and sensitivities.

## Mucous Membrane Barrier Default

The respiratory system is a complex and sensitive network of airways involving the nose, nasal cavity, pharynx, larynx, trachea, bronchi, and

# The Skinny on Skin

Two layers comprise the skin, the epidermis and the dermis. The epidermis, the outer layer of skin, is generally quite thin, less than 0.12 mm over most of the body. It consists of five levels. The outermost level is the stratum corneum, a network of cells on the surface of the skin that provides protection from the outside world and helps restrict the loss of water. The lowest epidermal level is the stratum basale. Found in the stratum basale are melanocyte cells, which produce the pigment melanin that protects us from ultraviolet radiation. Langerhans cells, which trap and help destroy viruses and antigens, and keratinocytes, cells that produce the protein fiber keratin (mostly found in hair an nails), are also found in the epidermis. Dead epidermal cells are constantly being shed, replaced by new cells that push up from the stratum basale approximately every 28 days.

The dermis is the second layer of skin, approximately 2 mm thick, containing blood vessels, lymph vessels, and nerves. The dermis is made up of two layers, the papillary dermis and the reticular dermis. The papillary dermis has projections (papillae) that protrude into the epidermis, making fingerprint patterns. This level also contains sensory receptors that respond to external stimuli such as temperature and pressure changes. The reticular dermis is the deeper level, consisting mostly of collagen, protein bundles arranged in wavy bands that provide structure and support to the skin. Elastin, a fibrous, elastic material that enables the skin to stretch, is also found here.

Throughout the dermal layers are eccrine (sweat) glands. Hair follicles are planted deep in the base of the dermis and contain sebaceous glands, which produce a greasy substance (sebum) that lubricates the skin and provides further protection against external substances. Beneath the dermis is the subcutaneous fatty tissue, where blood vessels connect the dermal layers to the circulatory system.

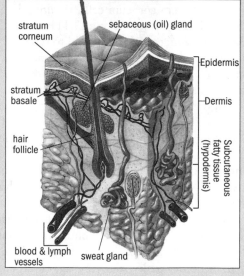

stratum corneum

sebaceous (oil) gland

Epidermis

stratum basale

Dermis

hair follicle

Subcutaneous fatty tissue (hypodermis)

blood & lymph vessels

sweat gland

lungs that supplies the body with oxygen and removes carbon dioxide. To perform these functions, the respiratory system is in constant contact with the outside environment—and with countless irritants and antigens. To prevent these foreign substances from entering the bloodstream, the respiratory network is equipped with specialized cleaning mechanisms. Air is filtered through nose hairs and lymph tissue in the throat, and then constantly refiltered through millions of tiny cilia (hairlike projections along membranous cell tissue) to remove any particles that could cause lung damage.

Particles that manage to bypass the respiratory defenses are trapped in the mucous membranes, the lining of our respiratory organs, particularly the nose and lungs, which is covered by a sheet of mucus. Cilia move particles, mixed with mucus, from deep in the respiratory system to the pharynx (part of the upper throat behind the tongue and nasal cavity). From there, the particles are expelled by coughing or swallowed, where they are destroyed by stomach acid. To trap the foreign substances, the mucous membranes must be kept moist to foster the integrity of mucus. Lack of humidity and environmental irritants can damage the mucous membranes and allow foreign particles entry into the bloodstream, leading to allergies.

**Lack of Humidity**—When you sleep, you breathe constantly, without taking in any fluids or food. If the heat is on or you live in a low-humidity climate, your mucous membranes will dry out in this period of time. Research has also shown that ciliary movement also slows down in a dry environment.[20] Without mucus and properly functioning cilia, you are at an increased risk for sensitizing to substances in your bedroom air.

**Environmental Irritants**—Re-search shows that inhalation of environmental pollutants, such as sulfur dioxide and tobacco smoke, alters and reduces mucus secretion and ciliary activity in all people, not just those who are deemed "atopic," or susceptible to allergies.[21] In a state of chronic exposure, the mucosa (mucous membranes) becomes inflamed, cilia move more slowly, and areas of abnormally thin or even broken epithelial lining develop. This condition is similar to leaky

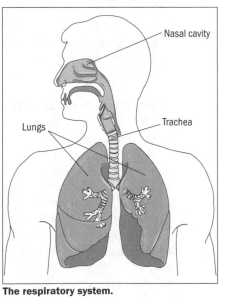

**The respiratory system.**

To learn **how to improve mucous membrane barrier function**, see Chapter 10: Supporting the Respiratory System, pp. 260-277. For information on **avoiding environmental pollutants**, see Chapter 5: Environmental Control, pp. 128-157.

gut, in that foreign particles are allowed entry into the blood-stream, increasing the risk of sensitization.

Most Americans are exposed to air pollution. Approximately 107 million people live in counties with unhealthy air, according to the U.S. Environmental Protection Agency.[22] However, if you work or live in a modern building, chances are you don't have to step outside to encounter air irritants. Approximately 30% of new or renovated buildings are "sick buildings," sealed, energy-efficient buildings with dangerously high volatile organic compound (VOC) levels constantly being re-circulated inside.[23] Common allergens such as dust mites and cockroaches are also trapped inside the air ducts of these sick buildings.

# Toxic Overload Impairs All Barrier Functions

As our food and environment become increasingly saturated with pollutants and chemicals, the body's mechanisms for elimination of toxins cannot keep up with the chemical deluge. All organs involved in detoxification, which include the allergy barrier systems of the intestines, skin, and respiratory system, can become overloaded. This overload weakens the barrier functions and can lead to sensitization. Furthermore, the constant circulation of toxins in the body taxes the immune system, which must continually strive to destroy or eliminate them. An overburdened immune system ultimately becomes hypersensitive, and allergies—to food, airborne agents, and chemicals—develop.

### The Detoxification Defense System

The body is equipped with a specialized detoxification system to handle toxins. The detoxification system has two lines of defense—specific organs prevent toxins from entering the body and others neutralize and excrete the poisonous compounds that get through this initial line of defense. When functioning properly, the body's defenses prevent toxic overload, keep the immune system regulated, and protect tissues from harmful free radicals (SEE QUICK DEFINITION) or circulating toxins. Key components of the detoxification system include:

- Gastrointestinal barrier, including the small and large intestines
- Liver
- Lymphatic system, which transports waste products from the cells to the major organs of detoxification

■ Kidneys, bladder, and other components of the urinary system

■ Skin, including the sweat and sebaceous glands

■ Lungs

The gastrointestinal system is typically the first line of defense against toxins and, when compromised, the first place to harbor seeds of disease. Within the 25 feet of the intestinal lining are many hiding places for disease-causing agents, which then break through the intestinal membrane and gain access to the bloodstream. This is one facet of how allergies and sensitivities, especially to foods, begin—once the bowel is toxic, the entire body soon follows. Undigested food materials, bacteria, and other substances usually confined to the intestines escape into the bloodstream and set off the immune system, and inflammation ensues. If the intestines are letting toxins through, then the liver, lymph, kidneys, skin, and other organs involved in detoxification become overwhelmed.

The liver bears most of the burden for eliminating toxins. All antigens and allergens are sent to the liver to be neutralized and expelled from the body The antigen-antibody complexes are eliminated intact in the urine. Through enzymes and antioxidants, the liver chemically transforms toxins into harmless substances that can be excreted via the urine or stool. Other toxins are eliminated through the lymphatic system, kidneys, the skin (by sweating), and respiratory system. When imbalances occur in this system, the result can be poor digestion, constipation, bloating and gas, immune dysfunction, reduced liver function, and a host of degenerative diseases.

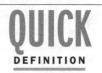

**QUICK**

**DEFINITION**

A **free radical** is an unstable, toxic molecule of oxygen with an unpaired electron that steals an electron from another molecule and produces harmful effects. Free radicals are formed when molecules within cells react with oxygen (oxidize) as part of normal metabolic processes. Free radicals then begin to break down cells, especially the cell membranes, often in a matter of minutes to an hour. Their work is enhanced if there are not enough free-radical quenching nutrients, such as vitamins C and E, in the cell. While free radicals are normal products of metabolism, uncontrolled free-radical production plays a major role in the development of degenerative disease, including cancer and heart disease. Free radicals harmfully alter important molecules, such as proteins, enzymes, fats, even DNA. Other sources of free radicals include pesticides, industrial pollutants, smoking, alcohol, viruses, most infections, allergies, stress, even certain foods and excessive exercise.

## How Toxins Become Harmful

While our emotional and physiological systems are remarkably resilient and adaptable by nature, they need to be maintained to adequately defend against outside contamination. When we undergo prolonged psychological stress without taking measures to alleviate it or expose ourselves involuntarily to pollution, when we eat foods that lack nutritional value on a regular basis or neglect to exercise or resign ourselves to chronic constipation, we essentially invite toxins to gain an upper hand. Once inside the body, toxins create or worsen a variety of negative conditions that con-

## Are Allergies an Attempt at Detoxification?

Some scientists contend that allergies are the body's last-ditch effort to eliminate toxins. When the body's natural detoxification system is overburdened with chemical pollutants and other toxins, the body responds with emergency cleansing measures—sneezing, coughing, watery eyes, even vomiting—to expel potentially harmful substances from the body. Leo Galland, M.D., of New York City, agrees with this theory, explaining that one of the functions of histamine, which is released during an allergic reaction, is to stimulate the liver's detoxifying enzymes.

But why does the body view seemingly harmless foods and pollens as toxic substances? Dr. Galland believes it's because allergens aren't as innocuous as they seem. "Pollen grains have some toxicity," he says. "They contain lectins [SEE QUICK DEFINITION] on their surface." Peanuts, another common allergen, contain aflatoxins, toxins excreted by molds, which can suppress the immune system. "A lot of substances to which people tend to be allergic are found in association with [toxic] molds," he explains. "There's something protective going on. The allergic system in the body is a backup to methods of detoxification to help you get rid of something toxic."

However, allergies are a high-cost way to eliminate toxins, as they further damage the immune system and make us feel sick. Unclogging and rebuilding the pathways of detoxification along with lightening our toxic load, are safer, healthier ways to address the problem of body toxicity.

## QUICK DEFINITION

**Lectins** are protein fragments of incompletely digested foods that bind with specific sugars on the surface of all cells of the body. They tend to stick like Velcro™ to the lining of the gastrointestinal tract, where they irritate the tissues and can destroy cell membranes. Most dietary lectins come from the indigestible fractions of plant products, often deriving from beans, grains, soy and wheat. Lectins cause food allergy and toxic reactions at the mucosal membranes in the intestines. In particular, soybean and wheat lectins can produce an increase in permeability in the cells they bind to, often leading to cell death. Lectins can cause the intestinal villi, are the fingerlike projections that afford the intestines its prodigious absorptive surface area, to atrophy.

For more about **lectins**, see Chapter 6: Therapeutic Diets, pp. 158-183.

tribute to the development of chronic allergies.

Studies by environmental scientists and physicians indicate that pollutants play a role in the creation of all allergies, as well as arthritis and autoimmune illnesses.[24] These reports corroborate the loading theory of toxicity. According to this theory's formulator, Serafina Corsello, M.D., director of the Corsello Centers for Nutritional Complementary Medicine in New York City and Huntington, New York, no single factor causes a disease. Rather, the cumulative load of multiple poisons creates allergies and other illnesses. People don't get most diseases—they develop them, Dr. Corsello explains.

In Dr. Corsello's view, multiple stressors weigh down the immune system and eventually throw it out of balance. Among the typical stressors are toxic metals (mercury leaching from dental fillings, copper, and aluminum), petrochemical residues (pesticides and fertilizers), chemical pollutants in the water and air, electromagnetic pollution (power lines), inappropriate foods (trans-fatty acids in many cooking oils and other foods), nutritional deficiencies, biochemical imbalances, insufficient exercise, and emotional stress (family, job, and personal). These factors impinge on the immune system's natural vitality to resist the downhill slide into illness. Dr. Corsello explains that "these stressors may be accumulating for years, over a lifetime, before they send the system into disrepair. One injurious effect is to lower the body's threshold of resistance to illness."

According to William Rea, M.D., an environmental physician in Dallas, Texas, when key detoxification organs become unable to fully detoxify themselves or the body, a pattern of chronic allergies may develop in which the immune system attacks its own unprocessed toxic load. This state of heightened allergic reactivity keeps the immune system on full alert and, eventually, makes it hyperactive. The constant circulation of toxins in the body taxes the immune system, which must continually strive to destroy them.

**The Damaging Effects of Free Radicals—**Free radicals create oxidation, which is why iron turns to rust and the exposed surfaces of sliced apples turn brown. They are "free" in the sense of being unattached: molecular loose cannons that combine with oxygen in the air to initiate the process of spoilage. Internally, the same sort of deterioration occurs. Free radicals attack cell membranes, often in a matter of minutes. To counter the effects of free radicals, our bodies manufacture or rely on outside sources of antioxidants, whose purpose is to scavenge for free radicals, bind with them, and eliminate them before they contaminate healthy cells. Toxins, however, impede this process by creating too many free radicals, which quickly deplete the body's reserve of antioxidant nutrients. Asthma is caused in part by free-radical damage to the bronchial passageways.[25]

For more on **how free radicals contribute to asthma and allergies**, see Chapter 10: Supporting the Respiratory System, pp. 260-277.

# Sources of Toxins

We are exposed to toxins every day of our lives, from chemicals and pesticide residues in the foods we eat, mercury amalgam dental fillings, biological contaminants such as pollen and parasites, and genetically altered foods, among other sources. Even our own bodies can produce toxins, called endotoxins, which can prove harmful to us if not properly controlled.

## Toxins in the Environment

Toxins emanate from a variety of noxious sources, but chiefly from environmental pollution. Unavoidably, many of us carry around an internal "chemical cocktail" derived from absorbing industrial by-products (coal tar or fuel exhaust), pesticides, herbicides, household contaminants (found in cleaners, paints, plastics, and solvents), and biological contaminants (pollens, molds, dust mites, and parasites). We are also exposed to toxins from processed or genetically altered and irradiated foods, alcohol or tap water (which usually contains heavy metals), and even the newspaper (from the inks used in printing). There are more than 3,200 chemical substances routinely added to various foods.

Since the 1980s, physicians began using the term *sick building syndrome* (SBS) to refer to a host of symptoms produced by sensitivities to low-grade toxic environmental conditions found in living or office spaces. SBS symptoms include respiratory, eye, and skin diseases, headaches, memory loss, fatigue, lethargy, temporary weight loss, infections, irritability, and impaired balance. All of these suppress the immune system, rendering the individual susceptible to long-term chronic illness.

Office workers are exposed to toxic air that is continuously recycled throughout sealed buildings. According to William Lee Cowden, M.D., a clinical researcher in Richardson, Texas, the air inside most modern buildings is five to 100 times more toxic than the outside air.[26] Since most people in industrialized nations spend more than 90% of the time indoors, these indoor concentrations of pollutants can lead to a permanent chronic exposure to toxic factors. This hazard received national publicity when CBS's *60 Minutes* disclosed that the head office of the Environmental Protection Agency in Washington, D.C., was environmentally unsafe for its workers. In most cases, problems with a building's engineering, construction, and ventilation system are the causes of SBS. Add to this the toxic vapors and fumes produced by construction materials, and the result is new, seemingly inexplicable illnesses that affect neurological and biochemical processes.

Environmental pollutants (called xenobiotics) can also disrupt the endocrine system (SEE QUICK DEFINITION), which provides the energy and regulatory hormones necessary to barrier function integrity as well as a smooth-running immune system. Evidence is accumulating that the 1,000 new chemicals introduced worldwide each year, even at very low concentrations and exposures, cause "hormone havoc"—autoimmune diseases, clinical depression, and reproductive system disorders, not to mention allergy and sensitivity. Xenobiotics have also been shown to activate T cell–mediated allergic reactions, such as allergic contact dermatitis.[27]

Toxins can enter the body in ways other than through breathing or swallowing—in particular, through the skin's pores. (Those same pores, of course, also facilitate the elimination of toxic chemicals.) Approximately 70% of the toxins from tap water enter the body through the skin; the remaining 30% of the toxins enter via ingestion. Tap water in the United States contains chlorine, aluminum, pesticides, lead, copper, and other toxic substances.[28]

## Harmful Metals and Chemicals

Mercury and other toxic metals increase free radicals, which attack cell membranes and initiate swelling and inflammation. Mercury fillings are the major source of mercury exposure for the general public,[29] at rates six times higher than those found in fish and seafood.[30] Conventional dental amalgams or "silver" fillings are actually made of only 25% silver, 50% mercury, and lesser amounts of tin, copper, nickel, and zinc. According to James Hardy, D.M.D., of Winter Park, Florida, and author of *Mercury Free*, approximately 100 million Americans have mercury amalgams. Mercury has been shown to be more toxic than arsenic.[31] Studies

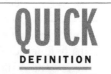

**DEFINITION**

**Endocrine glands,** including the testicles, ovaries, pancreas, adrenals, thyroid, parathyroid, thymus, and pituitary, are central to the regulation and normalization of all the body's complex, interconnected systems, from metabolism and heat production to spermatogenesis and uterine preparations for pregnancy.

An **antioxidant** (meaning "against oxidation") is a natural biochemical substance that protects living cells against damage from harmful free radicals. Antioxidants work against the process of oxidation—the robbing of electrons from substances. If unblocked or left uncontrolled, oxidation can lead to cellular aging, degeneration, arthritis, heart disease, cancer, and other illnesses. Antioxidants in the body react readily with oxygen breakdown products and free radicals, and neutralize them before they can damage the body.

by the World Health Organization show that a single amalgam can release 3-17 micrograms of mercury per day,[32] some of which travels into the body, affecting the bones, the joints, and the central nervous system and brain. Moreover, high levels of mercury inhibit metabolism of glutathione, an antioxidant (SEE QUICK DEFINITION) and free-radical scavenger. A depletion of this natural detoxifying chemical diminishes the liver's ability to eliminate xenobiotics and is implicated in the development of chemical sensitivities.[33] Signs of mercury poisoning include numbness, tingling, paralysis, tremors, and pain.

Copper-lined pipes in plumbing systems can be another source of toxicity. A greenish-brown ring around the tub, sink, or toilet can indi-

To find out **how doctors determine the levels of toxicity in your body**, see Chapter 3: Allergy/Sensitivity Testing, pp. 70-105. To learn **how to reduce your exposure to environmental toxins**, see Chapter 5: Environmental Control, pp. 128-157.

cate that your water is contaminated with copper, which is toxic at high levels. According to Paul C. Eck, Ph.D., and Larry Wilson, M.D., of the Eck Institute of Applied Nutrition and Bioenergetics in Phoenix, Arizona, many of the most prevalent metabolic dysfunctions of our time are in some way related to a copper imbalance and/or copper toxicity. Copper toxicity can cause osteoarthritis, liver problems, adrenal fatigue, and allergies.[34]

Individuals who drink unfiltered water, as well as welders, metal and construction workers, plumbers, and auto mechanics can be exposed to potentially toxic levels of copper.[35] Other sources of copper include birth control pills and intrauterine devices, and many fungicides and pesticides—all of which contain copper as a main ingredient. A thorough analysis from a health-care practitioner, including nutritional and heavy-metal assessment, can determine whether copper detoxification or supplementation is needed.

Chemicals found in dry-cleaning fluids (trichloroethylene), paint solvents (toluene), municipal water supplies (phenol and chlorine), carpets and flooring (formaldehyde), and some imported produce (DDT pesticide residues) are also potentially harmful, depending on your level of susceptibility. Studies have proven that these chemicals can interfere with proper nerve and muscle function, cause skeletal and muscular changes, and alter mental functioning, resulting in such allergy-related conditions as hyperactivity.[36]

## Inner Toxins

Environmental toxins are only one layer of the toxic load that our bodies must process. Endotoxins produced within the body are also present and are potentially dangerous if not efficiently eliminated. Endotoxins include uric and lactic acid, homocysteine, nitric oxide, intestinal toxins (indole, skatole, putrescine, cadaverine, spermadine, spermine), and cellular debris from dead microorganisms. These are normal by-products of metabolic processes that are typically broken down by the liver and excreted from the body. But in someone with a compromised immune system, they tend to accumulate in the blood (in the form of circulating immune complexes), where they burden the detoxification pathways or initiate an allergic reaction. For example, arginine and ornithine (important amino acids) enter the body in the course of a normal diet, but if your system is unable to digest them, they undergo unfavorable chemical changes. Ornithine is converted by bowel bacteria into a toxic substance called putrescine, which in turn, degrades into potentially harmful polyamines, such as spermadine, spermine, and cadaverine.

# Factors That Impair Support-Organ Function

Our adrenal, thyroid, and endocrine glands as well as our blood-sugar system (regulated by the pancreas) support our barrier functions and provide energy to the immune system. When these systems are overwhelmed by chronic stress or overconsumption of sugar, the immune system and barrier functions are suppressed, paving the way for allergy and sensitivity.

## Stress Debilitates the Adrenals and Immune System

Stress has been proven to depress the immune system, thus increasing your susceptibility to allergies and sensitivities. During a stress response, the adrenal glands release high amounts of cortisol, a natural hormone that prepares the body for fight or flight during a dangerous situation. Initially, cortisol actually stops an allergic reaction from occurring. But if stress becomes chronic, the adrenals can only produce this hormone at a certain rate and eventually fail to keep up with demand. The glands become exhausted and depleted of their natural cortisol, impairing the immune system's ability to stave off inflammatory reactions. Since allergies themselves are stressful, there is often a vicious cycle of allergies leading to weakened adrenals leading to more allergies.

To learn **how to reduce stress and its effects on allergy/sensitivity**, see Chapter 14: Mind/Body Approaches to Allergies, pp. 348-373.

Additionally, the adrenal glands play a central role in maintaining the body's energy levels and, when these glands are functioning poorly, the result can be allergic fatigue. The adrenals are also the place outside of the sex organs that produce all sex hormones (male and female). Adrenal exhaustion can negatively affect sexual function and other hormone-dependent processes.

## Sugar Overwhelms the Pancreas and Endocrine System

A frequently overlooked cause of immune problems such as allergy is sugar consumption. For our purposes, the term *sugar* refers to three main types of food-derived simple carbohydrates: glucose, found in some fruits, such as grapes; fructose, found in most fruits, fruit juices, honey, and some vegetables; and sucrose, found in sugar cane, sugar beets, maple syrup, molasses, sorghum, and pineapple (white table sugar is a sucrose). Glucose and sucrose are monosaccharides, the simplest carbohydrates in terms of molecular structure and the basic unit of energy for the body;

fructose molecules are disaccharides, two monosaccharides hooked together, and need to be broken down by special digestive enzymes into glucose. Refined white flour products (bread, cookies, cakes) and potatoes are not simple sugars per se, but they have a high glycemic index, meaning that they are quickly converted to glucose.

The average American consumes about 134 pounds of sugar per year; that's one pound every three days.[37] When you eat a carbohydrate, it is converted to glucose, which then enters the bloodstream. The pancreas gland then releases the hormone insulin to match the level of glucose. The insulin reduces the levels of circulating sugar by helping transfer it into the body's cells, where it is broken down and used as a fuel.

However, insulin is also required to transport vitamin C, a key antioxidant and anti-inflammatory, into the body's cells. Studies indicate that sugar takes precedence over vitamin C in securing the use of available insulin.[38] This results in a quick, and progressively more severe, impairment of phagocytes, white blood cells that engulf and immobilize antigens until other antibodies arrive to destroy the invaders.[39] In one study, eating a small amount of sugar (about two cans of soda) sparked a 92% drop in the phagocyte efficiency for up to five hours.[40] Such deregulation of phagocytes may result in hypersensitive reactions by the other white blood cells.

For tips on **how a whole-foods diet can minimize your intake of sugar**, see Chapter 4: Prevention of Sensitization, pp. 106-127.

Dr. Galland adds that high insulin levels also lead to increased production of pro-inflammatory prostaglandins by inhibiting the absorption of good fats. "Insulin alters the metabolism of the essential fatty acids in the direction of shifting towards those which promote inflammation [arachidonic acids] rather than those which suppress it [omega-3 fats]," he explains. A whole-foods diet, which avoids sugar, and omega-3 EFA supplementation are effective ways to reverse sugar-related problems.

# Eliminating Allergies with Alternative Therapies

Alternative medicine offers lasting relief from allergies. According to the alternative medicine approach, allergies/sensitivities result from multiple causes, many of them with a less-than-obvious connection to the disease or not easily detectable. As you learned above, a number of underlying imbalances, with accompanying physical, mental, and environmental factors, contribute to all forms of allergies.

It is essential to understand the factors that went into creating allergic reactions in each person, because allergies and sensitivities are never caused by one thing alone and no two people share exactly the same causal factors. Alternative medicine employs a battery of diagnostic tools—physical examination, dietary assessment, tests for immune, digestive, and detoxification function, and emotional evaluation—to build an individualized picture of the patient's condition. Skilled alternative practitioners take the time needed to find the root causes of allergies/sensitivities, and the patient also becomes actively involved in their treatment.

Alternative medicine not only respects differences between individuals, but concentrates its diagnosis and treatment plan around this "customized" approach. However, in the case of nearly all allergies and sensitivities—to food, chemicals, or aeroallergens—alternative medicine practitioners employ the same basic strategy: eliminate the allergen, alleviate the immuno-inflammatory action, and stabilize the barrier systems, whether gut, skin, or respiratory system.

To implement this strategy, physicians draw upon a wide range of therapies to help treat—and even prevent—allergies and sensitivities. The primary keys are proper diet and nutrition, detoxification, and stress reduction. Vitamins, minerals, herbs, and other natural supplements can provide effective relief without the side effects of conventional drugs.

Removing toxins from the body has shown to be remarkably therapeutic for allergy patients. Alternative medicine offers a number of safe and effective detoxification strategies. Meditation, biofeedback, hypnotherapy, and other mind/body techniques can help reduce stress (another key factor in allergies sometimes overlooked by conventional medicine). With alternative medicine, health is restored to the whole patient, rather than simply providing superficial symptom relief. The goal is to help each person achieve a balance among physical, the mental-emotional, and even spiritual aspects of their life.

**Testing**—In order to design an individual treatment program that will effectively eliminate allergies and restore you to health, it is necessary for a physician to determine what is happening inside your body. Chapter 3: Allergy/Sensitivity Testing covers the range of testing that alternative medicine physicians have found useful for pinpointing allergic triggers, including methods and self-tests that can identify allergens overlooked by conventional skin testing.

Also detailed are specific tests for discovering the underlying causes of allergies/sensitivities. These include identification of bacterial,

## How Fats Contribute to Allergic Inflammation

The kinds of fats that make up your diet directly affect the severity of inflammation and other allergy/sensitivity symptoms. There are "good" and "bad" dietary fats, and if your diet contains too many of the bad fats, it may be making your allergies worse or helping to create it in the first place. The inflammatory process can become over-reactive when certain dietary factors skew the delicate balance of inflammation-mediating substances. Prostaglandins (SEE QUICK DEFINITION), which can either cause or decrease inflammation, are composed of different fatty acids. The type of prostaglandins (anti- or pro-inflammatory) manufactured by the body depends upon what kinds of fats make up your diet, as well as the presence of enzymes and nutrients (vitamins C, B3, and B6, magnesium, and zinc).

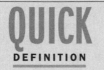

**DEFINITION**

A **prostaglandin** is a hormone-like, complex fatty acid that affects smooth muscle function, inflammatory processes, and blood vessel functions, particularly in the lungs and intestines. Eating too many trans-fatty acids (found in processed foods such as margarine) reduces production of helpful prostaglandins.

Prostaglandins that cause inflammation are formed when the diet is high in animal fats, which contain high amounts of arachidonic acid. Arachidonic acid is a long-chain polyunsaturated omega-6 fatty acid, found primarily in animal foods such as meat, poultry, and dairy products. When the diet is abundant in arachidonic acids, these are stored in cell membranes. An enzyme transforms these acids into prostaglandins and leukotrienes, which both instigate inflammation. If there is an overabundance of arachidonic acid, then more pro-inflammatory agents will be produced by the body.

For more on **how essential fatty acids can reverse inflammation**, see Chapter 11: Supplements for Symptom Control, pp. 278-303.

"Bad" fats called trans-fatty acids (found in hydrogenated oils) also promote production of pro-inflammatory prostaglandins. A diet containing high levels of omega-3 polyunsaturated fatty acids favors the production of anti-inflammatory prostaglandins. Dietary supplementation of omega-3 EFAs has been shown to minimize many allergy and sensitivity symptoms.

viral, parasitic, and yeast infections, immune system imbalances, heavy metal toxicity, and digestive function. Most of these tests involve a simple blood, urine, or stool analysis. When you have identified the primary causes of your allergies and sensitivities, you can use alternative therapies to free yourself of your health problems. A good strategy involves first eliminating the factors that cause hypersensitivity and then rebuilding and nourishing the immune system with supplements, herbs, and relaxation techniques.

**Prevent Sensitization—**Erroneous child-rearing practices, among other dietary and lifestyle choices, figure predominately in the development of allergies. To prevent allergies and sensitivities in children, mothers should breast-feed their infants. Additionally, parents should avoid early introduction of solid foods and early immunization. Drinking adequate amounts of fluids and decreasing intake of processed or "junk" foods are also imperative to preventing allergies. Some other recommendations include humidifying the sleeping space and protecting the skin. Chapter 4: Prevention of Sensitization details these and other suggestions.

**Avoid Allergens and Toxins**—To prepare the body for the healing process, allergy sufferers must practice avoidance strategies to reduce toxic load and body stress created by the allergic response. In Chapter 5: Environmental Control, you will learn how to reduce your exposure to aeroallergens and toxins in your home and on your food. In Chapter 6: Therapeutic Diets, you will learn special diets that avoid exposure to food allergens.

**Treat Barrier Function Defaults**—The way to an allergy-free life is through rebuilding your barrier functions, specifically the digestive tract, skin, and respiratory system. In Chapter 7: Healing Leaky Gut Syndrome, you will discover special healing methods for restoring intestinal wall function, eliminating parasites, and correcting enzyme and hydrochloric acid deficiencies. In Chapter 8: Intestinal Detoxification, you'll learn how to detoxify your colon and liver and restore balance to intestinal microflora. Chapter 9: Supporting the Skin delineates the importance of essential fatty acids and other skin therapies in repairing barrier damage. Chapter 10: Supporting the Respiratory System explains how to improve the function of your lungs and other key respiratory organs.

**Control Your Symptoms**—As you are treated for barrier function defaults and other underlying causes of allergies, it is very possible that you will still suffer from some symptomatic distress. Chapter 11: Supplements for Symptom Control offers valuable tips for relieving the discomfort of allergic reactions with nutritional supplements, essential fatty acids, and Western and Chinese herbs. You'll also learn about the dangers of conventional drugs commonly used to manage allergy/sensitivity symptoms. Chapter 12: Homeopathic and Physical Therapies provides suggestion about homeopathic remedies and physical treatments such as nasal irrigation, acupuncture/acupressure, and asthma-specific breathing techniques.

**Desensitize Your Immune System**—Desensitization is another control technique that provides allergy/sensitivity patients with a great degree of symptomatic relief while they're undergoing other therapies. In Chapter 13: Desensitizing the Immune System, we discuss the various treatments alternative medicine practitioners use to reprogram your immune system and make it less sensitive. Enzyme-potentiated desensitization (EPD), Nambudripad's Allergy Elimination Technique (NAET), and Natural Elimination of Allergy Therapy (NEAT) are among the therapies presented in this chapter.

**Heal the Psychological Side of Allergies**—In Chapter 14: Mind/Body Approaches to Allergies, you will learn how stress, suppressed emotions, and lifestyle choices can contribute to allergies, how to undo damaging thoughts, and how to incorporate habits for relaxation and increased confidence into your life.

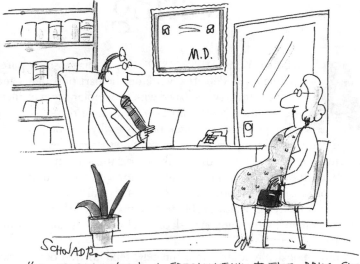

"I'M SENDING YOU TO A SPECIALIST WHO TREATS DRUG SIDE EFFECTS FROM DRUG SIDE EFFECTS."

CHAPTER

# 3

# Allergy/ Sensitivity Testing

**A**LLERGY AND SENSITIVITY diagnosis requires quite a bit of detective work on the part of patients and their doctors. When faced with the smoking gun of allergic reactions, both parties need to investigate not only what pulled the trigger but also why the bullets were loaded in the barrel to begin with. Discovering that ragweed pollen is inducing your hay fever or that milk is sparking your migraines is important, if only so you know to avoid ragweed or milk until your allergy or sensitivity subsides. However, it's crucial that a physician check for underlying health problems that may adversely affect your immune system, increasing your risk of developing these allergies and sensitivities.

Conventional physicians, unfortunately, tend to overlook barrier function defaults and other problems and test only for allergy triggers—and a fairly small number of total potential allergens at that, primarily pollen, animal dander, mold, and dust mites. Alternative medicine practitioners, however, recognize that there are thousands of possible allergy/sensitivity triggers—food, chemical, as well as airborne—and they employ innovative diagnostic methods to detect often overlooked allergens. Additionally, they focus on rooting out the underlying causes of allergies and sensitivities, such as barrier function defaults and co-existing disease, which must be corrected in order to stabilize and rebuild the hyperactive immune system. This chapter will help you understand the broad range of tests that alternative medicine physicians use to identify

## In This Chapter

- The First Step: Patient History
- Testing for Allergy/Sensitivity Triggers
- Testing for the Causes of Allergy/Sensitivity

not only the triggers but other factors that contribute to the development of allergies and sensitivities.

# The First Step: Patient History

Before embarking upon the often time-consuming and costly regimen of allergy tests, alternative medicine physicians typically begin the diagnostic process by conducting a comprehensive patient interview. The information disclosed during such discussions can help your doctor assess which tests are indicated in your particular case.

In her allergy-treatment practice in Buena Park, California, Devi Nambudripad, D.C., L.Ac., R.N., Ph.D., creator of Nambudripad's Allergy Elimination Technique (NAET), asks patients to carefully describe their symptoms, including when they first occurred, circumstances surrounding the original symptoms, and if there was any change in diet or environment at that time. Such meticulous questioning helped one patient who realized that she experienced her symptoms of allergic rhinitis only after reading the Sunday newspaper—the ink, it seems, made her sneeze.

When consulting his patients about possible food allergies, orthomolecular physician Abram Hoffer, M.D., of Victoria, British Columbia, Canada, asks his patients if there are any foods or combinations of foods that cause digestive upset or bloating. He also ascertains whether they have a craving for a particular food, which is often indicative of allergic addiction syndrome. He also requests a dietary history. "You have to look for the clues," says Dr. Hoffer of the allergy-testing process. "For instance, I had a patient who couldn't understand why she could eat steak at home without getting sick but not in a restaurant. A dietary history revealed that whenever she ate out, she ordered a large lettuce salad to accompany her steak, whereas at home she never touched lettuce. It wasn't the meat at all."

## Testing for Allergy/ Sensitivity Triggers

**CONVENTIONAL MEDICINE TESTS**
Scratch or Prick Skin Test
Patch Test
Serial Endpoint Titration (SET)
Radio Allergosorbent Test (RAST)
Enzyme-Linked Immuno-
    serological Assay (ELISA)
Cytotoxic Testing
Antigen Leukocyte Cellular
Antibody Test (ALCAT)

**ALTERNATIVE MEDICINE TESTS**
Provocative Neutralization (P/N)
Electrodermal Screening (EDS)
Applied Kinesiology
Traditional Chinese Medicine

**SELF-ADMINISTERED TESTS**
Elimination-and-Challenge Diet
Coca Pulse Test
Omura Bi-Digital O-Ring Test

For more information about **allergic addiction syndrome**, see Chapter 6: Therapeutic Diets, pp. 158-183.

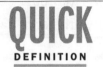

**DEFINITION**

Acupuncture meridians are specific pathways in the human body for the flow of life force or subtle energy, known as *qi* (pronounced CHEE). In most cases, these energy pathways run up and down both sides of the body, and correspond to individual organs or organ systems, designated as Lung, Small Intestine, Heart, and others. There are 12 principal meridians and eight secondary channels. Numerous points of heightened energy, or *qi*, exist on the body's surface along the meridians and are called acupoints. There are more than 1,000 acupoints, each of which is potentially a place for acupuncture treatment.

Finding out when symptoms appear can also be illuminating. Traditional Chinese medicine (TCM) says that there is a horary clock, whereby *qi* (vital life energy) passes through each of the 12 primary meridians (SEE QUICK DEFINITION) every two hours. Knowing the hours when certain symptoms arise helps the physician isolate the affected meridian. Furthermore, if a person becomes asthmatic when falling asleep or waking up, it's worth investigating the possibility of an allergy to something in the bedroom. Also, it is useful to know whether symptoms appeared after a major operation, personal loss, or following an illness such as a bacterial infection or pneumonia. Physiological and psychological traumas have an impact on the immune system and can render the body more vulnerable to allergic reactions.

# Testing for Allergy/Sensitivity Triggers

After your physician conducts a patient history, you will likely undergo allergy tests. Bear in mind that no allergy test correlates well with the symptoms or severity of allergic disease; these tests only detect what substances trigger allergic responses. Most tests require administration and diagnosis by a physician, allergy technician, or medical laboratories, but there are a few tests you can perform at home. The reliability of most tests depends on the skill of the technician and the strict regulation of the testing environment. Except for the self-administered exams, tests may cost as little as $100 or as much as $1,500 or more (for skin tests or blood tests).

### Conventional Allergy Tests

The scratch or prick skin test is the most common conventional allergy test. However, allergists may employ other methods to determine the substances that trigger allergic reactions. These tests are described below.

**Scratch or Prick Skin Test—**If you've ever been treated by a conventional allergist, you're probably familiar with scratch or prick skin testing. In each of these tests, the doctor lightly scratches or uses a needle to prick the surface of the skin, usually on the arm or back. Small dilutions of suspected allergens are then introduced on the pricked/scratched skin so that the substances can enter the body. If a

## Do You Have Allergies?

When assessing a new patient's allergy risks, alternative medicine doctors generally ask the following questions. With this information, physicians can predict potential allergens and perform appropriate tests to evaluate barrier function and other physiological conditions.

- Does your mother have allergies?
- Were you breastfed? If not, what type of formula were you fed?
- Did your parents have any difficulties feeding you?
- When were you introduced to solid foods? And what types of foods?
- Were you immunized as a child?
- Have you had any infections? If so, what types and how many times per year?
- Do you experience cravings for any foods?
- What types of foods do you like and dislike?
- Do you experience any reactions to foods, things in the air, or chemicals?
- Have you ever been exposed to unusual chemicals (e.g., drinking contaminated water) or exposed to high amounts of chemicals (e.g., in a chemical spill or industrial accident)?

wheal, a reddish inflammation resembling a mosquito bite, rises within 20 minutes, an allergy to the substance is confirmed. In conventional immunotherapy (SEE QUICK DEFINITION), extracts of the allergenic substances are then given as allergy shots in progressively stronger doses until a maintenance level is reached.

These tests are limited in that they only measure Type I, or IgE-mediated, allergic responses (asthma, allergic rhinitis, eczema, and hives), which are primarily triggered by inhaled allergens such as pollen, mold, dust, and animal dander. These procedures are only about 15% accurate in spotting food-induced allergic reactions.[1] Thus, delayed food allergies and chemical sensitivities often go undetected. Additionally, if more than ten skin tests are administered at a time, they may result in false positive due to too much histamine in the skin.

For more about **immunotherapy**, see Chapter 13: Desensitizing the Immune System, pp. 328-347.

**Patch Test**—In this conventional skin test, a patch containing a suspected

## QUICK DEFINITION

**Immunotherapy**, or "allergy shots," desensitizes an allergic person's body to its allergens. This type of therapy requires that patients receive injections containing extracts (minute amounts) of the reaction-inducing substance. The shots may be given as often as daily in the beginning of the program, decreasing to once or twice a month. Multiple shots may be required for multiple allergens. With each shot, the allergen is administered in progressively stronger doses until reaching the "maintenance level," the point at which the allergen is "neutralized"—that is, it no longer provokes an allergic reaction. It can take between one and five years—or never—to reach this level. Immunotherapy is used for immunoglobulin E–mediated allergies, primarily allergic rhinitis (hay fever). Allergies to food are not treated with immunotherapy. Response rates vary, with between 60% and 80% of allergy sufferers reporting relief of rhinitis/sinusitis symptoms from allergy shots.

# Pros and Cons of Allergy Tests

All allergy tests have benefits and drawbacks to their use. Here's a breakdown of the major advantages and disadvantages of some of these tests. Note that tests to detect IgE usually miss food allergies, which are primarily mediated by IgG antibodies.

| PROCEDURE | ADVANTAGES | DISADVANTAGES |
|---|---|---|
| Skin prick | Widely available; good for inhalants | Poor sensitivity; inconvenient |
| Cytotoxic/ ALCAT | Convenient; moderate cost | Poor reproducibility; limited availability |
| RAST | Convenient; good for inhalants; office kits available | Low sensitivity; expensive; detects IgE, IgG |
| Provocation Neutralization | Good for chemicals; office procedure | Expensive; time-consuming |
| EDS | Inexpensive; non-invasive; tests many items | Few clinical studies |
| Applied Kinesiology | Inexpensive; easily applied | Few clinical studies |
| Acupuncture | Easily applied | Few clinical studies |

allergen is applied to the skin and left in place for 24 to 48 hours. When the patch is removed, doctors check for a skin reaction, such as a rash, redness, lesions, or hardness. A reaction within one to two hours confirms a Type I (IgE-mediated) allergy to the substance; a reaction that appears up to three days later indicates a Type IV (T cell–mediated) allergy.

**Serial Endpoint Titration (SET)**—In a serial endpoint titration (SET) test, a physician injects a diluted amount of a potential allergen just below the skin. The ratio of dilution is up to the doctor; it may be as high as 1:5 or lower than 1:125. Each person's body will immediately react to the introduction of this foreign substance by forming a wheal of about 4 mm in diameter. Ten minutes after the injection, the wheal is measured again. A 5 mm diameter wheal indicates a nonallergic reaction to the dilution amount, while a wheal of 7 mm or higher is a sign that you have an allergy. Further testing (called progressive whealing) is done with incrementally weaker or stronger amounts of diluted substances to determine the endpoint, or the lowest concentration ratio at which a substance triggers a 2 mm growth in a wheal. In conventional immunotherapy, the endpoint concentration is used as the treatment dose for allergy shots. One advantage of this test is that it shows how strongly the body reacts to varying amounts of the substance; in other words, whether your allergy is mild, moderate, or severe.

Allergists generally consider the SET test to be more accurate than the scratch, prick, or patch tests. However, the SET method is similarly limited in scope, as it only detects IgE-mediated allergic reactions, not those induced by foods or chemicals.

**Radio Allergosorbent Test (RAST)**—In this test, a technician or doctor exposes a patient to a suspected allergen and then draws a sample of blood from the patient. A radioactive substance is then used to label the IgE and IgG antibodies in the blood specimen and the amounts of these antibodies are measured with a specialized instrument. RAST identifies classic allergens, such as pollens, animal dander, mold, or dust mites. Higher antibody amounts indicate the presence of an allergen. Since IgG is measured, RAST can detect food allergens. Extract doses for allergy shots are then derived from RAST results. However, RAST is expensive and sometimes faulty. Additionally, since it only measures antibody response, T cell–mediated allergic reactions and other non-antibody-mediated events cannot be identified with this test.

**ELISA Test**—Many alternative medicine practitioners consider the ELISA (enzyme-linked immunoserological assay) test to be among the most sensitive and useful blood tests in detecting delayed food allergies. The ELISA requires a small blood sample to be taken from the patient, then sent within 72 hours to any one of several specialized laboratories that perform this test. At the lab, technicians process the sample to collect the IgG antibodies, which are involved in delayed allergic reactions. A drop of this serum is placed in each of 102 tiny holding containers or "wells" in a laboratory testing plate. Each well contains a single potentially allergenic food or a component of highly

For **ELISA tests**, contact: Immuno Laboratories, Inc., 1620 West Oakland Park Blvd., Fort Lauderdale, FL 33311; tel: 800-231-9197 or 954-486-4500; fax: 954-739-6563; website: www.immunolabs.com. Meridian Valley Laboratory, 515 West Harrison Street, Suite 9, Kent, WA 98042; tel: 253-859-8700; fax: 253-859-1135; website: www.meridianvalleylab.com. MetaMetrix Medical Laboratory, 5000 Peachtree Industrial Blvd., Suite 110, Norcross, GA 30071; tel: 770-446-5483 or 800-221-4640; fax: 770-441-2237. Great Smokies Diagnostic Laboratory, 63 Zillicoa Street, Asheville, NC 28801; tel: 800-522-4762 or 704-253-0621; fax: 704-252-9303; website: www.gsdl.com.

allergenic foods, such as gluten, which is found in wheat. A computer then analyzes the samples.

The assay specifically looks for evidence of every IgG-mediated food allergy, including antibodies for IgG's subsets (components): IgG1, IgG2, IgG3, and IgG4. Each IgG subset is responsible for attacking specific kinds of invading protein molecules. John L. Rebellow, Ph.D., of Immuno Laboratories in Fort Lauderdale, Florida, emphasizes that testing for subsets allows the physician to precisely isolate food allergens. "If you only look for the presence of food-specific IgG1, you would identify approximately 50% of all IgG-mediated food allergies but you would miss IgG4, which encompasses 40%, and IgG2 and IgG3, which comprise the remaining 10%." It's important to note that any allergen, not just food, can prompt a reaction by any IgG subset or IgE. Hence, allergists using the ELISA make sure to test for all types of IgG and IgE presence.

**Cytotoxic Testing**—This procedure is commonly used by nutritionists to test for Type II allergic reactions to food and some chemicals. A technician mixes a suspected allergenic substance into a sample of the patient's blood and then examines the blood for white cell (lymphocytes, granulocytes, and platelets) changes under a microscope. Changes in the shape or amount of cells in response to the addition of the allergen, due to the cytotoxin being released by IgG and IgM antibodies, indicate an allergic reaction to the substance. Technician eye fatigue makes this test impractical; thus, it is infrequently used.

**The ALCAT**—A mechanized version of cytotoxic testing is called the ALCAT, or antigen leukocyte cellular antibody test. In this procedure, technicians use a specialized instrument to detect changes in the amount and size of a patient's white blood cells, after the introduction of a suspected antigen into the patient's blood sample. Significant changes in cell number and size point to an allergic reaction to the substance. Allergists prefer this test over manual cytotoxic testing.

## Alternative Allergy Tests

Alternative medicine tests to identify allergy triggers tend to be quicker and less invasive than the more conventional methods. In addition, these tests can accurately pinpoint food, chemical, as well as airborne allergens.

**Provocative Neutralization (P/N)**—This method of testing is similar to serial endpoint titration (SET) by its use of extracts, except they're usually administered sublingually rather than intravenously. In addition, some allergists find that P/N is more precise than SET and other conventional tests. It can be used to detect food and chemical sensitivities and takes into account a variety of patient responses, not just skin inflammation. In fact, patient complaints such as headaches or spaciness are often reproduced in a matter of minutes after receiving the extract; thus, symptoms can be linked directly to the specific allergen. Conventional allergists do not use this testing method, but alternative physicians find it to be both a highly accurate test for allergy triggers and remarkably effective treatment for symptomatic relief.

P/N is performed by introducing extracts of the suspected allergens either into the skin with an injection or as a drop of liquid under the tongue. The same substance is then given in weaker and weaker dilutions every ten minutes, starting with a 1:5 ratio and decreasing by a multiple of five each time, until a "neutralization" dose is reached. (Neutralization is determined when the symptoms disappear.) If a reaction is to occur, it most likely will do so at the strongest doses. In addition to measuring the size of a wheal's increase, a physician using P/N looks for changes in the patient's appearance, physical and mental functioning, pulse rate, breathing, and behavior. Some double-blind tests have shown that the P/N isn't very reliable, but many alternative allergists attest to its effectiveness.

To locate a **physician skilled in provocative neutralization**, contact: American Academy of Environmental Medicine, P.O. Box CN1001-8001, New Hope, PA 18938; tel: 215-862-4544.

**Electrodermal Screening (EDS)**—Electrodermal screening (EDS) involves the use of an electrical device that measures conductance. Conductance is how well energy moves through something. It is defined in terms of electrical resistances. It is a diagnostic tool—it doesn't treat allergies or sensitivities, but it is instrumental in the Natural Elimination of Allergy Therapy (NEAT).

In an EDS session, a trained practitioner places a blunt, noninvasive electric probe at acupuncture points on the patients hands or feet, corresponding to specific internal functions governed by acupuncture

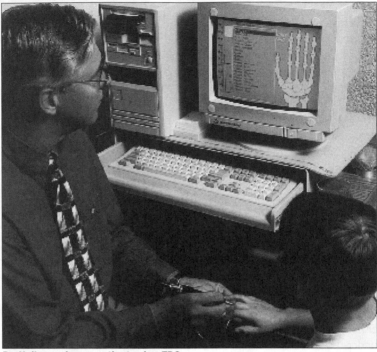

**Dr. Kail examines a patient using EDS.**

For information about **Natural Elimination of Allergy Therapy**, see Chapter 13: Desensitizing the Immune System, pp. 328-347.

meridians. Each acupuncture point has a specific "job" that it performs. Knowing what is happening with the energy of the point says something about that internal function or job. The EDS device emits a microcurrent that carries information (the electromagnetic spectrum of the allergen being tested) into the acupuncture point via the probe. If the patient's energy response (conductance) drops or does not reach a normal peak, then that response is interpreted as "positive," indicating a sensitivity or allergy to the allergen.

The EDS device registers the body's signals on a scale from 0 to 100. An EDS reading between 58 and 65 is generally considered normal, indicating that the body's organs and tissues are functioning properly despite the introduction of the substance's energy field. A measurement of 58 or less indicates that the tested substance is an allergen, its energetic properties causing impairment of energy to an organ associated with the meridian tested. A drop of more than two suggests organ degeneration or chronicity.

Some EDS devices do not require patients to physically hold potential allergens. The LISTEN system, the Omega Acubase, and the Acupro each contain an inventory of energy signals corresponding to several thousand different substances. The LISTEN system, for example, is programmed with information for about 4,000 substances, including various pollens, foods, chemicals, dental materials, molds, and bacteria.

Few clinical studies have tested the effectiveness of EDS as a tool for identifying allergy triggers. A 1997 double-blind, controlled study used EDS testing with 41 polysymptomatic allergy patients. In the first group of 17 patients, EDS correctly differentiated 82% of the time between house dust mite or histamine (allergens) and saline or

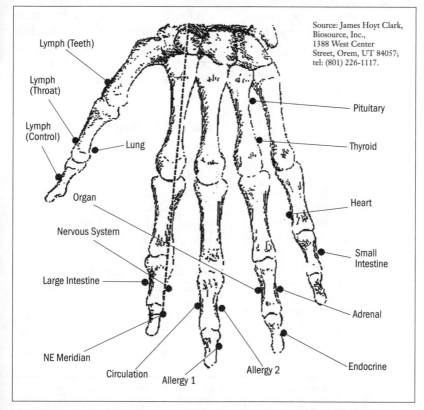

Source: James Hoyt Clark, Biosource, Inc., 1388 West Center Street, Orem, UT 84057; tel: (801) 226-1117.

Lymph (Teeth)
Lymph (Throat)
Lymph (Control)
Lung
Organ
Nervous System
Large Intestine
NE Meridian
Circulation
Allergy 1
Allergy 2
Pituitary
Thyroid
Heart
Small Intestine
Adrenal
Endocrine

**Electrodermal screening probes specific points on the hands (see black dots above) to gather information about the health, function, or possible toxicity of organs and body systems, as well as allergy/sensitivity triggers. These points are part of acupuncture meridians.**

# The Evolution of EDS

In 1945, a German doctor named Reinhold Voll accidentally stumbled upon a discovery that led to the development of electrodermal screening. While testing a patient for prostate problems with electroacupuncture (acupuncture performed with an electric probe instead of needles), Dr. Voll noticed the patient's electroacupuncture measurement dramatically declined when the patient held a bottle of a homeopathic remedy, and rose again when he put the remedy down. After studying this phenomenon with many other patients, Dr. Voll theorized that medicine, or any other substance, placed in contact with a patient's body affects the electroacupuncture measurement.

In the 1950s, Dr. Voll consolidated his findings and came up with a diagnostic tool called electoacupuncture according to Voll (EAV), which could record the effects substances had on a body's organs. Over the years, subsequent researchers expanded on Voll's findings and modified the electroacupuncture devices, resulting in the test now known as electrodermal screening.

water (nonallergens). In the second group of 24 patients, EDS discriminated 96% of the time between allergenic and nonallergenic substances, leading the researchers to state that EDS is a reliable method for detecting allergy triggers.[2]

Although EDS findings are accurate in diagnosis and in identifying food, environmental, and chemical allergy triggers, the physician should order additional blood, urine, or stool tests to confirm the EDS results in all cases. This information is not adequate for stand-alone diagnosis. Changes in energy may be present before any biochemical or physiological change can be measured.

**Applied Kinesiology**—Applied kinesiology, first developed by George Goodheart, D.C., of Detroit, Michigan, is the study of the relationship between muscle dysfunction (weak muscles) and related organ or gland dysfunction. In the case of allergies, when an allergen comes into contact with an allergic person, its energetic properties will block the body's flow of energy, resulting in weakened muscles.

To identify an allergen, whether food, chemical, or airborne, the practitioner has a patient lie down,

---

For **EDS devices and seminars,** contact: Biosource, Inc. (LISTEN system), 1388 West Center Street, Orem, UT 84057; tel: 801-226-1117. Vaughn Cook, L.Ac., Digital Health, Inc. (Omega Acubase), 1770 East Fort Union Blvd., No. 101, Salt Lake City, UT 84121; tel: 801-944-4070; fax: 801-944-4067. Doug Lieber, Computronix Electro-Medical Systems (Acupro), 145 Canyon Oaks Drive, Argyle, TX 76226; tel: 817-241-2768; fax: 817-455-2605. Jim Jose (EDMED), 1223 Wilshire Blvd. #321, Santa Monica, CA, 90403; tel: 310-394-6497. To find a **skilled EDS practitioner,** contact: American Association of Acupuncture and Bio-Energetic Medicine, 2512 Manoa Road, Honolulu, HI 96822; tel: 808-946-2069; fax: 808-946-0378.

holding a glass vial containing a suspected allergen in the less-dominant (non-writing) hand while raising the opposing arm to a 90° angle. The practitioner then gently pushes down on the raised arm towards the patient's side while the patient resists. A weak muscle response, shown by little resistance to the pressure, indicates an allergy or sensitivity to the substance in the vial. Dr. Nambudripad uses applied kinesiology to identify allergens as part of a total treatment protocol called Nambudripad's Allergy Elimination Technique (NAET).

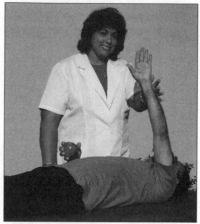

**Dr. Nambudripad demonstrates applied kinesiology testing.**

This test is very subjective but it can be accurate when employed by a properly skilled practitioner. It is also very difficult to reproduce results. EDS devices offer a more objective way of measuring the same phenomenon.

Form more about **Nambudripad's Allergy Elimination Technique**, see Chapter 13: Desensitizing the Immune System, pp. 328-347.

**Traditional Chinese Medicine**–Traditional Chinese medicine (TCM) views allergies as manifestations of blockages or imbalances of *qi* in different organs of the body. An allergy patient accustomed to Western medicine may be surprised that TCM diagnosis does not require procedures such as skin testing or blood tests. Instead, the TCM practitioner performs five noninvasive methods of investigation to assess the status of *qi* in the body:

To find a **practitioner skilled in applied kinesiology**, contact: International College of Applied Kinesiology, ICAKUSA Central Office, 6405 Metcalf Avenue, Suite 503, Shawnee Mission, KS 66202-3929; tel: 913-384-5336; fax: 913-384-5112; website: www.icakusa.com.

- Inspection of the complexion, general demeanor, body language, and tongue
- Patient history disclosing symptoms, medical history, diet, lifestyle, history of the present complaint, and any previous or concurrent therapies received
- Aural inspection of tone and strength of the voice
- Detection of odors from body excretions, breath, or body
- Palpation (feeling with the fingers) of the pulse at the radial arteries of both wrists (pulse diagnosis), the abdomen, and the meridians and/or acupuncture points

There are six pulses at each wrist, three deep and three superficial.

# The Principles of Traditional Chinese Medicine

In addition to *qi* and acupuncture meridians, traditional Chinese medicine is based upon a system called the Five Phase Theory. Under this system, the ten organs are arranged into a system that places each in one of five categories: fire, earth, metal, water, and wood. This categorization is based on the premise that each organ either nourishes or inhibits the proper functioning of another organ, just as the basic elements act either adversely or beneficially on each other. For example, as fire melts metal, the heart (associated with fire) controls the lungs (associated with metal). Likewise, as metal cuts wood, the lungs control the liver; as wood penetrates the earth, the liver controls the spleen; as the earth dams water, the spleen controls the kidneys; and as water quenches fire, the kidneys control the heart.

The organs are also divided into two groups of yin and yang organs, which complement each other's functions. Yin organs are associated with fluids, and have cooling or dampening energetic properties. Yang organs are associated with the heart, spleen, lungs, kidney, and liver. Each organ also has special energetic properties that keep the body's *qi* balanced and moving freely throughout the body. Yin organs are cooling; yang organs are heating. If a yin organ, such as the liver, becomes more yang (hot or agitated) either through diet or lifestyle choices, an imbalance in *qi*—and allergies—can follow.

In examining a patient with allergies, a TCM practitioner looks for patterns (behavior or appearance signs) reflecting an imbalance in the organs. Not all allergies are caused by the same *qi* imbalances. Conversely, people with different symptoms but the same pattern of disharmony can often be treated by the same therapies.

To learn more about **traditional Chinese medicine**, contact: American Academy of Medical Acupuncture, 5820 Wilshire Blvd., Suite 500, Los Angeles, CA 90036; tel: 323-937-5514; fax: 323-937-0959.

Through pulse diagnosis, a skilled practitioner can examine the strength or weakness of the *qi* and "blood," which in TCM thinking includes lymph and other bodily fluids, and assess how these affect each of the organs, tissues, and layers of the body. The practitioner will also look at the impact of a wide range of personal and environmental factors on *qi* mobility, including exposure to toxins, diet, mood, activity or inactivity, sex, drugs, weather, and seasons of the year.

For more on how **TCM is used to treat allergies/sensitivity**, see Chapter 12: Homeopathic and Physical Therapies, pp. 304-327.

### Self-Administered Allergy Tests

The following tests, which are used primarily to determine if a specific food is a potential allergen, can be undertaken at home, although appropriate professional supervision is advised. The Elimination-and-Challenge Diet is considered the "gold standard" for identifying reactions to foods.

**Elimination-and-Challenge Diet—**There are several variations of this diet developed by Albert H. Rowe, M.D., of Oakland, California, but the main idea in all of them is to abstain for four to seven days from eating foods that may be causing a delayed reaction. It takes an average of four days for the delayed reaction to a food to dissipate. Once the body is cleared of the test foods, and the patient's symptoms have disappeared, they are ready to proceed with the "challenge" phase. Reintroduce the test foods separately, as single-item meals. If you experience symptoms such as aches, pains, digestive difficulty, fatigue, an inability to think clearly, or any increase in any symptom within a few hours (although it may take up to 72 hours), it may be due to allergy. Ideally, one food is tested each day, and only organic foods are consumed to avoid mistaking a reaction to pesticide residues for a reaction to the food itself.[3] In some studies, electrodermal screening correlates with this test closer than any other allergy-testing method.

For more on **using the elimination diet to treat food allergies and sensitivities**, see Chapter 6: Therapeutic Diets, pp. 158-183.

If symptoms persist after seven days, Elson Haas, M.D., of San Rafael, California, recommends that you refrain from eating the foods being tested for several weeks before entering the challenge phase. If there is still no relief after that period of time, you may have inadvertently left allergenic foods in your diet or your symptoms are not sparked by food allergies.[4]

Some of the commonly allergenic foods that should be avoided during this testing period include dairy, wheat, eggs, corn and all its products (syrup, starch, and meal), tree nuts, peanuts, fish and shellfish, tomatoes, meat, chocolate, citrus, caffeine, sugar, yeast products, food coloring, and additives. Also, any foods you eat on a regular basis should be eliminated during the test, since people are often allergic to what they like best, crave, or consume frequently.

**Coca Pulse Test—**This is a relatively simple test developed by Arthur Coca, M.D., a pioneer in the field of environmental medicine. Dr. Coca based his test on many years of clinical observations of patients, during which he noticed that a common symptom of many food allergies is increased heart rate. Although the pulse test can help identify food allergies, you should not conclude that you are allergy-free if the foods you test do not affect your pulse rate. The problem is that not all food allergens will increase heart rate. "The weakness of this particular approach lies in the frank possibility that not every allergic reaction will necessarily produce the biochemical responses that result in a faster heartbeat," says Ralph Golan, M.D., a holistic physician

## How to Take the Coca Pulse Test

The pulse test is easy to self-administer and involves simply recording your pulse rate before and after meals. Stephen Langer, M.D., of Berkeley, California, observes that "certain of my patients who use the pulse test have seen their heartbeat raise from 72 to as high as 180 after they have eaten an allergenic food."[6] To take the test, follow these simple instructions:

■ Find the pulse point on your wrist by placing the second finger of the opposite hand on the inside of your wrist.

■ Count the beats (pulses) for six seconds and multiply the number by ten; this is your resting pulse.

■ Record your resting pulse first thing in the morning before getting out of bed.

■ Record your pulse 30 minutes before each meal, then 30 minutes and 60 minutes after each meal.

If the difference between the morning pulse and either of the two after-meal pulses is more than 12 to 16 beats, chances are you have a food allergy. Once you have identified a meal that triggers a rise in your pulse rate, you can begin testing individual foods eaten during that meal. However, in some cases, you may find that your resting pulse is higher than your after-meal pulse or that your before-meal pulse is higher than your after-meal pulse. If you observe such a pattern, it is possible that dust mites or some other airborne allergen is interfering with your test.[7]

from Seattle, Washington, and author of *Optimal Wellness*.[5] If you have no success in identifying a food allergen using the pulse test but still suspect that you are suffering from such an allergy, you should try one of the other tests.

**Omura Bi-Digital O-Ring Test—**The O-Ring test was developed by Yoshiaki Omura, M.D., an electrical engineer, in the late 1970s. It follows the same principle as that of applied kinesiology, except it uses a different test muscle. Dr. Omura recognized that a change in the body's electromagnetic field took place when a person came in contact with an unhealthy item (such as an allergen). The results of the contact, according to his experiments, showed up as weakened finger strength.[8] To conduct this test, follow these instructions:

Place the tip of your thumb against the tip of the index finger of the same hand to form an "O," keeping your elbows at least six inches from your body so the electromagnetic field around your kidneys does not influence the results. Try to separate the "O" with the index finger of your other hand. Repeat this demonstration three more times with the thumb and third, fourth, and fifth fingers in turn. Whichever combination produces an "O" that is resistant to being pulled apart, yet is not impossible to do so, is the best combination for the test.

Now, repeat the procedure while holding a test substance in the hand not forming the "O," making sure that your fingertips touch the suspected allergen. If the "O" separates easily, you probably have an allergy to the test object. If the "O" ring remains strong, you do not have an allergy.

# Testing for the Causes of Allergy/Sensitivity

For people who have never realized that their health problems are caused by allergies or sensitivities, identifying triggers is a major step toward well-being, if only to avoid exposure in the future. However, symptom control is not the aim of alternative medicine—disease reversal is. Curing allergy and sensitivity can be accomplished by detecting and correcting the underlying causes of barrier function defaults and immune stressors.

New York City–based allergy specialist Leo Galland, M.D., says that it is important to have more information than simply what allergen causes a person to react. "I want to know why this person is allergic and what factors are aggravating this person's allergy." He specifically looks for individual risk factors, such as parasitic infections and bacterial overgrowth. "Knowing the antecedents of an allergic condition," he explains, "allows me to help the person make more fundamental changes in their life so they are less sensitive to their allergic triggers."

Alternative medicine practitioners such as Dr. Galland employ various tests to uncover such antecedents. These include tests that screen for toxicity, liver and digestive tract malfunction, parasitic and bacterial infections, enzyme and nutritional deficiencies, and hormonal imbalances caused by stress. Electrodermal screening also is effective in pinpointing underlying causes. Test costs vary, from less than $100 to $300 each.

## Six Signs Suggesting Childhood Allergies

Some common allergy symptoms in children include the following, according to pediatric allergist Doris J. Rapp, M.D., F.A.A., F.A.E.M., F.A.A.P., author of *Is This Your Child?* and *Is This Your Child's World?*:[9]

- Dark circles or bags under the eyes
- Red earlobes or red cheeks
- Legs that wiggle
- A sudden adverse change in handwriting or drawing
- A "spacy" appearance accompanying misbehavior
- Grades that vary from day to day

## Immune System Function Tests

To get a basic overview of the immune system function, your doctor may order the T and B Cell Panel and Natural Killer Cell Function blood tests. These relatively expensive, standard tests detail the number and efficacy of 25 immune system components, including T cells and natural killer cells (cellular immunity), and B cells (humoral immunity). These tests do not provide answers as to why the immune system and its lymphocytes may be impaired, but it can give your physician important clues as to what additional tests—for nutrient deficiency, adrenal stress, leaky gut, and so forth—need to be performed.

To find out **how to reduce your exposure to heavy metals**, see Chapter 5: Environmental Control, pp. 128-157.

## Heavy Metal Toxicity Tests

Chronic low-level exposure to toxic heavy metals can cause or exacerbate allergies and allergy-related diseases. Testing can identify which metals are present and in what amounts. On the basis of this information, a physician is able to develop an individualized detoxification and nutritional prescription program.

**Hair Analysis—**Hair trace-mineral analysis allows physicians to measure critical mineral and toxic metal levels in the body's tissues. Hair is a soft tissue of the body; testing the hair is obtaining the equivalent of a soft-tissue biopsy, without any surgery. Although hair is technically dead, the minerals present in the hair cell during its formation are locked within the hair structure. Minerals as well as toxic metals in the hair are in a higher concentration than in the blood, making these elements easier to measure through hair analysis.

Hair analysis is an average reading over a several-month period; it gives a picture over time of the body's metabolic changes. A one-gram sample of hair (hair cannot be dyed, permed, bleached, or treated; pubic hair can be substituted) is cut and sent to the laboratory by the health-care practitioner. The laboratory then burns the hair and the elements are viewed and quantified via atomic spectroscopy. The results are returned to the practitioner for interpretation. Hair analysis and its diagnostic value were once considered controversial but due to stricter standards within the industry and better handling of samples, accuracy and reliability are now excellent. The U.S. Environmental Protection Agency states that hair analysis is an accurate, inexpensive screening tool for heavy metal toxicity.

**ToxMet Screen**–The ToxMet screen from MetaMetrix Medical Laboratory provides an inexpensive but detailed analysis of the levels of specific heavy metals in a patient's system, based on a urine sample. In most cases, the ToxMet results provide your physician with sufficient and accurate information about whether detoxification should be part of an allergy treatment.

ToxMet tests for levels of four highly toxic heavy metals, including arsenic, cadmium, lead, and mercury; it also reports on levels for ten potentially toxic elements, such as aluminum, bismuth, boron, nickel, and strontium. Finally, information is gathered on a patient's status regarding 14 essential metals and minerals, such as copper, calcium, chromium, molybdenum, selenium, and vanadium. When test results exceed limits believed to be safe, the report indicates a "high" concentration.

**EDTA Lead Versonate 24-Hour Urine Collection Test**–In this test, a physician intravenously administers EDTA (ethylene-diamine-tetra-acetic acid), a chemical that chelates or binds with heavy metals. EDTA pulls heavy metals out of the patient's system, which are then excreted in the urine. The urine is then collected over a 24-hour period and analyzed by a laboratory for proportions of heavy metals.

**DMPS Challenge Test**–This test is similar to the EDTA test, but it uses the chemical DMPS (2,3-dimercaptopropane-1-sulfonate) instead of EDTA. DMPS is orally administered and has been found to be more precise in measuring heavy metal toxicity because it can bind heavy metals lodged in hard-to-access tissues. One of DMPS's strengths is its ability to cross the blood-brain barrier. Many substances diffuse poorly from the blood into the brain. Those that do not easily pass into the

---

For more on **hair analysis**, contact: Analytical Research Labs, Inc., 8650 North 22nd Avenue, P.O. Box 37964, Phoenix, AZ 85069-7964; tel: 602-995-1580. For the **ToxMet Screen**, contact: MetaMetrix Medical Laboratory, 5000 Peachtree Industrial Blvd., Suite 110, Norcross, GA 30071; tel: 800-221-4640 or 770-446-5483; fax: 770-441-2237. To find a **physician in your area who can perform the EDTA Lead Versonate 24-Hour Urine Collection and DMPS Challenge Test**, contact: American College for Advancement in Medicine, 23121 Verdugo Drive, Suite 204, Laguna Hills, CA 92653; tel: 800-532-3688 or 714-583-7666; website: www.acam.org.

nervous tissue require the use of a protein carrier to get into the brain to chelate and remove any heavy metals found in the brain tissue.

## Detoxification Function Tests

Even if your body isn't overwhelmed by heavy metals, your allergies and sensitivities may still be caused by toxic overload if your body's detoxification system (organ processes that eliminate toxins from the body) isn't working properly. Here are two laboratory tests that can help determine how efficiently your body detoxifies itself.

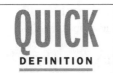

### QUICK DEFINITION

A **free radical** is an unstable, toxic molecule of oxygen with an unpaired electron that steals an electron from another molecule and produces harmful effects. Free radicals are formed when molecules within cells react with oxygen (oxidize) as part of normal metabolic processes. Free radicals then begin to break down cells, especially the cell membranes, often in a matter of minutes to an hour. Their work is enhanced if there are not enough free radical–quenching nutrients, such as L-glutathione and vitamins C and E, in the cell. While free radicals are normal products of metabolism, uncontrolled free-radical production plays a major role in the development of degenerative disease, including cancer and heart disease. Free radicals harmfully alter important molecules, such as proteins, enzymes, fats, even DNA. The glutathione peroxidase system (free radical–scavenging process involving L-glutathione) is an important pathway that has been found to be overwhelmed or impaired in most allergic patients.

**Detoxification phases** (Phase I and Phase II) in liver detoxification refers to the natural two-step process the liver conducts to rid the body of toxins. During Phase I, the liver converts toxic compounds into intermediate toxins. In Phase II, the liver converts these intermediate toxins into substances that can be eliminated from the body, delivering them to the colon (via the gallbladder) or bladder for excretion.

**Functional Liver Detoxification Profile**—If your liver is unable to adequately detoxify your body's store of toxins and waste products, this situation may contribute significantly to the emergence and continuation of your allergies. Excess free radicals (SEE QUICK DEFINITION) and by-products of incomplete metabolism resulting from poor detoxification can create problems in the cells. Specifically, they can interfere with the movement of substances across the cell membrane and induce damage to the mitochondria, the cells' "energy factories." The Detoxification Profile helps to identify places where your system is impaired in its ability to detoxify. It looks at the liver's ability to convert potentially dangerous toxins into harmless substances that can then be eliminated by the body; this conversion process occurs in two major chemical reactions referred to as Phase I and Phase II detoxification phases (SEE QUICK DEFINITION). The Detoxification Profile determines the presence of enzymes needed to start the conversion process and the rate at which Phase I and II detoxification are operating.

**Oxidative Stress Profile**—When your ability to detoxify is impaired and/or you are deficient in antioxidants (SEE QUICK DEFINITION), free radicals run unchallenged throughout the body, damaging cells. They tend to affect the immune, endocrine, and nervous systems, damaging mitochondria, interrupting communication among cells, and depleting key nutrients and antioxidants. This is called oxidative stress. The Oxidative Stress Profile assesses the degree of free-radical damage in the body and it measures the body's levels of L-glutathione, an amino acid–complex central to detoxification. Many asthma patients have been found to suffer from high oxidative stress, which contributes to mucous membrane barrier dysfunction.[10]

## Digestive Function Tests

Numerous factors may impair your digestive tract's ability to properly break down and assimilate your food, a condition that often leads to food allergies. The following tests determine how well or poorly you are digesting your food, and reveal specific problems, such as a leaky gut, bacterial imbalances, and other biochemical abnormalities, which may be causing your allergies.

**Comprehensive Digestive Stool Analysis**—The Great Smokies Laboratory in Asheville, North Carolina, offers the Comprehensive Digestive Stool Analysis, which consists of 18 tests. The test reviews the patient's overall gastrointestinal health by investigating the following areas:

Colonic Environment—To give a better picture of the overall colonic environment, the stool analysis measures indicators of intestinal dysbiosis (SEE QUICK DEFINITION). The main markers of imbalances in intestinal flora are deficiencies in *Lactobacillus* and *Bifidobacteria* "friendly" bacteria; an overgrowth of the yeast *Candida albicans*; an alkaline fecal pH, which promotes the growth of "unfriendly" bacteria; decreased levels of short-chain fatty acids (SCFA); and elevated levels of the enzyme beta-glucuronidase. Another indicator of intestinal health is the color of the stool. Yellow to green stools may indicate diarrhea and a bowel sterilized by antibiotics. Black or red may reflect bleeding in the gastrointestinal tract. Tan or gray can indicate a blockage of the common bile duct. Mucus or pus can point to irritable bowel syndrome, intestinal wall inflammation, polyps, or diverticulitis. Occult (hidden) blood might result from eating too much red meat,

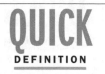

**QUICK DEFINITION**

An **antioxidant** (meaning "against oxidation") is a natural biochemical substance that protects living cells against damage from harmful free radicals. Antioxidants work against the process of oxidation—the robbing of electrons from substances. If unblocked or left uncontrolled, oxidation can lead to cellular aging, degeneration, arthritis, heart disease, cancer, and other illnesses. Antioxidants in the body react readily with oxygen breakdown products and free radicals, and neutralize them before they can damage the body. Antioxidant nutrients include vitamins A, C, and E, beta carotene, selenium, coenzyme Q10, pycnogenol (grape seed extract), L-glutathione, superoxide dismutase, N-acetyl-cysteine, bioflavonoids, and anthocyanidins (berries, cherries, etc.). When antioxidants are taken in combination, the effect is stronger than when they are used individually.

For the **Functional Liver Detoxification and Oxidative Stress Profiles**, contact: Great Smokies Diagnostic Laboratory, 63 Zillicoa Street, Asheville, NC 28801; tel: 704-253-0621 or 800-522-4762; fax: 704-252-9303; website: www.gsdl.com.

To learn how to **improve your detoxification function**, see Chapter 8: Intestinal Detoxification, pp. 212-235.

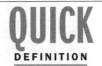

## QUICK DEFINITION

**Intestinal dysbiosis** refers to an imbalance of intestinal flora. These flora include "friendly" bacteria called probiotics (for example, *Lactobacillus acidophilus*) and harmful or "unfriendly" bacteria. At times, especially after the use of antibiotics, the balance of intestinal flora is skewed, allowing the unfriendly or pathogenic bacteria to flourish. These harmful bacteria include *Pseudomonas aeruginosa*, *Proteus vulgarus*, and *Klebsiella pneumoniae*. When the colonic environment favors unfriendly bacteria, known as a state of dysbiosis, the pathogenic bacteria begin to ferment, producing toxic by-products, which interfere with the intestinal pH, digestion and absorption, and the normal elimination cycle, all of which contribute to allergies.

hemorrhoids, or possibly colon cancer.

Digestive Abnormalities—Maldigestion, or incomplete digestion, is a common problem for many Americans, and poor digestion is both a primary cause and symptom of allergies. Often, due to an overgrowth of pathogenic bacteria, the production of hydrochloric acid (HCl) decreases, altering the stomach's pH and the release of digestive enzymes. This results in improper digestion, which impairs the body's ability to absorb nutrients (malabsorption) and gives pathogenic bowel bacteria fodder to multiply and crowd out the beneficial species. Different nutrients (fats, carbohydrates, and proteins) depend on different digestive processes and it is common for an individual to have malabsorption of one nutrient while adequately absorbing other nutrients.

The stool analysis determines how well fats, carbohydrates, proteins, and other nutrients are

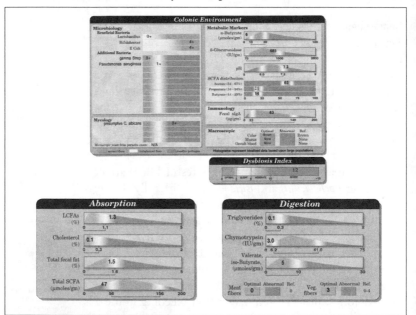

The stool analysis provides information about the health of the intestines and their function, particularly the levels of friendly and pathogenic bacteria, the degree of digestive dysfunction, and how well nutrients are being absorbed.

being digested and absorbed. This assessment is done by measuring the levels of triglycerides (fats), chymotrypsin (a digestive enzyme), valerate and iso-butyrate short-chain fatty acids, meat and vegetable fibers, long-chain fatty acids (LCFAs), cholesterol, and total fecal fat (the sum of all fats or lipids, except for SCFAs).

Integrity of Immune System—The largest part of the immune system is located just outside of the intestinal wall. Known as fecal secretory IgA (sIgA), these antibody proteins act as sentries against escaping food particles or other inappropriate, allergenic substances. A stool analysis can determine the level at which the fecal sIgA is functioning. Low levels of fecal sIgA mean an increased susceptibility to infection and food allergies, while high levels indicate normal activity or an active infectious process.

**Urine Analysis**—Many alternative health-care professionals rely on low-cost urine analysis (or urinalysis) to assess their patients' digestive function and enzyme status. The urinalysis provides information on what a person cannot digest, absorb, or assimilate, along with any nutritional problems one might have. A urinalysis can also reveal the degrees of kidney function, bowel toxicity, and pH (SEE QUICK DEFINITION); and show how the body is handling proteins, fats, carbohydrates, vitamin C, and other essential nutrients.

An individual's total urine output over a 24-hour period must be collected, not just periodic samples. The first morning collection of the Loomis 24-Hour Urine Test can also be used. This enables a physician to see how the concentrations of various substances in the urine change over time. The fluctuations are then averaged to give a complete picture of digestive problems.

**Gastric Analysis**—Many allergy and sensitivity patients are deficient in digestive factors (hydrochloric acid and pancreatic enzymes) needed to adequately break down food so that cells can absorb important nutrients. When digestion is incomplete or inadequate, food molecules can be inappropriately absorbed into the bloodstream, contributing to the onset of allergy and other diseases. Inside the stomach, a very low pH (acid level) is needed to break down food. To maintain the optimal pH (around 2, which is very acidic), the stomach secretes hydrochloric acid (HCl). With age, HCl levels tend to decline, leading to impaired digestion.

**QUICK DEFINITION**

The term **pH**, which means "potential hydrogen," represents a scale for the relative acidity or alkalinity of a solution. Acidity is measured as a pH of 0.1 to 6.9, alkalinity is 7.1 to 14, and neutral pH is 7.0. The numbers refer to how many hydrogen atoms are present compared to an ideal or standard solution. Normally, blood is slightly alkaline, at 7.35 to 7.45; urine pH can range from 4.8 to 7.5, although normal is closer to 7.0.

# Urine Analysis Terms and Measurements

The following specific values are measured in urine analysis. The most important is the indican value, since it checks for digestive barrier function. Urine analysis also measures total sediment in the urine, but this value is not useful for allergy treatment and is thus not described below.

■ Volume: the total urine output, either excessive (polyuria) or minimal (oliguria), in relation to the specific gravity. This indicates how well the kidneys are functioning.

■ Indican (Obermeyer test): indican comes from putrefying proteins in the large intestine, is extremely toxic, and may act as an allergen, sparking allergic reactions and inflammation. Indican levels in the urine indicate the degree of toxicity, putrefaction, gas, and fermentation in the intestines from undigested proteins (which escape from the gut due to function defaults). The higher the level, the greater the intestinal toxemia or inflammation in the digestive tract. Readings as close to 0.0 as possible are desirable.

■ Specific (SP) Gravity: measures the weight of total dissolved substances in the urine against an equal amount of water, such that a normal reading of 1.020 means that the urine is 20% heavier than water. Specific gravity shows the general water content (hydration) of the body. Values can typically range from 1.005 to 1.030, with normal at 1.020. A reading higher than 1.025 indicates solute (dissolved substance) concentrations and possible kidney stress. In terms of allergies, readings over 1.025 mean the mucous membranes are too dry, increasing the risk for inhalant allergies. Levels that are too low may indicate that the body is retaining too much fluid.

■ pH: this value indicates the degree of urine acidity versus alkalinity on a scale of 0 to 14, with urine pH usually ranging from 4.5 to 8.0 and with 7.0 being neutral.

■ Vitamin C: levels of vitamin C indicate body reserves of this key immune-boosting nutrient; a reading of 1-5 is normal and 6-10 deficient.

For more on **hydrochloric acid**, see Chapter 7: Healing Leaky Gut Syndrome, pp. 184-211.

In order to determine HCl levels, physicians use the Heidelberg Gastric Analysis. After a 12-hour fast, the patient swallows a Heidelberg capsule, a device about the size of a vitamin that has a pH meter and radio transmitter inside. Once the capsule is swallowed, the patient drinks a solution of bicarbonate of soda, which stimulates the stomach to secrete hydrochloric acid. The capsule measures and transmits the changing pH levels to a receiver placed over the patient's stomach, indicating whether or not they are producing adequate HCl. The capsule can easily pass through the gastrointestinal tract for excretion.

Another, less-expensive gastric test is called the string test, in which a capsule is supplied with a string inside it. Patients come in

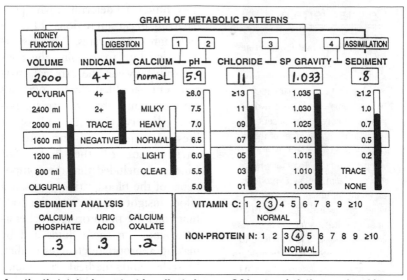

**GRAPH OF METABOLIC PATTERNS**

| KIDNEY FUNCTION | DIGESTION | | 1 | 2 | | 3 | | 4 | ASSIMILATION |
|---|---|---|---|---|---|---|---|---|---|
| VOLUME | INDICAN | CALCIUM | pH | CHLORIDE | | SP GRAVITY | | | SEDIMENT |
| **2000** | **4+** | **normal** | **5.9** | **11** | | **1.033** | | | **.8** |
| POLYURIA | 4+ | | ≥8.0 | ≥13 | | 1.035 | | | ≥1.2 |
| 2400 ml | 2+ | MILKY | 7.5 | 11 | | 1.030 | | | 1.0 |
| 2000 ml | TRACE | HEAVY | 7.0 | 09 | | 1.025 | | | 0.7 |
| 1600 ml | NEGATIVE | NORMAL | 6.5 | 07 | | 1.020 | | | 0.5 |
| 1200 ml | | LIGHT | 6.0 | 05 | | 1.015 | | | 0.2 |
| 800 ml | | CLEAR | 5.5 | 03 | | 1.010 | | | TRACE |
| OLIGURIA | | | 5.0 | 01 | | 1.005 | | | NONE |

| SEDIMENT ANALYSIS | | | VITAMIN C: 1 2 ③ 4 5 6 7 8 9 ≥10 NORMAL |
|---|---|---|---|
| CALCIUM PHOSPHATE | URIC ACID | CALCIUM OXALATE | NON-PROTEIN N: 1 2 3 ④ 5 6 7 8 9 ≥10 NORMAL |
| **.3** | **.3** | **.2** | |

A patient's total urine output is collected over a 24-hour period, then analyzed in a laboratory for the status of key biochemical factors.

exactly 25 minutes after finishing a fairly large protein meal. They swallow the capsule while holding on to the end of the string. The capsule goes down into the stomach and dissolves, leaving the end of the string in the stomach contents. After 10 minutes the string is pulled out, and the end that was in the stomach is painted with a chemical that changes color in acid. A color guide shows the pH of the stomach contents. Studies have shown that normally the body will make enough stomach acid within 30 minutes of even large meals to reduce the pH of their stomach contents to between 1 and 3. Betaine hydrochloride, a hydrochloric acid supplement, improves protein digestion, thus reducing the risk of food sensitization through digestive barrier dysfunction. Many doctors like this test because it is cheap ($25 or less) and noninvasive, and you get immediate results as well a direct measurement (the results need no interpretation).

For more about the **Heidelberg Gastric Analysis**, contact: Heidelberg International, Inc., 933 Beasley Street, Blairsville, GA 30512; tel: 706-745-9698; fax: 706-781-6229. For more about the **string test**, contact: Diagnos-Techs, 6620 South 192nd Place, #J104, Kent, WA 98032; tel: 425-251-0596; fax: 425-251-0637.

**Biological Terrain Assessment (BTA)—** French biologist Louis Claude Vincent, Ph.D., discovered that the key to healing was not the use of powerful drugs, but, rather, knowing the patient's biochemistry and the optimal conditions or "terrain" for body function. In 1958, Dr.

# A Primer on Cellular Terrain

**A**cid-base metabolism refers to the metabolic processes that maintain the balance of acids and bases (alkalines) in body fluids. Acids release hydrogen ions, while bases accept them. The total number of these hydrogen ions present determines the pH of a fluid. Too many hydrogen ions (a pH below 7) produce an acidic state called acidosis, while too few hydrogen ions (a pH above 7) cause an alkaline excess called alkalosis; both can lead to illness. **Oxidation-reduction** refers to a basic chemical mechanism in the cell by which energy is produced. Electrons (negatively charged particles in an atom) are removed from one atom, resulting in "oxidation" of this first atom, and then are added or transferred to another atom, resulting in "reduction" of this second atom. This continual process of energy metabolism is actually a flow of electrons, or a minute electrical current within the cell.

Vincent was hired by the French government to determine why people living in certain regions of France had high cancer rates. This assignment led him to examine the relationship between the external environment—molded by a person's emotional and physical stress exposure, dietary choices, and other lifestyle habits—and the internal environment of the body. Dr. Vincent concluded that the components of the blood, urine, and saliva afford insight into the way the body functions. By monitoring biochemical changes in these fluids and by making appropriate changes in diet, lifestyle, and medical treatment, health can be reestablished and disease processes, including allergies, retarded or possibly reversed.

*Biological terrain* is a phrase used to describe the conditions, general health, and activity level of cells. This includes the status of microorganisms at the cellular level—some are beneficial to life and health, others are not. Each type of bacterium, fungus, or virus thrives in a precise biochemical medium. Viruses require a fairly alkaline environment to function, whereas fungi favor a more acidic environment; bacteria can thrive under various conditions, but their growth is best stimulated in high-sugar conditions. An excess of toxins in one's diet and environment tends to increase the production of acid within cells, forcing the body to compensate by producing a strong alkaline chemical reaction in the blood, which, in turn, tends to favor the growth of fungi. Overgrowth of pathogenic bacteria and fungi is a major contributor to allergies/sensitivities.

The BTA tests for pH (acid/alkaline balance), resistivity (mineral "competency," or amounts), and redox (oxidation-reduction) values. The results help doctors determine the factors causing malabsorption and maldigestion, including bacterial overgrowth, parasitic infection,

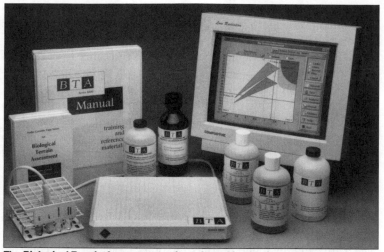

The Biological Terrain Assessment unit analyzes blood, urine, and saliva samples and displays information about an individual's cellular health on its monitor.

and enzymatic depletion. The analysis is performed on samples of blood, saliva, and first-morning urine, which are obtained following a 12-14 hour fast. The fast is necessary to assure that the test measures the body's baseline conditions and not recently eaten food.

The BTA test is carried out in only ten minutes by a computerized device called a BTA-S-1000. Using a pen-shaped microelectrode, the BTA-S-1000 analyzes biochemical factors in the blood, saliva, and urine. The reason for using all three bodily fluids is because urine is a good indicator of the body's secretory ability and toxic load on cells; blood is a good indicator of toxicity and oxygen balance; and saliva offers insight into a person's digestive capacities.

■ pH: the pH reading indicates whether the body's enzymes are being properly released and if digestion and absorption of vitamins and other nutrients is adequate. It also alerts doctors to the potential presence of environmental or industrial contaminants. In general, the urine is a better indicator of pH changes than the blood because the blood's pH level is very tightly controlled; however, both measures together, along with salivary pH, give a more complete picture of the body's chemical balance.

The acid/alkaline pH ratio indicates whether there may be an overgrowth of harmful microorganisms. An excess of toxins in your diet and surroundings tends to increase the production of acid within cells, forcing the body to compensate by producing a strong alkaline chemical reaction in the blood, which, in turn, favors the growth of fungi.

■ Oxidation-reduction potential: abbreviated as redox, this refers to the degree of oxidative stress on the body, or how much free-radical burden (oxidation of tissues) the body is exposed to. If the values are low, the person is susceptible to serious illnesses.

■ Resistivity: this is a measure of a tissue's resistance to the flow of electrical current, as opposed to conductivity, which indicates the ability to transmit an electrical current through a cell, nerve, or muscle. With low resistivity (high conductivity), there is typically a congestion or buildup of mineral salts. On the other hand, high resistivity (low conductivity) means a lack of minerals, which indicates the need to further evaluate the individual for specific deficiencies of these vital elements.

**Intestinal Permeability Test**—The Intestinal Permeability Test, or lactulose and mannitol test, requires a person to fast overnight and then drink a solution containing the sugars mannitol and lactulose, both of which are naturally found in fruits and other foods. Urine is collected over the next several hours and brought to the laboratory for analysis. Ordinarily, mannitol is easily absorbed; therefore a good amount should be present in the urine. Lactulose, on the other hand, is not easily absorbed and should pass out of the body with a bowel movement rather than through the urine. An indicator of a leaky gut is if the lactulose has managed to become absorbed and both sugars are found in the urine. On the other hand, if neither sugar is found in the urine in their expected ratios, digestive malabsorption may be an issue.

### Hypothyroidism Tests

For more on **how leaky gut causes allergies**, see Chapter 7: Healing Leaky Gut Syndrome, pp. 184-211. To learn more about **hypothyroidism and allergy**, see Chapter 7: Healing Leaky Gut Syndrome, pp. 184-211.

Hypothyroidism (SEE QUICK DEFINITION) can indirectly cause allergies. It often causes a sluggish digestive system, leading to a number of gastrointestinal problems, including constipation, gas and bloating, abdominal pain, and decreased absorption of nutrients, and if left untreated, may lead to leaky gut syndrome. Mainstream doctors generally test for hypothyroidism with the TSH (thyrotrophin-stimulating hormone) Test, but alternative medicine practioners prefer the TRH (thyrotrophin-releasing hormone)

For more about **Comprehensive Digestive Stool Analysis and Intestinal Permeability Test**, contact: Great Smokies Diagnostic Laboratory, 63 Zillicoa Street, Asheville, NC 28801; tel: 800-522-4762 or 704-253-0621; fax: 704-252-9303; website: www.gsdl.com. For **urine tests**, contact: 21st Century Nutrition, 6421 Enterprise Lane, Madison, WI 53719; tel: 800-662-2630; fax: 608-273-8110. For the **BTA test**, contact: Biological Technologies International, P.O. Box 560, Payson, AZ 85547; tel: 520-474-4181; fax: 520-474-1501. For more on **TRH Challenge Test**, contact: Meridian Valley Laboratory, 515 West Harrison Street, Suite 9, Kent, WA 98042; tel: 253-859-8700; fax: 253-859-1135; website: www.meridianvalleylab.com.

Challenge Test, which is described below. You can also test yourself for an underactive thyroid.

**TRH Challenge Test**—In this blood test, the physician measures the patient's level of TSH (thyroid-stimulating hormone), then gives an injection of TRH (a completely harmless synthetic hormone modeled after the TRH secreted by the hypothalamus gland in the brain), and finally draws blood 25 minutes later to remeasure the TSH. The TRH injection stimulates the pituitary gland, which produces thyroid-stimulating hormone; if the thyroid is underfunctioning, the pituitary gland will secrete excess TSH upon stimulation. If the second TSH blood test measures are high (above 10), it tells the physician that the patient's thyroid is underactive. A TSH reading of 15 is suspicious, while 20 strongly points to hypothyroidism.

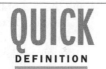

**DEFINITION**

**Hypothyroidism** is a condition of low or underactive thyroid gland function that can produce numerous symptoms. Among the 47 clinically recognized symptoms: fatigue, depression, lethargy, weakness, weight gain, low body temperature, chills, cold extremities, general inappropriate sensation of cold, infertility, rheumatic pain, menstrual disorders (excessive flow, cramps), repeated infections, colds, upper respiratory infections, skin problems (itching, eczema, psoriasis, acne, dry, coarse, or scaly skin, skin pallor), memory disturbances, concentration difficulties, paranoia, migraines, oversleep, "laziness," muscle aches and weakness, hearing disturbances, burning/prickling sensations, anemia, slow reaction time and mental sluggishness, swelling of the eyelids, constipation, labored or difficult breathing, hoarseness, brittle nails, and poor vision.

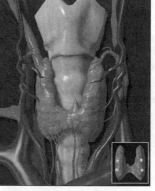

The thyroid gland, the largest of the seven endocrine glands, is located just below the larynx in the throat. The thyroid is the body's metabolic thermostat, controlling body temperature, energy use, and, for children, the body's growth rate. It affects the operation of all body processes and organs, including the immune system.

Copyright © 1989-97, TechPool Studios, USA

**Thyroid Function Self-Tests**—There are two simple tests you can do at home to check if you may have an underactive thyroid. To take the temperature test, measure your body temperature by placing an ordinary thermometer beneath your armpit; this is your axillary temperature. A resting body temperature below 97.8° F indicates hypothyroidism; menstruating women should take the underarm temperature only on the second and third days of menstruation. Another option is to take your oral temperature. A normal reading is 98° F in the morning before you become active and should increase to 98.6° F to 99° F for at least ten hours daily. The best time to do this test is about 20 minutes after lunch. A lower-than-normal temperature may indicate hypothyroidism.

Women should do this during their menstrual periods to insure missing the rise of temperature during ovulation.

You can also try the resting pulse test. Measure your resting pulse as described in the Coca Pulse Test for allergy triggers (see "Self-Administered Allergy Tests," p. 82). The healthy resting pulse should be about 85 beats per minute. If your pulse is less than 80, you may have an underactive thyroid. However, some people with low thyroid function have pulses over 100, so it's best to have your physician test you, too.

## Candidiasis Tests

In addition to causing leaky gut syndrome, an overgrowth of the *Candida albicans* fungus has been shown to confuse the immune system and lead to allergies on its own. The Comprehensive Digestive Stool Analysis (see "Digestive Function Tests," p. 89) can usually detect candidiasis, but there is another test that may assist your physician in pinpointing this imbalance as a primary cause of your allergies.

To learn **how eliminating candidiasis helps reverse allergies**, see Chapter 8: Intestinal Detoxification, pp. 212-235.

For more about the **Candida Antibody Titer Blood Test**, contact: Great Smokies Diagnostic Laboratory, 63 Zillicoa Street, Asheville, NC 28801; tel: 800-522-4762 or 704-253-0621; fax: 704-252-9303; website: www.gsdl.com.

**Candida Antibody Titer Blood Test**—This tests for the body's reaction to the presence of *Candida* as indicated by the levels of antibodies IgA, IgM, and IgG, rather than measuring the level of *Candida* directly. The test is useful, but not totally reliable. If positive, it can indicate past or present *Candida* infection somewhere in the body, but it may not indicate intestinal overgrowth. If negative, it may mean that although *Candida* is present, the body's immune mechanisms did not react appropriately to create the antibodies against *Candida*. This occurs in individuals with a compromised immune system.

## Parasitic Infection Tests

Parasitic infection, a frequent occurrence among allergy sufferers, can be as difficult to diagnose as hidden allergies. One of the main problems with parasitic infections and their link to systemic illness is the fact that many parasitology laboratories fail to find the majority of intestinal parasites in stool specimens submitted to them. David Casemore, M.D., of the Public Health Laboratories in Bodewuddan, Rhyh, Great Britain, adds that parasitic infection "is almost certainly underdetected, possibly by a factor of ten or more."[11] While the Comprehensive Digestive Stool Analysis can detect biochemical abnormalities indicating parasitic infection, doctors frequently overlook these clues. Steven Bailey, N.D., of Portland, Oregon, reports that one patient with AIDS required examination of 12 stool samples before giardiasis (infection with the protozoan *Giardia lamblia*) was diagnosed.[12]

According to Martin Lee, Ph.D., director of Great Smokies Laboratory in Asheville, North Carolina, many doctors, hospitals, and laboratories fail to diagnose parasitic infection because they rarely allow the time for careful analysis or multiple procedures using stool specimens collected over several days. Dr. Lee suggests that if you suspect you may have an intestinal parasite, or just want to be tested as a preventive measure, make sure your physician, hospital, or lab follows the guidelines set by the Centers for Disease Control and Prevention and the *Manual of Clinical Microbiology*. You can also ask your health-care practitioner to try one of these tests.

To learn how to **get rid of parasites**, see Chapter 8: Intestinal Detoxification, pp. 212-235.

■ Indirect Fluorescent Antibody (IFA): in this type of immunofluorescent testing, technicians tag special immune cells with fluorescent dyes, which make them highly visible under a darkfield microscope. As these cells specifically attack parasites, they will only show up where there is a parasitic presence.

■ Applied Kinesiology: this technique not only identifies allergy triggers, it also detects parasitic infections. When testing for parasites, the practitioner challenges a strong muscle while the patient holds a vial containing parasite specimens; the muscle will weaken if one of these parasites is causing their health problem.

■ Electrodermal Screening (EDS): in the search for parasites, practitioners use EDS similarly to the way they do allergy-trigger testing. EDS can use a computerized list or vials containing specimens of various parasites to test the meridians of the patient; if parasites are a factor, there will be a corresponding weakened EDS reading.

## Nutrient Deficiency Tests
Since digestive dysfunction, candidiasis, and parasitic infection, among other factors, result in the body not obtaining its full complement of nutrients, people with allergies often have vitamin and mineral deficiencies. There are numerous tests that claim to accurately analyze nutrient deficiencies, but some of them are not useful in clinically diagnosing and treating allergies. Below are select tests that may provide your health-care practitioner with detailed, practical information about your nutritional status. Note that these tests are not appropriate for all allergic patients; your doctor can discuss whether or not any of these tests would prove valuable for your condition.

### Functional Intracellular Analysis (FIA)—The Functional Intracellular Analysis

## QUICK
### DEFINITION

**Amino acids** are the building blocks of the 40,000 different proteins in the body, including enzymes, hormones, and the brain chemical messengers called neurotransmitters. Eight amino acids cannot be made by the body and must be obtained through the diet; others are produced in the body but not always in sufficient amounts. The body's main "amino acid pool" consists of: alanine, arginine, aspargine, aspartic acid, carnitine, citrulline, cysteine, cystine, GABA, glutamic acid, glutamine, glycine, histidine, isoleucine, leucine, lysine, methionine, ornithine, phenylalanine, proline, serine, taurine, threonine, tryptophan, tyrosine, and valine.

**Essential fatty acids (EFAs)** are unsaturated fats required in the diet. Omega-3 and omega-6 oils are the two principal types. The primary omega-3 oil is alpha-linolenic acid (ALA), found in flaxseed and canola oils, as well as pumpkins, walnuts, and soybeans. Fish oils, such as salmon, cod, and mackerel, contain the other important omega-3 oils, DHA (docosahexaenoic acid) and EPA (eicosapentaenoic acid). Linoleic acid is the main omega-6 oil and is found in most vegetable oils, including safflower, corn, peanut, and sesame. The most therapeutic form of omega-6 oil is gamma-linolenic acid (GLA), found in evening primrose, black currant, and borage oils. Once in the body, omega-3 and omega-6 are converted to prostaglandins, hormone-like substances that regulate many metabolic functions, particularly inflammatory processes.

is a group of relatively costly tests that can accurately measure the cellular function of key vitamins, minerals, antioxidants, amino acids (SEE QUICK DEFINITION), fatty acids, and metabolites (choline, inositol). Rather than simply measuring the levels of micronutrients in the blood (which may or may not provide useful information about actual cell metabolism), the FIA test measures how these micronutrients are actually functioning within the activities of living white blood cells. More specifically, FIA assesses the amount of cell growth for metabolically active lymphocytes, a type of white blood cell, as a way of identifying micronutrient deficiencies that are known to interfere with growth or immune function in the cell. These tests also assess the status of carbohydrate metabolism in terms of insulin function and fructose intolerance.

**Cell Membrane Lipid Profile**—This expensive but accurate blood test screens for adequate levels of essential fatty acids (SEE QUICK DEFINITION) by analyzing red blood cell membranes. The correct formation of cell membranes is dependent upon essential fatty acids. The test measures levels of omega-3 and omega-6 fatty acids that inhibit inflammation as well as toxic pro-inflammatory fatty acids. Correct fatty-acid content in the body has been shown to reduce the risk of allergic reactions. Dietary supplementation to correct fatty-acid imbalances can be accurately monitored through this profile.

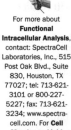

For more about **Functional Intracellular Analysis**, contact: SpectraCell Laboratories, Inc., 515 Post Oak Blvd., Suite 830, Houston, TX 77027; tel: 713-621-3101 or 800-227-5227; fax: 713-621-3234; www.spectracell.com. For **Cell Membrane Lipid Profile and Organic Acid Analysis**, contact: MetaMetrix Medical Laboratory, 5000 Peachtree Industrial Blvd., Suite 110, Norcross, GA 30071; tel: 800-221-4640 or 770-446-5483; fax: 770-441-2237.

For more on **how essential fatty acids relate to allergy/sensitivity**, see Chapter 9: Supporting the Skin, pp. 236-259, and Chapter 11: Supplements for Symptom Control, pp. 278-303.

**Organic Acid Analysis**—The levels at which organic acids (intermediate compounds of metabolism) appear in the blood or urine help determine how well energy production, enzyme reactions, and other chemical operations are functioning. Organic acid analysis is a costly test that may allow your doctor to peer into the energy cycles of the cell (also called the Krebs cycle) and pinpoint nutritional deficiencies as well as the presence of toxic chemicals. Low or high levels of a particular organic acid suggests a deficiency in a specific amino acid, vitamin, or mineral needed to "start" its corresponding biochemical reaction. Though this information may be of assistance in developing therapeutic programs of avoidance and nutritional support, its value is ultimately questionable.

## Enzyme Deficiency Tests

Enzymes are specialized living proteins fundamental to all processes in the body, necessary for every chemical reaction and the normal activity of our organs, tissues, fluids, and cells.

For more about **enzymes and allergies**, see Chapter 7: Healing Leaky Gut Syndrome, pp. 184-211.

Enzymes are essential for the production of energy required to run cellular functions. There are hundreds of thousands of these "Nature's workers." Enzymes enable the body to digest and assimilate food. There are special enzymes for digesting proteins, carbohydrates, fats, and plant fibers. Specifically, protease digests proteins, amylase digests carbohydrates, lipase digests fats, cellulase digests fiber, and disaccharidase digests sugars. Enzymes also assist in clearing the body of toxins and cellular debris. Enzyme expert Lita Lee, Ph.D., of Eugene, Oregon, says that food allergies are one of the more common disorders stemming from an inadequate supply of enzymes.

The 24-Hour Loomis Urine Test detects enzyme deficiencies and other digestive abnormalities by measuring specific gravity (body fluids), the indole (which measures protein maldigestion and level of toxification), calcium (minerals), vitamin C (water-soluble nutrients) and chloride (inversely related to adrenal function).

## Adrenal Hormone Level Tests

The adrenal glands play a central role in maintaining the body's energy levels. When a person is subject to stress, whether physical, psychological, or emotional, the adrenals release adrenaline, cortisol, and DHEA (SEE QUICK DEFINITION) to prepare the body for flight or fight. Constant stress exhausts the adrenals. When these glands are

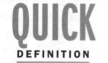

**DEFINITION**

**Cortisol** is a hormone secreted by the adrenal glands, which are located atop the kidneys. Cortisol secretion (as well as the adrenal gland's other hormones, DHEA, all sex hormones, adrenaline, and aldosterone) occurs in daily cycles, peaking in the morning and having the lowest values at night. Cortisol promotes protein building, regulates insulin and glycogen synthesis, and helps produce prostaglandins. Under conditions of stress, high amounts of cortisol are released; chronic excess secretion is associated with obesity and suppressed thyroid function. Imbalances in cortisol secretion are linked with low energy, muscle dysfunction, impaired bone repair, thyroid dysfunction, immune system depression, sleep disorders, poor skin regeneration, and decreased growth hormone uptake.

**DHEA** (dehydroepiandrosterone) is naturally produced by the human adrenal glands and gonads with optimal levels occurring around age 20 for women and age 25 for men. After those ages, DHEA levels gradually decline so that a person 80 years old produces only a fraction of the DHEA they did when they were 20. As an antioxidant, hormone regulator, and the building block from which estrogen and testosterone are produced, DHEA is vital to health. Low DHEA levels have been associated with cancer, diabetes, multiple sclerosis, hypertension, obesity, AIDS, heart disease, Alzheimer's, and immune dysfunction illnesses.

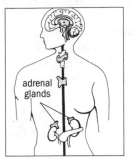

The adrenal glands, part of the body's endocrine system, are located atop the kidneys. The glands are composed of two types of tissue: the adrenal medulla and the adrenal cortex. The adrenal medulla, comprising 10%-20% of the gland, is located in the interior portion and is responsible for the production of the hormones epinephrine (adrenaline) and norepinephrine (noradrenaline). These hormones are released in direct respons to the sympathetic nervous system, which is responsible for the fight-or-flight response to stress or physical threat. The adrenal cortex, the outer layer, surrounds the medula and accounts for 80%-90% of the gland. It is responsible for the production of corticosteriods (also called adrenal steroids). More than 30 different steroids have been isolated from the adrenal cortex, including cortisol and cortisone.

---

functioning poorly, the result can be fatigue, a signal that you may need your adrenal hormones tested. Normal antibody production is also dependent upon healthy adrenal glands. Since allergic reactions themselves cause stress to the body, there is often a vicious cycle of allergies leading to weakened adrenals leading to more allergies.

The following tests measure specific hormone levels in the blood and provide guidelines for supplementation should you find your measures out of the normal range.

**Aeron LifeCycles Saliva Assay Report—**The Aeron LifeCycles saliva assay report, which can be ordered by both patients and physicians, provides graphs of individual hormone levels. Changing levels can be plotted over time on the same graph if supplementation or subsequent testing is done. Although hormones are present in saliva only in fractional amounts compared to the blood, "clinically relevant and highly accurate levels of hormones can be determined in saliva," says John Kells, president of Aeron LifeCycles in San Leandro, California, a laboratory that offers the saliva-based test for measuring levels of eight different hormones. "Saliva testing provides a means to establish whether or not your hormone levels are within the expected normal range for your age."

The saliva assay has several advantages over traditional blood testing for hormones. It is painless and noninvasive, and tests can be performed simply at any time or place. As DHEA, cortisol, estrogen, progesterone, and testosterone levels are highest in the morning, it is far more convenient to be able to test them at home (and then immediately ship the saliva sample to Aeron's laboratory) than to drive to a physician's office possibly at a later time when their levels have naturally fallen off a little.

# Do-At-Home Nutrient Testing

The Vitamed Test offers allergy sufferers a low-cost alternative to finding out precisely what nutrients their body needs. You send a urine sample to the laboratory and, in about ten days, you receive test results showing your specific levels of vitamins, minerals, and other nutrients. Based on this information, an effective supplementation program can be implemented. It is best to determine supplementation requirements under the guidance of a qualified health-care practitioner and needs to be used within context of other tests to verify accuracy. The kit contains the following three tests, which can be ordered separately or together:

For the **VitaMed Test**, contact: Medical Direct Corporation, 22722 Vistawood Way, Boca Raton, FL 33428; tel: 800-658-2227 or 561-483-0375; fax: 561-483-1969.

■ Oxidative Stress Test: this test is discussed in detail under "Detoxification Function Tests," this chapter, p. 87.

■ Mineral Component Test: this test is similar to the ToxMet Screen (see p. 86). Test results are displayed on an easy-to-read bar graph, showing your actual level of each element and designating it as high, normal, or low.

■ Vitamin Deficiency Test: this test looks at four indicators in the urine that point to metabolic deficiencies: cysteine, L-glutathione, creatinine, and homocysteine. Cysteine, an amino acid, is important in a number of body processes including immune stimulation, protein synthesis, and tissue healing. Glutathione is a complex of amino acids that is essential for the proper operation of the immune system and has important antioxidant functions. Creatinine is a waste product produced in the course of muscle activity and excreted through the kidneys. A high level in the urine could indicate several problems, including a diet too high in meat proteins, muscle atrophy, and kidney dysfunction. Homocysteine, an amino acid, is the normal by-product of protein metabolism, specifically of the amino acid methionine. A high level in the urine indicates a deficiency of B vitamins and folic acid, necessary to the healthy production of antibodies, along with other functions.

As the test is less expensive than blood testing, you can do frequent testing to monitor changes (brought on by interventions such as diet, exercise, herbs, stress reduction, allergy desensitization, or acupuncture) and to adjust dosages of over-the-counter hormones such as DHEA or melatonin, Kells says. In general, Kells explains that it is best to establish a baseline level of saliva hormones first, then after intervention (which can include hormone supplementation), test a second time to measure the changes.

**Adrenal Stress Index (ASI)—**This simple, noninvasive saliva test, can pinpoint whether an imbalance in the adrenal glands might be contribut-

For information on **reducing adrenal stress**, see Chapter 14: Mind/Body Approaches to Allergies, pp. 348-373.

ing to your allergies or allergy-related condition. As mentioned, the adrenal glands do not secrete their hormones at a constant level throughout the day; instead, hormones are released in a cycle, with the highest volume in the morning and the lowest at night. This 24-hour cycle, known as circadian rhythm, can influence a variety of body functions, from immune response to quality of sleep.

The ASI saliva test evaluates how well your adrenal glands are functioning by tracking the 24-hour cycle. Four saliva samples taken at intervals throughout the day are used to reconstruct the adrenal rhythm in the laboratory and determine whether the three main stress hormones, cortisol, adrenaline, and DHEA, are being secreted in proper proportion to each other, and at the right times. Based on the results, a physician can prescribe the appropriate treatment to restore the balance of hormones and correct the circadian rhythm.

**DHEA Challenge Test—**Some people have been helped with their allergies through taking the supplement DHEA when the hormone proves to be deficient. However, while many people taking DHEA report improvement in allergies, sleeping patterns, energy level, and ability to cope with stress, some people actually experience the opposite effect.

For information on **hormonal supplements for allergy**, see Chapter 11: Supplements for Symptom Control, pp. 278-303.

Depending upon a person's genetic makeup, a certain amount of DHEA from a supplement may be converted by the body into the hormones testosterone and estradiol, a type of estrogen. If you are one of those people who are genetically predisposed to convert DHEA, you may experience unwanted side effects with supplementation as a result of increased amounts of testosterone and estradiol (one of the female hormones). These side effects can include fatigue, insomnia, irritability, acne, oily skin, deepening of the voice, and an increase in body hair.

For the **Aeron LifeCycles Saliva Assay Report**, contact: Aeron LifeCycles, 1933 Davis Street, Suite 310, San Leandro, CA 94577; tel: 800-631-7900 or 510-729-0375; fax: 510-729-0383. For the **DHEA Challenge Test**, contact: Diagnos-Techs, 6620 South 192nd Place, #J104, Kent, WA 98032; tel: 425-251-0596; fax: 425-251-0637.

Through a simple saliva sample, the DHEA Challenge Test determines whether, in your particular case, DHEA supplements will improve—or worsen—your health. The test works by measuring levels of the two hormones (testosterone and estradiol) in the saliva both before and after a five- to seven-day treatment with DHEA (15 mg for women, 25 mg for men). If your testosterone and estradiol levels are too high following the "challenge" to the system, continuing to take DHEA supplements is probably not advisable.

Everyone who suffers from allergies also
suffers from varying degrees of compromised barrier functions
in the intestines, skin, and mucous membranes.
Prevention strategies can help strengthen and condition these
organs. Becoming allergy free can begin as early
as infancy and involves common child-rearing strategies:
prolonged breast-feeding, later introduction of solid foods,
and the avoidance of early immunizations.

# CHAPTER

# 4

# Prevention of Sensitization

**E**VERYONE WHO SUFFERS from allergies and sensitivities also suffers from varying degrees of compromised barrier functions in the intestines, skin, and mucous membranes. The prevention strategies discussed in this chapter can help strengthen and condition these organs so that they function properly without irritation and sensitization. Becoming allergy free can begin as early as infancy and involves what were once common child-rearing strategies: prolonged breast-feeding, later introduction of solid foods, and the avoidance of early immunizations. The other strategies discussed in this chapter are applicable to all age groups and include eating a healthy diet (free of allergenic foods), drinking adequate fluids, avoiding harmful environmental allergens, and protecting the skin. These strategies are complements to one another and should be practiced together.

## Breast-Feed Your Infant

One of the best ways to decrease the likelihood of developing allergies later in life, according to most alternative medicine practitioners, is to feed an infant mother's milk. Breast-feeding builds a strong immune system equipped to deal with infection, environmental toxins, and food allergens. Lendon Smith, M.D., a pediatrician in Portland, Oregon, and author of numerous books on children's health, emphasizes that nursing contributes to the child having fewer allergies. He states, "If babies are given anything other than breast milk in the first few months of life, food sensitivities may develop. Their intestines are not meant to digest anything other than breast milk. The immature cells lining the intestines will allow foreign food particles to pass through undigested. These bits are antigenic [material that causes immune reactions] and may set up an allergenic or antibody response that the child will never outgrow."

A recent Finnish study revealed that breast-feeding in infancy lowered the risk of allergic symptoms by one-third in children by the age 17.[1] In another study, high-risk (atopic) infants were less likely to develop allergic eczema if they were breast-fed for more than four months.[2] In addition, a recent study published in the *British Medical Journal* reports that babies who are breast-fed during their first six months of life have a significantly lower risk of developing childhood asthma.[3]

Human breast milk contains nutrients that are easily digested, contribute to healthy brain development and growth, and provide immunity to infectious agents that the mother (and also the infant) will encounter in their environment. In building an infant's immune system, breast milk acts on many levels. It contains anti-inflammatory substances that infants cannot manufacture on their own; stimulates the production of IgA, which can neutralize a substance foreign to the body before it becomes an allergen; and populates the child's immature intestinal barrier with beneficial microflora, which blocks the growth of disease-causing bacteria. A protein called lactoferrin—which makes up 20% of the total protein in human colostrum (breast milk secreted immediately after delivery)—seems to have an inhibitory effect on "unfriendly" bacteria such as *Staphylococcus aureus*, *Escherichia coli*, and *Helicobacter pylori*, all of which are increasingly identified as contributing to numerous health problems, including allergies.[4] According to researchers at the Shanghai Institute for Pediatric Research in Shanghai, China, breast-fed, full-term children had healthier intestinal bacteria than formula-fed infants. Furthermore, their findings supported the claim that factors in breast milk prevent intestinal pathogens from developing.[5]

Most researchers and medical experts have found that children who are breast-fed for at least six months or more experience greater health benefits and fewer episodes of common childhood illnesses, such as ear infections, than do children who are not breast-fed or are breast-fed for less than four months. Dr. Smith recommends that infants be breast-fed for at least eight to ten months. The American Academy of Pediatrics recommends that children be breast-fed for six to 12 months. The academy suggests that parents can begin to introduce age-specific solid to the child at age six months but the child should continue nursing for at least the first year of life.

If the mother has allergies or sensitivities, breast-feeding alone will not protect a newborn from developing allergies. As discussed in Chapter 2: Causes of Allergy and Sensitivity, mothers can inadvertently pass food antigens and their associated antibodies to their children through nursing or even prior to birth through the wall of the placenta. Antibodies to cow's milk protein, a common trigger of atopic eczema, were detected in breast milk samples taken by German researchers in a study at the Universitats-Kinderklinik in Wien, Germany. The researchers found that infants produced the same type of antibodies to cow's milk that their mothers did even if the children's diet consisted solely of breast milk. But, the researchers found, if foods that trigger an immune response in the mother are avoided both during pregnancy and lactation, infants experience a lower incidence of sensitivity to cow's milk and thus a lower incidence of atopic eczema than infants whose mothers were on an unrestricted diet.[6]

The most common allergy-producing foods are cow's milk, peanuts, eggs, wheat, soy, chicken, turkey, beef, and pork. A study appearing in the *American Journal of Clinical Nutrition* found that exclusive breast-feeding and elimination of peanut, egg, fish, and dairy products from the mother's diet during lactation reduced the occurrence of food sensitivity in the infant.[7] James Braly, M.D., author of *Dr. Braly's Food Allergy and Nutrition Revolution*, recommends that women predisposed to allergies discover what foods they are allergic to before pregnancy and eliminate them from their diet. They should then breast-feed their babies without consuming dairy products for a minimum of six months while still refraining from the foods they are allergic to. According to a French study, eliminating only cow's milk from the mother's diet did not result in reduced allergic episodes. Elimination of two to four foods, however, did prove sufficient.[8]

To learn about **testing for individual food allergies or sensitivities**, see Chapter 3, Allergy/Sensitivity Testing, pp. 70-105.

## Breast Milk Alternatives

If a mother is unable to breast-feed, for whatever reason, one recommendation by Dr. Smith is to see a lactation consultant who can help design a nutritionally balanced substitute to breast milk or discuss ways for the women to encourage lactation. The breast milk substitutions provided in this chapter are as good an approximation of breast milk that can be obtained without going to a commercial formula.

# Breast Milk Substitutes

Here are three infant formulas to use if you cannot breast-feed your infant. Add commercial colostrum supplements soon after birth to more closely approximate natural breast milk. Joanne Sanchez is an herbalist based in Phoenix, Arizona, who developed a special formula in conjunction with a local lactation consultant. Note: Do not substitute honey for molasses, maple syrup, or cane sugar. Children under one year of age who eat honey are at risk for contracting botulism, a serious paralytic disease.

## GOAT MILK FORMULA

⅔ qt goat's milk
½ qt pure spring water
3 tbsp lactose
After three months of age, add:
½ tsp blackstrap molasses
½ tsp brewer's yeast

## WRIGHT-LAUFFER FORMULA

1 qt soy milk
1 cup carrot juice
¼ tsp barley greens
¼ tsp nutritional yeast
200 mg vitamin D (grind with a mortar and pestle)
100 mg ascorbate (vitamin C) powder
1 tbsp safflower oil (pure, expeller-pressed)
3 tbsp pure maple syrup or lactose

## JOANNE SANCHEZ FORMULA

1 gallon soy milk
2 tbsp oil (flaxseed, olive, or safflower; expeller-pressed)
1 tbsp lecithin
400 IU powdered vitamin D
1 tsp *Bifidobacterium bifidum* crystals
700 mg calcium lactate
100 mg ascorbate (vitamin C) powder
1-3 tbsp rice protein powder
8 tbsp organic cane sugar

Dr. Smith has found that goat's milk can be a good replacement for breast-feeding for the first 10 to 12 months. He suggests diluting it with pure water (three parts goat's milk to one part water). He also cautions parents to be sure to use goat's milk that is supplemented with folic acid, as goat's milk has been associated with a type of anemia related to low folic acid content in the milk. The label on the carton will reveal if the milk contains folate.

Soybean milk is another popular alternative to cow's milk but, because of the popularity of soy, it has become a common food allergen, so caution is advised. Other options are amino acid milk, almond milk, and rice milk. However, Eric Jones, N.D., a naturopathic pediatrician in Seattle, Washington, cautions that these milks by themselves do not provide full nutrition to infants so you will have to supplement them with nutrients (see "Breast Milk Substitutes," p. 109).

Unfortunately, none of these milks are guaranteed to be non-allergenic. Dr. Smith has seen babies who have developed eczema from cow's milk, asthma from soy milk, diarrhea from almond milk, and irritability from goat's milk. Therefore, he suggests rotating them to prevent babies from developing an allergic reaction to any particular one.

## Introduce Solid Foods Later

Postponing the introduction of solid foods and prolonging breast-feeding gives an infant's immune system enough time to adequately mature. Studies suggest that a later introduction of solid foods, in particular peanuts, eggs, wheat, and fish, may reduce the incidence of allergies.[9] A study published in the *British Medical Journal* found that children who were started on solid foods before the age of four months were more likely to experience chronic or recurrent episodes of eczema than children of the same age who were not introduced to solid foods.[10] When a child is ready to eat solid foods, usually after six months, parents can give them a healthy start by designing a diet made up of fresh fruits and vegetables, legumes, and low-fat proteins like chicken and fish, recommends Dr. Smith. Organically grown products are the best choice as they contain fewer environmental toxins that can put a young immune system at risk of developing an allergic response. It is also a good idea to avoid foods that are high in processed sugars, fats, or other additives, such as many baby foods, most breakfast cereals, candy, soda, and fast foods.

Wheat, eggs, and fish should not be introduced until the infant is older than 12 months of age, especially if either parent has food sensitivities or allergies.[11] Hugh Sampson, of Johns Hopkins University School of Medicine in Baltimore, recommends that peanuts (a legume) and tree nuts be avoided until the child is three years old or older.[12] A recent study suggests that the rise in peanut and nut allergies might be due to the trend of giving peanut butter and other nuts to very young children. Pamela W. Ewan, of the Medical Research Council Centre in Cambridge, England, studied 62 nut-sensitive patients (11 months to 53 years old) and found peanut allergies in 76% of the patients, with Brazil nuts the second most common nut allergy at 30%. Interestingly, most of the people had developed their nut allergies by age three; 97% of allergies were evident by age seven.[13]

## Avoid Early Immunization

Currently in the United States, conventional doctors require that a series of immunization shots be started when an infant is two months old. The first vaccines given are hepatitis B, DPT (diphtheria, tetanus,

# Food Introduction Schedule

Introduce foods one at a time (one new food every three days). Discontinue if allergy/sensitivity symptoms occur—rash, hyperactivity or lethargy, tantrums, runny nose, infections (especially ear), mucus in stools or diarrhea, red cheeks, or changes in drawing ability in older children. Provide a variety of foods and don't give each food often. The most allergenic foods (wheat and dairy) should be introduced late. Also, watch for reactions with meats, corn, and peanuts.

**6 MONTHS**
banana
cherries
prunes
blackberries
carrot (cooked and
   mashed)
sprouts
broccoli (cooked and
   blended)
applesauce
grapes
yams
pears
cauliflower

**9 MONTHS**
oats
lima beans
split peas
potato (cooked and
   mashed)
basmati rice
brown rice
artichoke
cabbage
millet
string beans
papaya
nectarine
blueberries (frozen
   helps teething)

**12 MONTHS**
squash
tofu
asparagus
avocado
barley
swiss chard
parsnips
blackstrap molasses
yogurt (if no reaction)
goat's milk (fresh)

**18 MONTHS**
eggs
kelp
beets and beet greens
chard
beans
eggplant
lamb
chicken
fish
other greens (lettuce,
   mustard, etc.)
rye
buckwheat
tahini
goat milk yogurt
garbanzo beans

**21 MONTHS**
beef liver
cashew butter
almond butter
salmon
orange
turkey
pineapple
brewer's yeast
wheat

**2–3 YEARS**
sunflower seeds
peanut butter
lentils
cottage cheese
hard cheese
soy clams
corn (if no reaction)

and pertussis), influenza type B, and polio. In total, an average American child is vaccinated against ten childhood diseases and receives up to 21 shots over the first 15 months of life. It is well documented that certain vaccines can cause immediate allergic reactions in some children; these reactions range from temporary discomfort to death. For example, the MMR (measles-mumps-rubella) vaccine can cause swelling of the neck glands, rash, joint aching or swelling, arthritis, slight fever, anaphylaxis, and encephalitis. Neurological problems (including brain damage) have been reported after individuals received the pertussis vaccine (part of DPT).[14] The vaccine for hepatitis B (a disease spread in body fluids) was discontinued in France in 1998 after recently vaccinated school-aged children developed arthritis and multiple sclerosis symptoms. In 1998, the National Vaccine Injury Compensation Program in the United States was created to award compensation to people who had suffered adverse reactions to vaccines. Within the program's first year, 5,000 claims were filed and more than 1,100 awards totaling $800 million in compensation were disbursed.

More recently, vaccines are suspected cofactors in the development of allergies, AIDS, SIDS (Sudden Infant Death Syndrome), and developmental delays including autism and attention deficit disorder. A study at the Karolinska Institute and Hospital in Stockholm, Sweden, found that children who had not received the full spectrum of vaccinations had a lower incidence of allergies than children who had been fully vaccinated. Researchers surveyed 675 children between the ages of five and 13 for prevalence of allergies and a correlation to certain lifestyle factors. The first group consisted of 295 children who were being raised with an Anthroposophic (SEE QUICK DEFINITION) lifestyle—restricted use of antibiotics, few vaccinations, and diets high in *Lactobacilli* bacteria; the second group (380 children) had been vaccinated against measles, mumps, rubella, received antibiotics in the past, and ate little to no foods containing beneficial bacteria. Skin-prick and blood tests found that the prevalence of atopy was lower in children from Anthroposophic families than in children from conventional families.[15]

The risks and side effects of vaccines have sparked much debate in the medical community. The majority of conventional doctors maintain

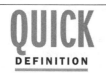

**DEFINITION**

**Anthroposophic medicine** is an extension of conventional Western medicine developed by Austrian scientist Rudolf Steiner in the 1920s, in conjunction with other European physicians. It is based on a spiritual model of the human being and its medicines are extensions of homeopathic remedies. In the U.S., there are about 60 practitioners, all M.D.s or D.O.s, plus many hundreds of nurses and adjunctive therapists, but in German-speaking countries, there are thousands of practitioners plus several hospitals in Germany and Switzerland devoted exclusively to this medical approach.

that the adverse effects of vaccines are rare and a small price to pay for eradicating diseases that are capable of epidemics. In the U.S., support for vaccinations is so great that increased research dollars are spent on developing new vaccines (from chicken pox to AIDS) but little has been done to investigate the possible correlation between vaccines and developmental problems (as in the possible connection between the MMR vaccine and autism).

Detractors suggest that today's vaccine policy is indifferent to the individual and may hinder some children with lifelong, yet nonfatal, diseases. Better nutrition and improved sanitation, vaccine reform advocates maintain, played a larger role in the eradication of disease than vaccines. Scarlet fever, for example, is now relatively unheard of in the U.S., but a vaccine was never created for it. Furthermore, some childhood illnesses may be important to the development of the immune system. According to the Medical Working Group, which consists of 180 Swiss doctors, childhood illnesses spur the immune system into defending itself against allergies, infections, asthma, eczema, and even cancer.[16] The following statistics serve to highlight the shortcomings of modern vaccination: the death rate in children under 15 has declined since 1900, but the rate of chronic disease (asthma, diabetes, autism, etc.) is 3.7 times higher than it was in 1960. From 1960 to 1980, the number of chronically disabled children doubled, and it has nearly doubled again since 1982. In 1960, the incidence of asthma, allergies, and autism in children was 1.8%; in the most recent study in 1994, it was 6.7%.[17]

As a parent, you have the right to choose whether or not your child will be vaccinated, at what age, and for which diseases. In order to make these decisions, you should be informed of the vaccines' negative effects and weigh those against the vaccines' benefits. It is also highly advised to delay immunization until the child is six months old (rather than two months) and to only give one vaccination at a time. Giving vaccinations to older children allows for greater immune system maturity; staggering vaccines allows the immune system to recover and makes it easier to determine which vaccine may be responsible for an adverse reaction.

If your child has chronic or severe asthma or food allergies to eggs or gelatin, it is advisable to forego the administration of the MMR and DPT vaccines. MMR vaccines are grown in cultures from chick cells and bovine gelatin is often added to the MMR and DPT vaccines as a stabilizer. Studies have found a correlation between children who experience adverse reactions to these vaccines and the presence of

For information on the controversy and legal implications of vaccination and the National Vaccine Injury Compensation Program, contact: National Vaccine Information Center, 512 West Maple Avenue, Suite 206, Vienna, VA 22180; tel: 800-909-SHOT or 703-938-DPT3; fax: 703-938-5768; website: www.909shot.com.

allergies to eggs and/or gelatin, or asthma. Researchers at the UCLA School of Public Health found that DTP or tetanus vaccination increased the risk of allergies and related respiratory symptoms in children and adolescents.[18]

If you choose not to have your child vaccinated, you must obtain an exemption (medical, religious, or philosophical) since immunization is compulsory in many states in the U.S. A medical exemption, obtained from a doctor, usually applies to just one vaccine and is given following a previous adverse reaction. Religious exemptions are available in 48 states (exceptions are Mississippi and West Virginia) and require legal documentation of your decision. Your state's health department can provide you with information on the state's immunization regulations and requirements. Obtaining a philosophical exemption follows the same procedure as obtaining a religious exemption.

## Success Story: How Measles Cured Eczema

Now let's see how undergoing childhood measles may actually improve a child's health, both immediately and in the long-term. Consider the case of Kurt, whom Philip Incao, M.D., of Denver, Colorado, first treated for measles when Kurt was nine.

Philip Incao, M.D.: Gilpin Street Holistic Center, 1624 Gilpin Street, Denver, CO 80218; tel: 303-321-2100; fax: 303-321-3737. For Anthroposophic medicines and home remedies, contact: Weleda USA, P.O. Box 249, Congers, NY 10920; tel: 800-241-1030 or 914-268-8572; fax: 914-268-8574; website: usa.weleda.com. Raphael Pharmacy, 7597 California Avenue, Fairoaks, CA 95628; tel: 916-962-1099; fax: 916-967-0510. For doctor referrals, contact: Physicians Association for Anthroposophic Medicine, 7953 California Avenue, Fairoaks, CA 95628; tel: 916-966-1417; fax: 916-966-5314.

Kurt did not receive the measles vaccine because he was allergic to eggs (the measles vaccine contains an egg product and is not recommended for children with this allergy). When he was nine, he came down with the measles, which is a bit late for children. Of considerable interest here is the fact that, for years, Kurt had suffered from severe eczema; his skin was dry and cracked, particularly behind the elbows and knees, and occasionally it bled. In fact, Kurt often could not straighten his legs because the eczema made it too painful.

His measles produced a strong rash and a fever of 104° F, yet Dr. Incao did nothing to suppress these reactions with Tylenol or Advil, for example, as conventional medicine would recommend. Instead, Dr. Incao gave Kurt Anthroposophic remedies to support him through the measles process. Specifically, Dr. Incao gave him low potencies of *Apis, Belladonna, Argentum/Carbo/Silicea, Ferrum Phosphate, Prunus Spinosa* (from the sloe plum), and *Echinacea*.

These remedies do not suppress the fever, but allow the constitution to tolerate it better. The important concept here is that the fever is a natural, useful, necessary process

## Vaccines and Allergy: The Odds Are Against You

Children who receive the following vaccines are more likely to experience asthma and allergic disorders than unvaccinated children. Children between the ages of five and ten appear to be the most at risk. Note that in the MMR vaccine study, older immunized children had a greater risk of developing hay fever than their younger vaccinated siblings, possibly because the younger children had been cumulatively exposed to more infections from their older siblings. Additionally, a recent report contradicts the MMR findings, saying that measles infections and allergy occur together more frequently than the researchers had expected.[19]

| VACCINE | RISKS |
| --- | --- |
| DPT (diphtheria, tetanus, and pertussis) | 200% greater risk for asthma and 63% greater risk for allergy-related respiratory disorders (rhinitis, sinusitis)[20] |
| Pertussis | 500% greater risk for asthma and 200% greater risk for otitis media (ear infections)[21] |
| Measles | 200% greater risk for allergy-related respiratory disorders[22] and hay fever[23] |

for a child's health. The child must be closely observed by a medical professional during the illness to be sure the course of illness is benign. It is important to find out if complications like encephalitis or pneumonia are developing. These rarely occur, however, and are not directly linked to the degree of the fever.

The remedies Anthroposophic doctors use for children make the body more permeable to allow the toxicity or fever process to flow through it without getting stuck. If you suppress the fever with drugs or antibiotics, you block this flow. How long a child has the disease is not as important as avoiding complications. The length of time depends on how much toxicity the body needs to discharge through the fever. Care should always be taken, however, to see that children have warm feet, especially during a fever.

When Kurt's measles were over, his eczema had almost completely disappeared. Kurt is now in his twenties and has never had a recurrence of eczema. This is a typical example of how stimulating the immune system can help the body overcome an allergic problem. The measles process enabled Kurt's system to stop reacting allergically and producing eczema symptoms. In a sense, you could say that the fever burned the allergic reaction out of his body.

## Remedies for Dealing with Childhood Illnesses

Vaccination is not a sure guarantee against childhood illness. In the first part of 1987, more than half of the reported cases of measles were in children who had been fully vaccinated, according to the Centers for Disease Control and Prevention.[24] The mumps and pertussis vaccines are similarly ineffective. These diseases, however, are not as deadly as they were in the past. Dr. Incao has found that over a 20-year period, he has seen approximately 100 cases of whooping cough (pertussis), which were treatable and did not require hospitalization. He maintains that childhood diseases such as measles and pertussis are much milder, due in part to the sanitation improvements of a modernized nation, and that a bout with these illnesses actually strengthens a child's immune system.

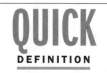

For **referrals to home-paths in your area**, contact: National Center for Homeopathy, 801 North Fairfax Street, Suite 306, Alexandria, VA 22314; tel: 703-548-7790; fax: 703-548-7792; website: www.healthy.net/nch.

To avoid the use of antibiotics or drugs, Anthroposophic medicine offers many remedies to parents to support the discharging—or the "expressing"—of the illness, driving it out of the body, according to Dr. Incao. He asserts that most of childhood illnesses can be helped with low-potency home remedies, including 13 Anthroposophic or homeopathic medicines. Classical homeopathic remedies (SEE QUICK DEFINITION) include *Ferrum phosphate*, which is effective for relieving colds, flu, sinusitis, or any upper respiratory infection such as bronchitis; *Cinnabar*, for sore throats and swollen lymph glands; and *Apis Belladonna* (a homeopathic combination of the honey bee and deadly nightshade), for fevers and pain.

## QUICK DEFINITION

**Homeopathy** was founded in the early 1800s by German physician Samuel Hahnemann. Today, an estimated 500 million people worldwide receive homeopathic treatment; in Britain, homeopathy enjoys royal patronage. Homeopathy is now practiced according to two differing concepts. In classical homeopathy, only one single-component remedy is prescribed at a time, in a potency specifically adjusted to the patient; the physician waits to see the results before prescribing anything further. In complex homeopathy, typified by *Hepar compositum*, multiple substances are given at the same time, usually in low potencies.

Among specifically Anthroposophic medicines is *Infludo* for flu, bronchitis, or pneumonia. This formula contains phosphorus, *Aconite*, *Bryonia*, eucalyptus, *Eupatorium*, and *Sabadilla*. For earaches, capsicum (red pepper) can be used or the herb lovage, given orally or directly into the ear where it has a gentle warming effect that relieves the pain.

Anthroposophic, homeopathic, and other natural medicines have enabled Dr. Incao for the last 20 years to avoid using antibiotics in treating children. The aim of treatment is to support the externalizing and discharging of the illness process—to get it out of the body—so that no residual illness remains to become a chronic problem later in life.

For more on **homeopathy**, see Chapter 12: Homeopathic and Physical Therapies, pp. 304-327.

Suppression of illness in childhood is likely to result in more chronic illness in adulthood.

## Preventing Allergic Vaccination Reactions with EDS

If you do choose to have your child vaccinated, the risks associated with immunizations can be reduced through more sophisticated approaches to vaccination. Harold Whitcomb, M.D., an internist with more than 45 years of medical experience, now practicing in Aspen, Colorado, finds that sophistication in the use of electrodermal screening (EDS). This is a way of determining in advance whether a child is likely to have an allergic reaction to a vaccine and, therefore, whether it is advisable to give the immunization at all. "I do this with all the young children I see," he reports.

EDS enables Dr. Whitcomb to assess how a child's system will react to each of the main elements in the DPT vaccine before giving it. In about 50% of his cases, Dr. Whitcomb finds that young children do not tolerate the pertussis component and he eliminates it from the vaccine mixture, giving only the diphtheria and tetanus components. "The risk of getting whooping cough [pertussis] is a lot less than the overt risk of taking a vaccine that will cause a problem," he notes. There are several reasons why a young child cannot handle pertussis or other vaccines, explains Dr. Whitcomb. In some cases, the child is simply too young and has an immature immune

## Hering's Laws of Cure

Constantine Hering was a German homeopath who immigrated to the United States in the 1830s and promoted the practice of homeopathy in America. He proposed three general laws of the homeopathic healing process. These tenets provide a general guide to determine whether patients, especially children undergoing illnesses such as measles and whooping cough, are healing with homeopathy.

**Law 1:** Healing progresses from the deepest part of the organism (mental and emotional levels and the vital organs) to the extremities, such as skin and appendages. A cure is happening when a patient's psychological symptoms diminish while their physical symptoms increase ("healing crisis"), but not to a dangerous degree. Ultimately, the deep healing spreads outward to the physical level. If the physical improves but the psychological weakens, then health is deteriorating.

**Law 2:** As healing progresses, the symptoms appear and reappear in the reverse order to which they first appeared. During the healing period, patients will re-experience symptoms from past conditions.

**Law 3:** Healing progresses from the upper to the lower parts of the body. Healing is occurring if symptoms in the head and neck disappear while symptoms in the lower extremities persist.

system; in Japan, DPT vaccinations are not given until the child is two years old, while in the U.S., they are given at two months. In other cases,

For more on **electro-dermal screening,** see Chapter 3: Allergy/Sensitivity Testing, pp. 70-105, and Chapter 13: Desensitizing the Immune System, pp. 328-347.

a child's health history, diet, or family history may preclude an early vaccination.

"If I have a child with recurrent ear infections, which is very common, I will never approve a vaccination," Dr. Whitcomb states. Other immune stressors contraindicating vaccines, he says, are if the child is not well-nourished, has a diet of sugar and processed foods, or lives in a non-nurturing home environment. "If you give a child living under these conditions a vaccination, they will have more trouble with that vaccine than healthier, stronger children. In such a case, I would delay the vaccine until, according to EDS, the child could handle it."

Another option, using EDS results, is to reduce the vaccine dosage. Dr. Whitcomb cites an example of a child whose EDS evaluation indicated a problem with all three components of DPT. Dr. Whitcomb cut the dose of each in half so that the vaccine produced only a small reaction, which he neutralized with low potencies of *Aconite* and *Bryonia,* two homeopathic remedies that counteract the negative effects of the vaccine. The ideal approach, made possible by EDS, he says, is that instead of giving every child the same dose at the same age, doctors can adjust, or titer, the dose to suit the individual child, or they can wait until the child's immune system is more able to deal with the stimulus of the vaccination. However, it should be noted

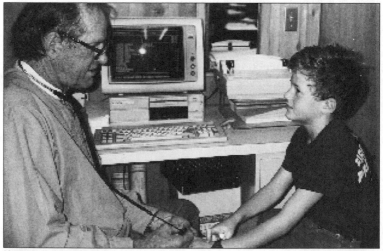

**Harold Whitcomb, M.D., uses an electrodermal screening probe to painlessly gather information about this child's health based on energy signals from acupuncture points on his fingers.**

that there are no studies to support the hypothesis that low-dose inoculation confers immunity.

**Harold Whitcomb, M.D.**: Aspen Clinic for Preventive and Environmental Medicine at Internal Medicine Associates, 100 E. Main Street, #201, Aspen, CO 81611; tel: 970-920-2523 or 970-925-5440; fax: 970-920-2282.

The skillful use of EDS also enables Dr. Whitcomb to antidote vaccine damage after the immunization. For example, Scott had a strong reaction to his second DPT shot and, after his third, failed to thrive and did not grow for almost two years. Dr. Whitcomb used EDS to prepare a homeopathic remedy that would neutralize the effect of the disabling DPT vaccine. The EDS computer draws on its large repertory of substances, drugs, and natural medicines, which are stored as information or energy signals (virtual remedies), to identify a remedy that will reverse the reaction in question and undo its damage. Dr. Whitcomb relates that this allows him to make a remedy, or information signal, that balances the energy field (in this instance, of the DPT vaccine) that created the problem. In the case of Scott, after Dr. Whitcomb neutralized the pertussis, "he came out of it and started to grow again."

# Drink Adequate Fluids

As the regulator of all physiological functions, water is equated with life. Comprising 75% of our bodies, water is the main source of energy for every cell of the body, generating electrical and magnetic energy—literally, the power to live—through its breakdown, or hydrolysis. Water aligns microscopic solid particulates en route to our cells, just as a magnet aligns metal filings.

Water also activates all the nerve endings and sensors in the skin. Facial skin has many photosensitive and energy-sensitive nerve endings that receive and transmit signals. Water energizes the nerve endings so that they become more responsive, thus enhancing the skin's vitality. It also contributes to protecting both the skin and mucous membrane barrier functions.

Water also acts as an antioxidant by flushing oxidants and other toxins out through the kidneys. This is the basic way the brain cells get rid of the excess hydrogen ions produced by hydrolysis and maintain an alkaline environment. Dehydration contributes to toxic overload, which in turn can lead to a hyperactive immune system and allergies.

In addition, the sinuses drain better when they are well hydrated and their mucous membrane is more resistant to infection.[25] A lack of water allows toxins to overload the system, and may result in allergic reactions. The U.S. Surgeon General's Office recommends three quarts of water a day for adults of average size, with average activity, in average humidity.

For people with allergies and sensitivities, it is particularly important to keep well hydrated. Most alternative medicine physicians generally recommend eight to ten 8-ounce glasses daily, with little or no fluid intake at meals, since it may dilute the stomach's hydrochloric acid, making it difficult to absorb minerals and digest protein. Thirty minutes before or two hours after meals is commonly advised before drinking other than a few sips of water. Additional water is needed if you consume coffee, alcohol, or caffeine products, or eat heavy meats. Exercise is one of the keys to good health because it helps redistribute water, but you'll also need to drink more to compensate for your sweat.

It's advisable to drink only water that has been reliably purified through reverse osmosis, activated charcoal, de-ionization, ultraviolet light, or distillation; these filtration methods remove chlorine and fluoride from tap water. Fluoride can deactivate many enzymes that might provide protection against possible allergens. Chlorine is a skin irritant and depletes the body's friendly intestinal flora and levels of polyunsaturated fats and vitamin E, two important nutrients in the prevention of eczema. Patients suffering from eczema have often recovered once unfiltered water was eliminated from their diet and supplements of *Lactobacillus acidophilus* and *Bifidobacterium bifidum* were taken.[26]

Water can also be absorbed through the skin. Showers and baths are excellent ways of hydrating the body and variations in water temperature can provide therapeutic benefits. Showering with water at higher temperatures helps drains clogged sinuses; alternating to cold water before the end of a shower reduces inflammation and sinus irritation.

# Allergy-Proof Your House

Early exposure to indoor environmental factors, such as dust mites, molds, smoke, formaldehyde from building materials, and high levels of radon, can act directly by blocking a person's airways or indirectly by causing sensitivities to allergens. By reducing exposure to air pollutants, the likelihood of developing allergies/sensitivities or suffering chronic allergic reactions can be reduced. Environmental control can be especially helpful in preventing the development of asthma in infants.[27]

The following suggestions can reduce a person's exposure to common household allergens by up to 95%:

## Allergies May Be a Sign of Dehydration

Allergies and pain may be indicators of water shortage. The neurotransmitter histamine has a major role in regulating water retention and redistributing the amount of water in circulation or determining when it can be drawn away from other areas. As such, it can create signs such as swelling, allergies, asthma, and chronic pains in different parts of the body. It's better to heed histamine's red flags rather than block them continuously with medications such as antihistamines.

Ironically, edema or puffiness can appear when there is severe dehydration. When water is not available to get into the cells freely, it is filtered from the salty supply outside the cells and injected into overworked cells resulting in edema.

Other water intake and distribution regulators (which are also mediators in allergic reactions), such as prostaglandins, kinins, and PAF (platelet activating factor, another histamine-associated agent) can cause pain when they come across pain-sensing nerves in the body. Therefore pain—other than that caused by injury—can also be a crisis signal of water shortage in the body. Headaches are a common sign of dehydration.

In the bedroom—

■ Wash pillows, blankets, and other bedding monthly in hot water.

■ Use foam pillows and enclose mattress and box spring in plastic mite-proof covers.

■ Remove stuffed animals from bed.

■ Remove bedroom carpeting or treat carpet with tannic acid, which denatures allergens.

■ Eliminate exposure to pets or at least restrict your pets' access to the bedroom.

In the house—

■ Keep windows closed, especially during "allergy season."

■ Avoid tobacco smoke.

■ Achieve ideal relative humidity: use air conditioning and dehumidification to help reduce mold production if your home is too damp; if your home is too dry, use a humidifier.

■ Use air filters (electrostatic precipitators and high-efficiency particulate air—HEPA) and purifiers (ionizers and ozone) to remove particulate matter and odors from the air.

■ Use mite-specific exterminating chemicals, such as tannic acid, but be wary of commercial products. The Environmental Protection Agency recently pulled a dust mite product from the market. Although it was "allergist approved," it caused terrible reactions in people with allergies. Your best bet is to make your own tannic acid spray.

## Humidify the Sleeping Space

Sleeping in a room with dry air dehydrates the sinuses and can cause irritation of the mucous membranes. Dry air can trigger asthma and nasal congestion and contribute to sinusitis and allergies, according to Marchall Plaut, M.D., Section Chief of Allergic Mechanisms at the National Institute of Allergy and Infectious Diseases.

Adding moisture to the air is very helpful, and studies have found that warm, moist air improved nasal congestion and allergies in patients with allergic rhinitis.[28] Indoor air should be between 35% and 45% relative humidity for maximum health benefits; however, indoor air is much drier due to heating and cooling systems. Room humidifiers can add moisture to a room; running water fountains can also increase humidity. (As long as the water is kept flowing, you don't have to worry about molds growing in your humidifying device.)

For more information about **avoiding environmental allergens**, see Chapter 5: Environmental Control, pp. 128-157.

# Adopt a Healthy Diet

A healthy, whole-foods diet will help keep your barrier functions in optimal condition, preventing sensitization and the development of allergies. Of course, there is no ideal diet for everyone; your individual needs should be assessed by a qualified alternative medicine practitioner. However, for most people, a whole foods diet is low in unhealthy fats, animal protein, and processed foods, and high in complex carbohydrates, especially whole grains rich in fiber, essential fatty acids, and at least five servings daily of fruits and vegetables.

Timothy Birdsall, N.D., at Cancer Centers for America, suggests a maximum of 25% of the daily food intake be in the form of fat; in particular, foods containing omega-3 and beneficial omega-6 (linoleic acid and/or gamma-linolenic acid) essential fatty acids. In general, this amounts to 45-50 grams per day and represents about 450 calories. A whole foods diet is generously filled with a wide variety of different colored vegetables, fruits, and grains; raw seeds and nuts and their butters; beans; fermented milk products such as yogurt and kefir; and fish, poultry, and bean products such as tofu. It should also be lower in animal meats, fats, and cheeses. Eating well-balanced meals at regular times during the day (four to five hours apart) will stabilize your blood sugar, which is particularly important for your support organs.

### Making the Transition to Whole Foods

Eating better means living better. The types of dietary changes that you make should not be threatening, limiting, or difficult to live with.

Most Americans were raised eating meat and the transition to a more vegetable-oriented, whole foods diet may seem daunting. However, this change may be easier and more pleasurable than imagined and, considering the enormous health benefits, is worth it. Here are some tips:

■ Eat more high-fiber plant foods such as grains, legumes, nuts, and seeds.

■ When dining out, try more exotic vegetarian dishes. Most ethnic restaurants—Indian, Chinese, Thai, Japanese, Mexican, Latin American, African, Middle Eastern—offer wonderful dishes with vegetables and grains. You can also prepare many of these at home. Experiment with spices and seasonings and invest in vegetarian or ethnic cookbooks for the secrets to the exotic flavors found in vegetarian cooking.

■ Choose range-fed, hormone-free, additive-free meats.

■ Cook protein foods by one of the following methods: bake, broil, poach, stir-fry, saute, or steam. Avoid frying as much as possible, as it requires using bad fats and may add to the toxic load in the body. Do not overcook meats, which diminishes their nutritional value.

## Don't Forget to Chew Your Food

Proper digestion begins in the mouth, not the stomach, with the activation of salivary enzymes. But most people don't take enough time to thoroughly chew their food, allowing enzymes to break down tough food molecules, such as protein, before sending it to the stomach. If the stomach and pancreas do not have enough enzymes to do the mouth's work, metabolic enzymes (that are used for other functions in the body such as immunity) are called upon to fill the digestive need, putting the body at greater risk for illness. And if you have a leaky gut, errant undigested food molecules can escape and set you up for food allergies. One of the most basic things you can do to prevent this cascade of allergy-inducing problems is to chew your food, up to 50 or more times, until the food is liquid. This process may conflict with our fast-paced lifestyle, but it is one sure way to boost your digestive—and immune—functions.

■ Don't be rigid about your diet. Move toward a whole foods diet gradually.

■ Achieve rhythm in your diet. Eating regularly provides your body with a consistent intake of nutrients and avoids the stress associated with skipping meals and overeating.

■ Use a lot of herbs and spices. These add flavor, which tends to diminish when you remove the fat.

### At the Market
Choosing the ingredients for an ideal diet in today's marketplace requires a healthy dose of skepticism, diligence, and a certain amount

# Guidelines for Healthy Eating

| Avoid These Foods | Use These Foods Instead |
|---|---|
| Refined sugars: white sugar (sucrose), fructose, corn syrup, sorbitol, mannitol. Synthetic sugars: NutraSweet™ and saccharin. | Natural sweeteners: fruit juice, raw honey, organic maple syrup, molasses, barley malt, sucanat (organic sugar cane), *Stevia raubundia*. Avoid if diabetic or sugar intolerant. |
| Refined flours: white, unbleached, bleached, enriched flour and products containing these flours. | Organic whole grains: best are heirloom (genetically unaltered) grains such as kamut, quinoa, amaranth, and spelt. Grain-intolerant people may do well on heirlooms. Spelt has the texture most like wheat, but often it and other grains will cross-react with wheat. |
| Synthetic fats: margarine, hydrogenated or partially hydrogenated oils, vegetable shortening, Mocha Mix™, Olestra™. | Unsaturated oils (olive, flaxseed, safflower); butter, preferably raw and organic. |
| High levels of saturated fats (from meats, butter, palm and coconut oils). | Use unsaturated oils such as cold-pressed grapeseed, olive, corn, canola, and safflower oils. Oils must be fresh and cold-pressed; rancid oils can be harmful. Refrigerate all oils, nuts, and grains. |
| Homogenized, pasteurized, nonfat, or *acidophilus* milk, and processed cheese. | Raw, whole milk (contains vitamin A), cultured milk products (kefir, yogurt, buttermilk), and goat's milk; unprocessed cheese. Use in moderation if you are lactose intolerant. |
| Nuts and seeds: commercial, oiled, sugared, and salted. Beware of aflatoxin, a toxin secreted by a fungus found on peanuts. | Organic nuts and seeds. Must be soaked (6 hrs), blanched, or roasted to destroy enzyme inhibitors. |
| All commercial red meat and poultry. | Lamb or organic beef, organic free-range poultry. Fish is fine if it is not from polluted waters, especially deep cold-water fish like salmon and halibut. |

| **Avoid These Foods** | **Use These Foods Instead** |
|---|---|
| Commercial eggs or egg substitutes. | Organic eggs (no chemicals, drugs, or hormones) from free-range chickens or ducks. |
| Canned, pre-cooked, microwaved, or processed fast foods, and junk foods. | Buy fresh, organic foods first, fresh nonorganic second, frozen third, and canned if that is the only food available. |
| Drinks: commercial, sugared fruit juices, juice drinks, and soft drinks (both diet and regular). | Raw juices: juice your own or buy 100% juice, preferably raw and organic. Natural spritzers containing only fruit and carbonated water. |
| Canned coffee and commercial decaffeinated coffee. | Grind your own beans, preferably organic. Use only Swiss water-processed decaffeinated beans. Don't exceed three cups daily. Try organic black, green, or herbal teas. |

of fortitude to resist slipping into old convenience patterns. But the improvements you make in your food choices will pay off in better health. Here are some shopping guidelines:

■ Read labels—The package label is the last place one is apt to find the truth about a product. Bold statements such as "100% Natural" or "98% Fat-Free" might be legal, but could be deceiving. Go directly to the ingredient list and nutritional analysis. In particular, look for clues indicating the use of trans fats (shortening, partially hydrogenated, and hydrogenated oils).

■ Think complex carbohydrates—The "main dish" approach centering on protein and a high-fat sauce is out. Replace those large portions of meat loaf and baby back pork ribs with whole grains, beans, and fresh vegetables, balanced with moderate amounts of lean animal proteins.

■ Buy organic foods—Organic farming doesn't use artificial fertilizers, pesticides, herbicides, growth regulators, and livestock feed additives. Crop rotations, animal and "green" manures, organic wastes, mineral-bearing rock, and biological pest controls are used by organic farmers to raise whole, natural foods.

■ Buy seasonal foods—By definition, foods grown out of season must be treated or manipulated to grow using artificial means. Often, the foods are imported from countries where pesticides banned in the United States continue to be used. Seasonal foods are healthier, more abundant, and less expensive.

■ Eat colorfully—Instead of being concerned with getting all the right vitamins and minerals in perfect ratios, focus on eating a colorful diet. "Variations in color are due to various minerals, vitamins, and other nutrients in the body that perform important health-promoting functions in the body," explains nutritionist Lindsey Berkson, M.A., D.C., of Santa Fe, New Mexico. By making an effort to get at least three different colored vegetables or fruits at both lunch and dinner, you will ensure the best exposure to appropriate nutrients.

## Avoid Lectins

Lectins are proteins that occur in many foods, germs, and our own immune system. They act like glue and are used to bind one surface to another surface—a basic and benign chemical function. Certain lectins, however, are incompatible with a person's blood type and can cause cells to bind together where they irritate the tissues and can destroy cell membranes. In the lining of the gastrointestinal tract, for example, lectins can cause inflammation of the mucosal lining and mimic food allergies. Lectins can also cause the intestinal villi (the fingerlike projections that afford the intestines its absorptive surface area) to atrophy, as well as other degenerative changes.

To determine which **lectin-containing foods should be avoided based on your blood type,** see Chapter 6: Therapeutic Diets, pp. 158-183.

Most dietary lectins come from the indigestible fractions of plant products, often deriving from beans, grains, soy, and wheat. In particular, soybean and wheat lectins can produce an increase in permeability in the cells they bind to, often leading to cell death. It is almost impossible to eliminate lectins from your diet, but it is important to avoid the lectins that will negatively react to your blood type. Wheat and grain products, which are high in gluten, can cause substantial inflammation, especially in people who have type O blood.

# Protect Skin

Specific nutrients and precautions can help protect the skin and ensure that this organ functions properly as one of the main barriers to toxins and allergens. The integrity of the skin can be maintained by eating foods rich in essential fatty acids (EFAs—SEE QUICK DEFINITION) and avoiding foods that contain trans-fatty acids (TFAs), which deplete EFAs. If you're like most Americans who buy commercially processed foods, eliminating TFAs from your diet won't be easy—but the health rewards are worth it. Many commercial breakfast cereals, baked snacks and breads, corn chips, salad dressings, margarine spreads, French fries, and other convenience foods contain high amounts of TFAs. Food manufacturers aren't required to identify trans-fat content on their labels, although the FDA is currently considering a proposal that would do just that. Read labels carefully for trans-fat terms: "shortening," "partially hydrogenated oils," and "hydrogenated oils."

Also, avoid long-term or excessive use of aspirin and other nonsteroidal, anti-inflammatory drugs (NSAIDs), as they have been shown to deplete gamma-linolenic acid (GLA) and inhibit the production of anti-inflammatory prostaglandins.

Additionally, do not use any oils (except olive oil) for cooking, as the heated oils form toxic byproducts. High cooking temperatures can destroy the EFA content in fish as well, so baking or grilling fish is a preferable cooking method to frying. Purchase oils that are "expeller-pressed," not just "cold-pressed." Check the expiration date and adhere to it; keep oils refrigerated, especially flaxseed oil.

Also, protect the skin from sun damage by staying indoors during the hottest part of the day (between 11 a.m. and 3 p.m.), wearing protective clothing that covers the arms and legs, and using a broad-spectrum sunscreen product that blocks both ultraviolet A and B rays at SPF 40 or higher. When choosing a sunscreen, rub a sample on a small patch of skin to ensure that its ingredients aren't irritating. Lotions and creams are recommended for sensitive skin.

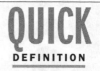

## DEFINITION

**Essential fatty acids (EFAs)** are unsaturated fats required in the diet. Omega-3 and omega-6 oils are the two principal types. The primary omega-3 oil is alpha-linolenic acid (ALA), found in flaxseed and canola oils, as well as pumpkins, walnuts, and soybeans. Fish oils, such as salmon, cod, and mackerel, contain the other important omega-3 oils, DHA (docosahexaenoic acid) and EPA (eicosapentaenoic acid). Linoleic acid is the main omega-6 oil and is found in most vegetable oils, including safflower, corn, peanut, and sesame. The most therapeutic form of omega-6 oil is gamma-linolenic acid (GLA), found in evening primrose, black currant, and borage oils. Once in the body, omega-3 and omega-6 are converted to prostaglandins, hormone-like substances that regulate many metabolic functions, particularly inflammatory processes.

For more on how to **improve your skin barrier function**, see Chapter 9: Supporting the Skin, pp. 236-259. For more on **essential fatty acids**, see Chapter 11: Supplements for Symptom Control, pp. 278-303.

# 5 Environmental Control

**T**OXINS—AND POTENTIAL ALLERGENS—are everywhere in our environment: pesticides in our food, mercury in our mouth, industrial waste in our water, carbon monoxide and other chemicals in our air. In the past 50 years, production of synthetic organic (carbon-containing) chemicals has risen from one billion pounds to more than 400 billion pounds each year,[1] with only a fraction of the 70,000 chemical compounds in production tested by the U.S. Environmental Protection Agency for acute toxic or chronic effects.[2] Approximately 107 million Americans live in areas that exceed smog standards; most drinking water contains more than 700 chemicals, including excessive levels of lead, and one in four municipal water facilities violates the federal standards for tap water. In addition, some 3,000 chemicals are added to the food supply, and as many as 10,000 chemicals are used in processing and storage.[3] It seems that nothing is safe from potentially harmful contamination—not our food, water, air, homes, schools, or workplaces.

According to Walter J. Crinnion, N.D., a naturopathic doctor and researcher on environmental medicine in Kirkland, Washington, runaway chemical technology is directly related to the rising surge of allergies around the world. Studies confirm that an overload of food and environmental toxins overwhelms the immune, endocrine, and adrenal systems and contributes to barrier function defaults. Allergies and sensitivities are but two of the many adverse health consequences of toxicity. The link between widespread chemical use and allergic conditions is evident around the world. For instance, before 1960 asthma was virtually non-existent in sub-Saharan African countries; today, having turned to chemical agents in agriculture and industry, these countries now have asthma rates equal to those in many industrialized countries.[4]

The evidence linking environmental toxicity to allergy is damning, but what may be even more unnerving is the thought that we cannot avoid allergy-promoting pollutants. However, there are many simple and affordable ways to reduce our exposure to harmful substances, thereby preventing allergies and sensitivities from developing or helping to alleviate those that already exist. Some of these environmental controls may be time-consuming and tedious, but the benefits outweigh the inconveniences. This chapter presents numerous strategies to detoxify your environment, as a means of both allergy prevention and allergy treatment.

# Sources of Environmental Toxicity

It's almost impossible to enumerate all of the toxins and irritants in our environment. In Chapter 2, we briefly discussed the major agents that contribute to toxic overload and allergy, including pesticides, heavy metals, and petrochemicals. Common household substances such as personal-care products, molds, and animal dander have also been shown to act as allergy/sensitivity irritants.

Air pollutants such as diesel and gasoline fumes and tobacco smoke inflame the mucous membranes in the respiratory tract, impairing mucus secretion and ciliary activity, and causing barrier default and sensitization.[5] Other contaminants in the air, including cockroach and dust mite casings, animal dander, and pollens also exert irritant effects on the airways, contributing to the onset of reactive airway disease and asthma. Air pollution also exacerbates existing cases of reactive airway disease and asthma, and increases in pollution correspond to jumps in asthma attacks and related emergency room visits.[6]

However, not all toxins are in our air. Cleaning agents, personal-care products, even foods contain high levels of potentially harmful chemicals that have been shown to impair barrier functions and immune strength, leading to allergy, chemical sensitivity, and a vast array of other health problems.

## Vehicle Emissions

Gasoline exhaust contains many virulent toxins—carbon monoxide, sulfur dioxide, tar, small amounts of lead and lead bromide, ammonia,

# Common Environmental Hazards

**Formaldehyde:** A highly toxic known carcinogen (causes cancer) derived from methanol, a natural gas, or other petroleum products. Gaseous emissions ("outgassing") of this chemical irritate the mucous membranes of the eyes, nose, and throat, as well as skin. It may cause nausea, headaches, nosebleeds, dizziness, memory loss, and shortness of breath. Formaldehyde is found in pressed wood products (particleboard, plywood), textile products (permanent-press clothing, bedding, drapery), glue, and paint preservatives. Outgas levels are highest in new products. Low-level exposure to formaldehyde is linked to increased rates of asthma and upper respiratory allergies, especially in children.[7]

**Lead:** Lead is a naturally occurring metal that has been used in various household products, including paint, dinnerware, pottery, and toys. While lead is no longer recommended for use in these items, traces of it can still be found in homes, as well as in contaminated air, drinking water, and food. Pottery from Mexico and other foreign countries is highly suspect for lead contamination. Lead can damage the kidneys, liver, and nervous, reproductive, cardiovascular, immune, and gastrointestinal systems, and cause fetal defects. Children absorb four times more lead than adults.

**Organocholorine Compounds (OCC):** Types of chemicals found in many pesticides and herbicides, including DDT, and dry-cleaning solvents. These chemicals have been found to impair cell-mediated immunity, alter the spleen, thymus, and lymph glands, cause fetal immune defects, and damage the endocrine system. They are also associated with significantly increased risks of cancer, leukemia, and soft-tissue sarcomas.

**Organophosphates:** These chemicals, found in pesticides, are toxic to the immune system. They cause decreased cell-mediated immunity, resulting in increased incidences of allergy and autoimmune disorders.

**Phenol:** Phenol occurs naturally, in the toxic oil in poison ivy, sumac, and oak, and is also synthetically derived. It is used in the manufacture of plastics and is found in computers, televisions, plastic goods, and waterbeds; cleaning products and newsprint emit phenol gases. Phenol from coal tar is also used to make aspirin and sulfa drugs and preserve injectable medicines, including some allergy shots. Phenol is quickly absorbed through the skin and in high amounts causes various skin disorders, hives, burning, nausea, vomiting, headache, cold sweats, irritability, and respiratory distress.

and various organic acids. Not only do these agents irritate the mucous membranes in our respiratory system, but many of them can also cause damage to the nervous system.[8]

Carbon monoxide contributes to the creation of ozone, a greenhouse gas. In a 20-year study in Reno, Nevada, researchers found that emergency room visits for asthma jumped 33.7% for each 100 ppb (parts per billion) increase in ambient ozone levels.[9] (Note that 100 ppb is equivalent to 100 blades of grass on a football field.) While federal and state governments are working to reduce ozone pollution, even concentrations below federal standards have been shown to spark asthma attacks. Diesel exhaust contains nitrogen dioxide, sulfuric acid, formaldehyde, phenol, and other chemical by-products that also cause respiratory inflammation.

In one recent study, high outdoor levels of nitrogen oxides emitted from vehicles corresponded to an increased incidence of allergic rhinitis in 317 children.[10] Of note is that these children were not sensitized to the particles in air pollution, but to other substances they encountered often, such as pollen, animal dander, dust mites, milk, and eggs. Similar studies report the same results, suggesting that constant exposure to traffic emissions causes barrier function defaults, setting the stage for allergy.[11]

## Commercial Waste

Many types of businesses and industries release potentially harmful and irritating compounds into the air, land, and water. Among the more toxic enterprises are oil refineries, which emit chlorine gas and harmful petrochemicals; dry-cleaning businesses, which use formaldehyde- and glycerine-based cleaning solutions; beauty salons, which use products containing formaldehyde, phenols, and various petrochemicals; and building material manufacturers, which rely heavily on formaldehyde (especially in plywood and particleboard) and assorted petrochemicals in solvents. All of these chemicals may leak from products that contain them. Formaldehyde is particularly toxic; as little as 0.1 ppm (part per million) in the ambient air can irritate the mucous membrane barrier functions, leading to or exacerbating asthma and other respiratory problems.[12] Gas stations are also notorious for releasing petrochemicals and volatile organic compounds (VOCs) from the gasoline and diesel fuels.

## Pesticides

Pesticides are routinely sprayed on lawns at golf courses, government buildings, and many school grounds. They also follow us into our homes and can be found in such diverse products as cotton sheets, disposable diapers, rubber bands, flea collars, no-pest strips, lanolin skin creams, swimming pool chemicals, floor and carpet dust (often tracked in from pesticide-laced lawns), latex paint, deodorant soaps, and pressure-treated wood. They are also found in our food ("conventionally," not organically, grown) and water (due to agricultural run-off). According to Dr.

**Walter J. Crinnion, N.D.:** Healing Naturally, 11811 Northeast 128th Street, Suite 202, Kirkland, WA 98034.

Crinnion, strawberries, bell peppers, spinach, cherries, Mexican cantaloupe, celery, apples, apricots, green beans, Chilean grapes, and cucumbers are the most pesticide-laden fruits and vegetables.[13] Pesticide exposure has been shown to cause barrier function default of the intestines and respiratory tract; impair immune, neurological, and endocrine function; and dramatically increase cancer risk.

## Tobacco Smoke

The dangers of smoking tobacco are well documented—lung, throat, and other cancers, emphysema, cardiovascular disease, miscarriage, and increased risks of premature birth and birth defects. Secondhand smoke comes with its own dangers, among them respiratory function defaults and a significant increase in reactive airway disease/asthma and ear infections. In fact, several studies show that children exposed to secondhand smoke from their parents are more at risk than other children for developing asthma.[15] Secondhand smoke contains many toxins that impair barrier and immune functions, including ammonia, carbon monoxide, formaldehyde, hydrogen cyanide (a poisonous gas that attacks respiratory enzymes), nitrogen dioxide, nicotine (which aggravates respiratory disease), phenols, cadmium (a heavy metal), and other carcinogens.

## Household Appliances and Products

Common household appliances, cleaning agents, and paints emit noxious gases and compounds. Gas and kerosene heaters and ranges emit potentially lethal, often irritating petrochemical fumes. Most cleaning supplies, such as oven cleaners, tile cleansers, laundry detergents, and aerosol disinfectants, contain phenol, petrochemicals, and glycerin, which are not only detrimental to mucous membrane integrity but also irritate the skin barrier. While lead is no longer used in paints and gasoline, we are still being exposed to the toxic metal in old paint and pottery ware, as well as through contaminated drinking water and food. In 1995, University of Missouri researchers studied 144 children, aged 9 months to 6 years, and found that 50% had blood levels of lead exceeding federal safety standards.[16] These children also had higher than normal levels of IgE antibodies, indicating that their bodies were responding to the lead exposure with an allergic reaction.

## Personal-Care Products

Every day, millions of Americans are unaware that they are using potentially harmful ingredients on and in their bodies, all in the name of personal hygiene. Mouthwash, toothpaste, soaps, shampoo, conditioner, bubble bath, shaving gels and creams, deodorants, feminine products, cosmetics, perfumes, and nail polishes all contain known environmental toxins and irritants. Among the most dangerous is sodium lauryl sulfate (also known as sodium laureth or lauryl sulfate), which can dry out the skin; in fact, this chemical is used in clinical studies to disrupt skin barrier function. It also may damage children's teeth, disrupt the endocrine system, and lead to eye problems and cataracts, among other disorders. Another detrimental chemical is bentonite or kaolin, which may act as a suffocating barrier to the skin. (This chemical is also found in many bowel detoxification formulas.) Most perfumes, aftershave lotions, deodorants, hand lotions, shampoos, hair dyes, hair sprays contain phenols. Many feminine hygiene products, including tampons and sanitary pads, outgas formaldehyde and can contain other dangerous toxins, such as bleaches.

Many cosmetics and skin-care products also contain glycerin. This chemical occurs naturally in any foods from which oil can be extracted. Synthetic derivatives are used in many foods as a preservative, since it prevents moisture loss, but it is also used in personal-care products for these properties. External use of glycerin-containing products, however, is detrimental to skin barrier function, because the chemical draws moisture from the skin's underlying tissues to keep the surface moist, ultimately damaging the barrier integrity.

## Are You Having a Toxic or Allergic Reaction?

There is a difference between a toxic reaction and an allergic reaction, although the two are not mutually exclusive. A toxin, by definition, is a substance poisonous to the body, and everyone reacts adversely to it when it enters their system. For instance, a chemical spill in the neighborhood might provoke a toxic reaction in both you and your neighbors, most likely with symptoms resembling the flu, headaches, weakness, nausea, dizziness, and muscle and joint aches. A chemical sensitivity, on the other hand, is a more individual response, says Doris Rapp, M.D., F.A.A.A., F.A.A.P., of Scottsdale, Arizona, "and is more prone to affect those who have allergies, allergic relatives, or damaged immune systems."[14] A second distinction between allergies and chemical toxicity, according to Dr. Rapp, is that a tiny amount of the chemical may be all that is required to spark an allergic response, whereas a larger or cumulative exposure is usually necessary to set off a toxic reaction.

For more about the **dangers of personal-care products**, see Chapter 9: Supporting the Skin, pp. 236-259.

### Dental Fillings

Dental amalgam fillings can release mercury, tin, copper, silver, and sometimes zinc into the body. All of these metals have varying degrees

## Are "Hypoallergenic" Products Safe?

Conscientious shoppers may feel that personal-care products labeled "hypoallergenic" won't trigger allergic reactions, and it's true that manufacturers generally avoid using common allergens and irritants in hypoallergenic products. However, they may still use potentially harmful chemicals, such as glycerin or sodium lauryl sulfate, which contribute to barrier function defaults. Hypoallergenic products are certainly less likely to trigger adverse reactions, but be sure to read labels to avoid buying items that use other damaging substances. Even the most natural and hypoallergenic substance can become an antigen/allergen if your barrier functions and normal biochemical functions can't handle it. It has little to do with quality and much to do with exposure when you are vulnerable. (The U.S. Food and Drug Administration provides tips for reading cosmetic ingredient labels at www.vm.cfsan.fda.gov/~dms/cos-bal.html.)

of toxicity and, when placed as fillings in the teeth, can corrode or disassociate into metallic ions (charged atoms). These metallic ions can then migrate from the tooth into the root of the tooth, the mouth, the bone, the connective tissues of the jaw, and finally into the nerves. From there, they can travel into the central nervous system, where the ions will reside, permanently disrupting the body's normal functioning if nothing is done to remove them.

Mercury has been recognized as a poison since the 1500s, and yet mercury amalgams have been used in dentistry since the 1820s. They are still being used today even though the EPA declared scrap dental amalgam a hazardous waste in 1988. According to the German Ministry of Health, amalgam is considered "a health risk from a medical viewpoint due to the release of mercury vapor."[17] Everyday activities such as chewing and brushing the teeth have been shown to release mercury vapors from amalgams.[18] Amalgams can also erode and corrode with time (ideally they should be replaced after seven to ten years), adding to their

toxic output. For the allergy/sensitivity sufferer, mercury amalgams add to the toxic overload, overwhelming the immune system and adjunct organs that provide barrier and support functions.

### Tap Water

According the EPA, the tap water of 30 million people in the United States contains potentially hazardous levels of lead. In addition, one out of every four public water systems has violated federal standards for tap water.[19] Americans' water supply can contain many different contaminants, including pathogenic (disease-causing) bacteria, radioactive particles, heavy metals (such as mercury and lead), industrial wastes (such as solvents), and chemical residues. Even chlorine and fluoride, intentionally added to public water supplies, are considered by many to pose risks to health. While adding chlorine-type compounds to drinking water protects the public from several kinds of potentially deadly bacteria such as typhus, chlorine has been proven to form cancer-causing compounds. Fluoride added to water to prevent tooth decay seems to have negative effects on the bones and even the teeth. Studies suggest that fluoride can cause mottling of the teeth[20] and can make bones more brittle in the elderly, leading to an increased rate of fracture.[21] All of these chemicals contribute to toxic overload and support-organ dysfunction, paving the way to sensitization.

## Fabrics and Plastics
Formaldehyde is used extensively in textile manufacturing, specifically to make wrinkle-free (permanent press) and waterproof fabrics and to set dyes. Additionally, formaldehyde is used in tanning and preserving animal hides; leather apparel contains formaldehyde residues. New clothes, drapery, and upholstery fabrics are significant sources of formaldehyde emissions; bed sheets may also outgas this toxin.

This chemical is also used to make plastic coatings, such as those found on electronics equipment and appliances, toilet seats, utensil handles, waxed paper, razor blades, and water filters, among other household items.

## Carpeting
Carpets not only harbor biological pollutants (see below) in your home, they also emit dangerous substances. Rosalind Anderson, Ph.D., of Anderson Laboratories in Dedham, Massachusetts, analyzed the effects of gas emissions on laboratory mice from more than 300 carpet samples obtained through retail stores, carpet mills, or from chemically sensitive patients' homes. All carpets had been in use from one week to 12 years and none were older than 40 years. Dr. Anderson performed more than 500 different experiments and found that carpet emissions decreased the breathing rate of mice immediately on contact, from a norm of 280 times per minute to a low of 235 after eight minutes of exposure. When the mice were removed from exposure to the carpet emissions, their respiration rates became normal again.

Dr. Anderson next learned that exposure to the carpet samples produced a range of alarming symptoms, including swollen faces, hemorrhaging beneath the skin surface, altered posture, loss of balance, hyperactivity, tremors, limb paralysis, convulsions, even death. Then, she analyzed 125 carpet samples for signs of neurotoxicity, that is, emissions that harm brain cells or the nervous system. Dr. Anderson found that 90% produced at least one toxic effect and 60% produced three or more "severe neurotoxic effects" in at least 25% of the mice.

More than 200 different chemicals have been identified in the typical modern carpet, according to Dr. Anderson, and these can produce "diverse toxic effects" in humans, including flu-like symptoms, muscle pain, fatigue, tremors, headaches (lasting up to 16 weeks after exposure), memory loss, and concentration difficulties. When it comes to negative health effects from carpets, "this is not a psychological phenomenon," says Dr. Anderson.[22]

## Biological Pollutants

Biological pollutants come from living, or formerly living, organisms. Pollen is a notorious outdoor pollutant, triggering hay fever in millions of Americans each year. But biological pollutants are often found indoors, too. Every home, no matter how clean, contains some of these substances, even pollen, as the particles are small (between 15 and 50 microns in diameter) and light enough to be carried by the wind. With the exclusion of molds, these substances are not toxic; it is only when individuals suffering from barrier function default inhale these particles that they experience adverse reactions. However, constant exposure to pollens, animal dander, and insect parts, along with other toxins, can overwhelm the detoxification pathways and impair immune and barrier functions.

**Pollen**—Every seed-bearing plant generates pollen, powdery male reproductive cells. Approximately 100 plant species, including trees, weeds, grasses, and some flowers, produce pollen small enough to be carried by the wind for pollination, for as far as several miles. (Bees and birds are responsible for carrying heavier pollens.) These pollen grains are then inhaled, sparking allergic reactions in sensitized individuals. Up to 75% of hay fever sufferers are sensitized to ragweed pollen. Heavy morning rains and frost curtail the release of pollen, which occurs usually between 6 a.m. and 10 a.m. Pollen activity dates vary according to geographical location and plant species. In general, pollen season starts in January or February and can last until October. Tree pollen is released earlier than weed, grass, and other pollens. Many county health departments publish local pollen count information.

**Molds**—Molds are microscopic fungi that grow both indoors and outdoors. Outside, mold is mostly found in the soil and on leaves, trees, and rotting wood. Inside, molds generally grow in bathrooms, basements, attics, refrigerators, garbage containers, carpets, and upholstery—we often refer to these molds as "mildew." Molds thrive in moist conditions at room temperature, though some types can survive in subfreezing or hot environments. Molds go into a spore form when it is too dry in order to survive. Mold spores (reproductive cells) found in the tomb of King Tut were found to grow living molds when hydrated, even after thousands of years. The EPA reports that 30% to 50% of all structures (public buildings and homes) have damp conditions that may encourage the growth and buildup of mold.

People who suffer from mold allergy usually are not sensitized to the molds themselves, but rather to the inhaled airborne spores, which are released year-round outdoors and indoors, except in very cold conditions. Mushrooms, other fungi, and seaweed may also cause cross-reactions in mold-allergic individuals. These mold spores may colonize the nasal passages and lungs, causing respiratory problems; people experiencing chronic sinus problems and asthma should probably be checked for fungal growth in their respiratory tract.[23] Note that poisonous molds can grow on certain foods, including peanuts, rye, and wheat, sometimes causing toxic reactions characterized by convulsions, dizziness, rashes, swelling of the heart, hemorrhage, blood vessel and liver damage, and possibly death.

**Animals—**Up to 10 million Americans suffer allergic reactions, including eczema, rhinitis, and asthma, to animals.[24] But it's not the animals' fur that triggers allergic reactions but rather their dander (skin debris and dandruff shed by all animals) and saliva. Cat dander and saliva are the most allergenic of animal substances and can become lodged in carpeting and furniture for years after the cat is removed. Since cat dander is so lightweight, it is easily carried by the wind and deposited in homes, schools, and offices that have never had feline occupants. Other allergenic animals include dogs, horses, rabbits, and various livestock. Bird feathers can also trigger allergic reactions; down pillows and comforters may be a source of allergy for many people who suffer from respiratory problems at night or upon awakening.

**Dust Mites and Cockroaches—**Even the most spotless home can have dust mites, microscopic insects related to ticks and spiders that feed off dead human skin scales. As indicated by their name, dust mites live in specks of dust, and thrive in warm, humid environments. They cannot exist in dry or hot climates or at high altitudes. Dust mites colonize everyday items—stuffed toys, upholstery, carpets, and mattresses. Live dust mites do not trigger allergic or asthmatic reactions, because they are able to cling to surfaces and avoid inhalation. Dead dust mites and their excrement are the main sensitizing culprits.

Cockroaches, or rather dead cockroach parts and their feces, are also major indoor biological pollutants. Cockroaches are a main trigger of childhood asthma, affecting children of all social classes, and in both urban and rural areas.[25] One study found that 75% of asthmatic children living in non-public housing and 30% of asthmatic children in public housing tested positive to cockroach allergy.[26] Some studies estimate that the average inner city room has about 3,000 cockroaches and that an inner city mattress could contain up to three pounds of cockroach feces and body parts. No wonder there is an epidemic of childhood allergy and asthma in the inner cities. Cockroach allergens are often found in kitchens but can be spread throughout the house by heating and air-conditioning systems.

# Chemical Sensitivity and Chronic Fatigue Syndrome

Theron G. Randolph, M.D., a pioneer of environmental medicine (SEE QUICK DEFINITION), first described chemical susceptibility. Today, it is commonly accepted that herbicides and pesticides, among other environmental toxins, in the food supply and environment pose a hazard to human health. Even low-level exposure to chemicals can cause a wide variety of chronic diseases, including cancer, endocrine disruption, and chemical sensitivity.[27] Many patients reporting chemical sensitivity exhibit abnormalities of brain metabolism indicating neurotoxicity, or brain damage caused by toxic exposure.[28]

Chemical sensitivity has been a subject of much contention in the past two decades, with some doctors dismissing related complaints as psychological in nature. The existence of multiple chemical sensitivity (MCS) has been particularly controversial. However, the EPA and U.S. Consumer Product Safety Commission, among other organizations, have ruled that MCS, also known as environmental illness, is not a psychosomatic disease and should be diagnosed and treated as any other health disorder;[29] MCS is now covered under the Americans With Disabilities Act. The prevalence of chemical sensitivity and MCS is hard to pin down, because diagnostic tools are still in development (though researchers have created questionnaires to screen MCS).[30] However, a 1995 survey conducted in California reported that 6.3% of subjects had been diagnosed with MCS, while 15.9% reported being "allergic or unusually sensitive to everyday chemicals."[31] Women are more likely than men to suffer from chemical sensitivity.

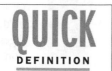

**QUICK DEFINITION**

**Environmental medicine** explores the role of dietary and environmental allergens in health and illness. Dust, molds, chemicals, certain foods, and many other substances can cause allergic reactions, which can be linked to disorders such as chronic fatigue, asthma, arthritis, headaches, depression, gastrointestinal problems, and environmental illness. Environmental medicine physicians identify and treat patients' allergies as a means to resolve their health condition. Environmental medicine also addresses "sick building syndrome," which is when the physical environment of a building—its construction materials, furnishings, paints, lighting, ventilation—directly contributes to the ill health of those living or working in it.

Chemical sensitivity, like other forms of intolerance, varies in intensity. Some patients note mild irritation or headaches with exposure to certain perfumes, disinfectants, paints, tobacco smoke, or automobile exhaust. Others experience MCS, or environmental illness, a multiple-symptom, debilitating, chronic disorder involving prolonged, heightened, and often incapacitating sensitivities to numerous common substances found in one's environment. Symptoms may include headaches, fatigue, muscle pain or weakness, coughing or wheezing, asthma, weight loss, infections, and emotional fluctuations, depression, or irritability. Some patients suffering from MCS are so sensitive to nearly all synthetic chemicals, such as car exhaust, synthetic carpets, plywood and other building materials, cleaning agents, office machines, and plastics, that to minimize their reactions, they leave their troubling environment and move to clean housing in less-polluted, rural areas.

As the symptoms of chemical sensitivity and MCS often resemble the symptoms endemic to reactive airway disease/asthma and other respiratory allergies, researchers have conducted studies to see if environmental toxins similarly impair the barrier functions of chemically sensitive patients. These studies have found that these patients experience airway constriction analogous to asthma attacks,[32] and that chemical sensitivity, like allergy, can be acquired in association with irritant exposures.[33] The main difference is that chemical sensitivity reactions do not involve antibodies as allergic reactions do. Additionally, recent research indicates that people who suffer from antibody-mediated allergies, such as asthma and hay fever, may be more susceptible to acquiring chemical sensitivities.[34]

## The Chronic Fatigue Syndrome Link

Chronic fatigue syndrome (CFS) is an umbrella term for a multiple-symptom disorder characterized most commonly by the sudden onset of extreme, debilitating fatigue, pain in the muscles and joints, headaches, and poor concentration. The fatigue is not alleviated by rest and results

To learn more about the **connection between chronic fatigue syndrome and chemical sensitivity**, see *Alternative Medicine Guide to Chronic Fatigue, Fibromyalgia, and Environmental Illness* (Future Medicine Publishing, 1998; ISBN 1-887299-11-4); to order, call 800-333-HEAL.

in a substantial reduction in previous levels of daily activity. CFS is often cyclical, with periods of relative health followed by debilitation. Other symptoms include depression, anxiety, digestive disorders, memory loss, allergies, recurring infections, and low-grade fever. According to the U.S. Centers for Disease Control, CFS predominantly affects white women between the ages of 25 and 45.

The symptoms of CFS bear a striking similarity to those of multiple chemical sensitivity. Some alternative medicine practitioners believe that MCS is an extreme extension or outcome of prolonged chronic fatigue syndrome. Shari Lieberman, Ph.D., C.N.S., a nutritional specialist based in New York City, is among them. She has treated hundreds of people with CFS and reports: "I see patients with environmental sensitivities who have come to me after three to five years of chronic fatigue. If they've only had CFS for six months, they don't tend to have environmental sensitivities."

According to recent research, chronic fatigue syndrome, like chemical sensitivity, may be induced by repeated low-level exposure to chemicals. In a 1995 study, 22 patients with diagnosed CFS were found to have significantly higher organochlorine levels than the control group of 34 non-CFS subjects. The researchers concluded that toxic chemical exposure may play a causal role in CFS.[35]

Patients with CFS will often find that the same therapies recommended for chemical sensitivity will relieve, even reverse, their symptoms. Detoxification, environmental control, enzyme supplementation, and mind/body therapies are particularly recommended for people with CFS.

## What Causes Chemical Sensitivity?

How do people become sensitive to common chemicals? Scientists mostly agree that a two-step process, called "toxicant-induced lack of tolerance," underlies chemical sensitivity, as well as other disorders such as chronic fatigue syndrome.[36] In the first step, indoor air contaminants, chemical spills, or pesticide applications cause certain susceptible people to lose their prior tolerance for common chemicals and other substances. Subsequent exposure to these chemicals trigger chemical sensitivity reactions. Chemical spills occur infrequently and primarily affect those in hazardous occupations. Pesticide application makes people who work or live near farms and forests particularly vulnerable. But as we spend up to 90% of our time inside buildings, indoor air contamination makes nearly every American susceptible to acquiring chemical sensitivities. The main culprit in indoor air contamination is a "sick building."

*Sick buildings* refer to the tightly sealed, energy-efficient buildings that became popular in the 1970s as a response to the energy crisis in the United States. While these structures may save money on gas bills, the downside is that various toxins and biological pollutants are trapped inside, repeatedly circulated throughout the building via central heating and cooling systems. Sick buildings also have high, potentially dangerous levels of volatile organic compounds (VOCs) released from particleboard desks, furniture, carpets, glues, paints, and office machine toners, including those from printers and photocopiers.[37]

Chronic low-grade exposure to these chemicals and debris leads to "sick building syndrome" (SBS), a condition characterized by mucous membrane irritation of the eyes, nose, and throat, chest, tightness, skin complaints (dryness, itching, redness), headaches, fatigue, lethargy, coughing, asthma, chronic nasal stuffiness, infections, and emotional irritability.[40] Several studies have analyzed these complaints and confirmed that sick building syndrome can lead to full-blown MCS and even asthma.[41]

Additionally, children are more likely to suffer from allergic respiratory diseases if they attend schools that ineffectively control indoor pollutants. In one study, schools that were larger, had more open shelves, lower room temperature, higher relative air humidity, higher

## What are Volatile Organic Compounds?

Volatile organic compounds (VOCs) are dangerous chemicals that often enter the body as vapors, although VOCs may also be liquid or solid in form. VOCs as vapors easily evade respiratory defense systems, passing by nose hairs, mucous membranes, and cilia until they reach the lungs. From there, VOCs enter the bloodstream. Symptoms of VOC exposure include eye and respiratory tract irritation, headaches, dizziness, visual disorders, memory impairment, and asthma attacks. VOCs also escape into the air, exacerbating ozone and smog pollution. Atopic (susceptible to allergy) people appear to be more sensitive than nonatopic individuals to the effects of VOCs.[38]

VOCs are commonly emitted from adhesives, caulking compounds, carpeting, particle board, tile, linoleum, other floor coverings, wall coverings, paints, stains, varnishes, waxes, and cleaning fluids (especially dry-cleaning fluids). The VOC benzene (found in tobacco smoke, stored fuels, and paint supplies) is known to cause cancer in humans. Other VOCs, including perchloroethylene (common dry-cleaning solvent) and methylene chloride (in paint strippers, adhesive removers, aerosol spray paints, and pesticide bombs), have been shown to cause cancer in animals. Low/no VOC products include Benjamin Moore and Best Paints, Bon Ami abrasive, and water-based glues.[39]

concentrations of formaldehyde or other volatile organic compounds, molds, bacteria, or more cat allergen in the settled dust had more asthmatic students than did other schools.[42] The workplace is also implicated in adult-onset asthma. A recent survey showed that 15.4% of all cases of asthma in the U.S. are due to work-related exposure to approximately 250 chemicals.[43]

## The Root of Sick Building Syndrome

According to Michael Hodgson, M.D., M.P.H., of the School of Medicine, University of Connecticut Health Center in Farmington, in most cases, problems with a building's engineering, construction, and ventilation system make a building "sick." Studies suggest that symptoms occur 50% more frequently in buildings with mechanical ventilation systems. Among 2,000 office workers in Germany with work-related symptoms, there was a 50% higher rate of upper respiratory tract infections that were directly traceable to problems with mechanically ventilated buildings, reports Dr. Hodgson.

For more information on the **health effects of sick building syndrome**, contact: Environmental Detoxification Consultants, 413 Grassy Hill Road, Woodbury, CT 06798; tel/fax: 203-263-2970.

Besides ventilation problems, other sources of indoor toxic pollution include volatile organic compounds. All contribute to "a complex mixture of very low levels of individual pollutants," states Dr. Hodgson. Bio-aerosols are also indoor contaminants and originate as biological agents from mold spores, allergy-producing microbes, mites, or animal dander; then they are distributed through an indoor space by ventilation, heating, or air conditioning systems.

Of buildings classified as sources of SBS, one study showed that 70% have inadequate flow of fresh outside air. It also found that 50% to 70% of such buildings have poor distribution of air within the occupied space; 60% have poor filtration of outdoor pollutants; 60% have standing water that fosters biological growths; and 20% have malfunctioning humidifiers.[44]

# Success Story: A Doctor Reverses Sick Building Syndrome

Susan Lange, O.M.D., L.Ac., a specialist in reversing the debilitating effects of MCS, and co-founder of the Meridian Center in Santa Monica, California, knows firsthand what it is like to become severely sensitive after working in a "sick building." In the early 1980s, she worked in a clinic that had kerosene gas stoves and small cubicles with no ventilation.

"This was a major source of petrochemical poisoning for me," she notes. In 1985, Dr. Lange did postgraduate acupuncture study in China in a hospital that was rife with allergy-provoking mold and fungus. "You could actually see the mold running down the walls," she recalls.

After that, Dr. Lange's occupation brought her to a clinic in Los Angeles where the air-conditioning filters had not been cleaned or replaced for years, so the system was venting dirty air and microbial contamination. On reflection, she realizes that she may have been carrying petrochemical residues in her system since birth. Her mother lived above a gas station and inhaled diesel fumes every day while she was pregnant. "She was throwing up all the time. It was a toxic womb—my cellular terrain (the biochemical condition and vitality of her cells) was damaged at an early age."

Dr. Lange's system was further compromised in her early twenties when she picked up intestinal parasites (SEE QUICK DEFINITION) in India. According to one diagnosis at that time, she had amoebic hepatitis. Years of diarrhea, cramps, and pain ensued. Her doctors gave her a battery of tests, X rays, and conventional drugs such as Flagyl and cortisone, not understanding that what she most needed was a rebalancing of her intestinal flora with "friendly bacteria," or probiotics.

While the antibiotics were unsuccessful in killing the parasites, they did kill the beneficial microbes, allowing the "unfriendly," pathogenic bacteria to thrive. Then, a friend introduced Dr. Lange to acupuncture. "That helped me survive, but it didn't clear up everything," she comments. (However, it did lead to her studying acupuncture professionally.) Unfortunately, Dr. Lange found her system was too weak to handle the Chinese herbs prescribed for her parasites.

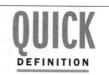

**DEFINITION**

A **parasite** is any organism that lives off another organism (called a host), and draws nourishment from it. Specifically, parasites are the protozoa (single-cell organisms), arthropods (insects), and worms that infect the body and cause serious damage to tissues and organs. Common forms of the protozoan parasites are *Giardia lamblia*, which causes giardiasis; *Entamoeba histolytica*, which causes dysentery; and *Cryptosporidium*, which causes diarrhea, particularly in people with immunologic diseases such as AIDS. The most common arthropod parasites are lice, mites, ticks, and fleas. Worm parasites include pinworms, roundworms, tapeworms, whipworms, hookworms, and filaria (threadlike worms that inhabit the blood and tissues).

## Sickened by Her House

The combination of environmental sensitivities left Dr. Lange "incredibly ill" and her condition worsened over time. She had frequent heart palpitations and her ability to concentrate on her studies began to wane. She was allergic to about 70% of all foods and many other substances—gas fumes and perfume nearly made her faint. "The term 'environmental illness' wasn't in use then," she recalls, "but when I walked into my own house, I felt like passing out."

Fortunately, Dr. Lange found that her system could handle homeopathy, so she used a series of homeopathic remedies to start detoxifying her system of all its poisons, starting with petrochemicals. According to electrodermal screening, these were the key toxins. She used *Petrochem Antitox* and *Mercury Antitox*, which are both complex homeopathic remedies; she also had the classical homeopathic remedy *Sulphur*, in doses ranging from 6C to 200C, to help drain toxins and chemicals from her organs.

At the beginning, the most she could handle of the detoxification remedies was one drop daily in water (a normal dosage for *Mercury Antitox* and *Petrochem Antitox* is ten drops, three times a day). Any more than that and "my heart and head would pound." Gradually, Dr. Lange started feeling better and was able to increase the dosages to five drops a day. She also took a complex homeopathic remedy called *Ribes Nigrum*, which helps the kidneys to detoxify and drain their toxins. For this, her dosage was two to three drops a day.

Electrodermal screening also indicated that she was seriously allergic to the mercury in her dental fillings. Complicating this was the fact that when she was 16, major dental work had misaligned her bite. As she had grown up in Hong Kong and Malaysia, she had received numerous vaccinations for cholera, smallpox, and other tropical infections. These factors weakened her body's "terrain," leaving her vulnerable to illness. "Electrodermal screening enabled me to look back through my health history to see how my immune system had been damaged," she says. It also showed her the way to restore her health.

For more on **electrodermal screening**, see Chapter 3: Allergy/Sensitivity Testing, pp. 70-105, and Chapter 13: Desensitizing the Immune System, pp. 328-347. For information on **eradicating parasites**, see Chapter 8: Intestinal Detoxification, pp. 212-235. For more on **homeopathic remedies**, see Chapter 12: Homeopathic and Physical Therapies, pp. 304-327. For more on the **psychological side to healing allergies**, see Chapter 14: Mind/Body Approaches to Allergy, pp. 348-373.

Eventually—it took three years to build up her system's vitality sufficiently to handle such a procedure—Dr. Lange had her mercury fillings removed and her dental bite corrected. To rebuild her immune system, she received two daily intravenous infusions of vitamin C (up to 10 g) combined with B complex (2 cc) and B12 (500 mg). She also took homeopathic *Mercury Antitox* to facilitate the removal of the mercury from her tissues. Within three weeks of removing the mercury fillings, her heart palpitations stopped and the chronic diarrhea began to lessen. "On a misery scale of one to ten, I had been a ten, the highest. After this, I went down to a two. That's dramatic."

Next to go were the parasites. Dr. Lange discovered she still had the amoebae from her time in India, along with *Helicobacter pylori*, bacteria she had picked up in China and which is associated with stomach ulcers and chronic gastric pain. A combination of Chinese and other herbs (including artemisia, coptis, philodendron, isatis, grapefruit seed extract, black walnut, and garlic) and an antibiotic eliminated the bacteria and, finally, the amoebae. After the parasites went, Dr. Lange steadily began to regain her health.

There was one more piece Dr. Lange had to address to fully heal and that was the psychological and emotional component of her illness. Looking back, Dr. Lange comments: "What kept me going was my commitment to getting well, but my biggest shift came when I faced and let go of the belief I was carrying that the world is dangerous and everything I put in my body is going to damage me."

## Building an Allergy-Free Clinic

Today, Dr. Lange's patients benefit from her prolonged bout with allergies and sensitivities. When she and her husband, Julian Lange, O.M.D., L.Ac., designed and launched the Meridian Center, she kept in mind that "sick patients require extra-special surroundings because they are so sensitized." A doctor's office should not make patients feel sicker from spending time there, she says. "Being environmentally ill was a large motivation for me in putting the clinic together the way we did. Now that I am well, I am acutely aware of the quality of energy in a building that is necessary for comfort and optimum health."

During her real-life tutorial in illness and healing, Dr. Lange came across Bau-Biologie, the art and science of the "biological building." Well-established in Germany, Bau-Biologie is about the impact of building environments on human health and how to use this knowledge to construct environmentally friendly interior spaces that support, not deteriorate, the health of those using them.

The Meridian Center, down to the finest detail, is a perfect demonstration of Bau-Biologie. Carpets are made of hypoallergenic nylon, free of formaldehyde, moth proofing, stain repellents, pesticides, and other toxic materials typically found in carpets. Dr. Lange also took great care to avoid using any products containing formaldehyde or other injurious chemicals. Similarly, the Meridian Center was designed to minimize indoor air pollution. "All aspects of the clinic's interior—furniture, walls, paint, ceiling tiles, treatment tables, doors, fabrics, lighting, water, electrical installation, gowns, paper and cleaning products, even the plants—were selected for having the lowest environmental toxicity and for their ability to contribute to, not detract

**Susan Lange, O.M.D., L.Ac.**: Meridian Center for Personal and Environmental Health, 1411 5th Street, Suite 405, Santa Monica, CA 90401; tel: 310-395-9525; fax: 310-395-9235. For **Bau-Biologie**, contact: Bau-Biologie and Ecology, Inc., P.O. Box 387, Clearwater, FL 33757; tel: 727-461-4371; fax: 727-441-4373; website: www.bau-biologieusa.com. For **Mercury Antitox** and **Petrochem Antitox,** contact: Apex Energetics, 1701 East Edinger Avenue, Suite A-4, Santa Ana, CA 92705; tel: 800-736-4381 or 714-973-7733; fax: 714-973-2238.

from, human health," says Dr. Lange. "Our facility and Bau-Biologie's principles demonstrate that it is possible to use materials that are environmentally safe and easily available."

Staff, patients, and visitors enjoy—relish—the clinic because "it's so free of the external disturbances experienced in ordinary living environments. The moment patients walk through the door, the healing process begins," she says. "To support the healing of the patient, we need facilities that are designed not to damage the environment, but to bring positive regeneration to it—facilities that are not sick, but which are healing places for the body, mind, spirit, even the planet."

# Eliminate Toxins in Your Environment

Numerous scientific reports advocate detoxifying the environment to prevent and treat allergies and sensitivities.[45] Many alternative medicine physicians concur with this recommendation, bearing in mind that it's nearly impossible to eliminate toxins outside, in the workplace, and in schools. The home is where most people will be able to effectively reduce their exposure to irritants and pollutants. "I try to teach my patients to create a safe haven within their own environment," says Abram Ber, M.D., of Scottsdale, Arizona. "You cannot just purchase things and bring them into the house and hope that everything will be fine. You have to live with consciousness."

Russell Olinsky is an environmental engineer who works with Dr. Ber, Dr. Rapp, and other alternative medicine physicians in the Phoenix-Scottsdale area to uncover hidden sources of allergens in the homes of patients. The following incorporates his recommendations for a cleaner home.

### Select an Environmentally Friendly Neighborhood
Be aware of the outside environment. Is your home near the following health hazards?
- Restaurants that emit smoke
- Dry cleaning or industrial facilities that give off chemicals
- A freeway where high amounts of soot from fuel exhaust can be inhaled
- Right-of-way areas near water where defoliant is sprayed to keep weeds down
- Schools, golf courses, and parks, which are often sprayed with pesticides
- Open fields where dirt can easily become airborne

Also, try to buy or rent housing that was built with the fewest environmentally toxic substances. Mobile homes, for example, outgas high levels of formaldehyde.

## Create an Oasis in Your Bedroom

■ Do not smoke in your bedroom or in any other room in your house.

■ Animal dander easily becomes an airborne allergy so, if you have a pet, set aside your bedroom as a pet-free zone. You will also want to bathe your pet regularly. Keep litter boxes out of the bedroom and as close to the outside of the house as possible.

■ Avoid plastic window blinds that may contain lead.

■ Use a good high efficiency air purifier, with at least four changes an hour and a flow pattern that directs the air up and away from the unit. The filter should contain activated carbon to reduce or remove chemicals, solvents, odors, exhaust fumes, pesticides and other allergens larger than one microgram from the room. High-efficiency particulate air (HEPA) purifiers are recommended, as are ionizers and ozonators.

For **air filtration devices**, contact: Fresh Air Company, 1181 North Hollywood Drive, Reedley, CA 93654; tel: 800-860-4244; fax: 619-723-0603. Environmental Detoxification Consultants, 413 Grassy Hill Road, Woodbury, CT 06798-3129; tel/fax: 203-263-2970. U.S. Complementary Health, Inc., 3441 E. Tierra Buena Lake, Phoenix, AZ 85032; tel: 602-493-1637.

■ Keep closet doors closed to separate your clothes from dust in the room.

■ Rid the bedroom of dust collectors. If you keep stuffed toys, dust can be reduced by putting them in the dryer on fluff cycle with a tennis ball to help puff them out.

■ Remove carpeting, or treat it with tannic acid, which denatures allergens; or replace with washable area rugs.

■ Synthetic pillows and comforters are better for people with allergies than are down or feathers, which are highly allergenic. (Products labeled "hypoallergenic" simply mean that most people will not have a reaction to the product; it does not mean you won't.)

■ Machine-wash pillows, blankets, and comforters monthly. The water should be at least 130° F to kill dust mites, a potent allergen.

■ Dust mites hang out in box springs as well as mattresses. Encase both with special protective vinyl coverings.

## Make Your Carpeting Less Allergenic

The first and best choice for people with allergies is to remove all carpeting. Washable throw rugs are a better option.

■ If you want carpeting, the best choice is a short-fiber carpet laid down with water-based adhesives as opposed to solvents. The short fibers release allergens to vacuuming more readily than the more complex fibers.

# Houseplants: Nature's Afir Filters

Common houseplants can be used as filters to remove pollution from indoor air, an idea that first came out of NASA space research in the 1970s.[46] Scientists discovered that not only could plants recycle oxygen, but they seemed to be able to remove air pollutants, too. According to Dr. Crinnion, the following plants are highly effective for removing benzene, formaldehyde, and trichlorethylene (a petrochemical) from indoor air.[47]

- Gerber Daisy (*Gerbera jamesonii*)
- Pot/Florist Mum (*Chrysanthemum morifolium*)
- English Ivy (*Hedera helix*)
- Mother-in-Law's Tongue (*Sansevieria trifasciata*)
- *Dracaena deremensis*
- *Dracaena marginata*
- Peace Lily (*Spathiphyllum araceae*)
- Chinese Evergreen (*Aglaonema modestum*)
- Bamboo Plant (*Chamaedorea seifrizii*)

For **nontoxic carpets** (100% wool, free of chemical or synthetic materials, almost completely biodegradable), contact: Nature's Carpet Environmental Home Center, 1724 Fourth Avenue South, Seattle, WA 98134; tel: 800-281-9785 or 206-682-7332; fax: 206-682-8275.

- Solid foam carpet pads are a better choice than the multicolor pads of recycled material, which are pieced together with glue; they are also less expensive.

- Watch out for wool carpets; some people are allergic to the lanolin they contain.

- Before installing a carpet, have the floor cleaned thoroughly and seal any cracks in the foundation and exterior walls. This prevents insects, pollution, dirt, and mold from accumulating on the carpet.

- Lift your carpet and inspect underneath for mold growth from water leaks. Signs that you might have mold are stains and rusty nails on the tack strips. Mold on floors can be removed with a 10% bleach solution and water. If you are the one with allergies, it is preferable to have someone else do it.

- Never carpet the bathroom. Mold flourishes with moisture. Also, dust mites prefer warm temperatures and 50% or greater humidity. When you take a bath or shower you are inviting them to enjoy ideal conditions as well as providing them with food in the form of skin cells that drop to the floor when you towel yourself off. Carpeting becomes a breeding ground.

- Have your carpet cleaned with a professional truck-mounted, high-suction, external vacuum so that the dirt is removed from the house. A safe detergent would be an unscented emulsifier. You can use natural enzymes for stains. A professional will hand-spray the carpet, then use pure hot water and extract the debris. Do not use too much water or you can saturate the carpet and pad, attracting mold.

- Remove your shoes outside so that you don't trap toxins and allergens from outside in your carpet. This is particularly important if you have a baby crawling on the carpet.

■ Vacuum at least once a week. A central vacuum with good air-flow and rotating brush and head is recommended so that the dander and dust are beat out of the carpet and forced outside. Another good choice is a heavier vacuum with rotating brushes and high-efficiency filter bags. True HEPA filter vacuums are good. The seals should be checked on all filters to make sure they are tightly fitted.

## Clean Your Heating and Cooling Systems

A major problem for people with allergies is dirty air ducts, which can harbor all sorts of allergens and debris. Additionally, air leaks allow in pollen, chemical exhaust from outside, and insects (which are very allergenic to some).

■ If your heating system is natural gas, propane, or other fuels, it is critical to make sure that there are no leaks and you have good ventilation. All heating systems should be cleaned annually.

■ Use high efficiency, pleated (or corrugated) filters for air systems.

## Purify Your Water Supply

■ In older homes, check to make sure you do not have lead solder on your water pipes, which can contaminate your water.

For information on **home water purifiers**, contact: Environmental Detoxification Consultants (solid block carbon filters), 413 Grassy Hill Road, Woodbury, CT 06798-3129; tel/fax: 203-263-2970. NSF International (certifies home water purifiers), P.O. Box 130140, Ann Arbor, MI 48113-0140; tel: 800-NSF-MARK or 734-769-8010; fax: 734-769-0109; web-site: www.nsf.com. U.S. Complementary Health, Inc., 3441 E. Tierra Buena Lake, Phoenix, AZ 85032; tel: 602-493-1637.

■ Make sure that your hot water is at least 130° F, so that it is hot enough to kill bacteria such as *Legionella*.

■ Purify your water with activated carbon filters, reverse osmosis systems, or ultraviolet (UV) light systems, all of which remove parasites, organic chemicals such as chlorine and chlorine by-products, pesticides, and heavy metals.

■ Old water filters can breed bacteria or leach out some of the chemicals they were supposed to be removing. They should be serviced every six months to a year. Contact the manufacturer to find out the appropriate disinfectant.

■ A refrigerator with an icemaker and water dispenser is difficult to clean and it is advisable to have a professional do it. The nozzles on refrigerator water dispensers can be disinfected with vinegar water. Inspect the flap where the ice cubes come out because it can be a source of mold growth.

## Clean Without Toxic Chemicals

The key to cleaning surfaces is to get rid of the dirt. Once the surface is washed clean, it will no longer support the growth of microorganisms.

■ Remove chemical contaminants and toxic household cleansers from your home, or at least limit your exposure to them.

■ Substitute natural cleaning products, such as distilled white vinegar, baking soda, borax, lemon juice, citrus cleaners (non-petroleum-based), Castille soaps, and safe commercial products, for the toxic ones. These products are available in many health food stores or through mail-order services provided by environmentally concerned companies.

■ Vinegar and water with a couple of drops of dish soap will get a window clean and the bacteria will be gone.

■ Baking soda is a good abrasive. In bathrooms, you can sprinkle a little baking soda on the surface and wipe it with a damp sponge. You can also use it as a scouring powder as opposed to a chlorine-based products. Vinegar will remove soap scum in tubs and sinks.

For **environmentally friendly cleaning products**, contact: Seventh Generation, One Mill Street, Box A-26, Burlington, VT 05401-1530; tel: 800-456-1191 or 802-658-3773; fax: 802-658-1771; website: www.seventhgen.com.

■ Dust with a damp cloth. A couple of drops of unscented dishwashing detergent will act as an emulsifying agent.

■ Switch from aerosol products to hand pumps. Whenever you use an aerosol you can wind up breathing in the chemicals in the product.

■ Avoid scented products.

## Practice Integrated Pest Management Techniques (IPM)

■ Avoid using pesticides inside and outside the home.

■ Seal cracks where insects can come in; make sure you don't see daylight at the bottom of doors or windows; check cracks in duct work and the exterior of the house.

■ Look for outside breeding grounds such as stagnant water, debris piles, and plants adjacent to the house.

■ Use safer products outside such as diatomaceous earth, microscopic plankton that suffocates insects when they walk on it (available in health food stores). Natural pyrethrin, a chrysanthemum derivative, can be used outside the house.

■ Clean up food sources that attract pests, such as sugar and cookie crumbs.

■ If ants are coming in during heavy rains, check your drainage.

■ Pea-sized balls of borax mixed with chopped onion, sugar and flour can be placed in out-of-the-way places (away from pets) to kill cockroaches.

## Prevent Water Damage and Stop Mold Growth

Molds are not only allergenic but they produce toxins. They thrive in damp areas, especially inside walls and behind baseboards. Sources of water leaks are flat roofs, poor drainage, water heater leaks, water from washing machines, dishwashers, refrigerators, sinks, air-conditioners, drain pans and drain lines, showers, and bathtubs.

■ Any water leak should quickly be cleaned up to prevent mold growth. If allowed to remain wet for five days, mold growth is encouraged.

■ Check under the bathroom sink for water damage and note whether or not the cabinets are warped.

■ Make sure showers and bathtubs do not have water leaking out of the sides into the walls and floors. The areas are usually stained so you can see them. Check around the fixtures for water leaks and at bottom of shower. Caulk areas around fixtures.

■ Make sure bathrooms have a good fan that will provide enough ventilation to get rid of moisture after taking a shower or bath. Once you get mold around showers and tubs, it's very hard to eliminate since these areas tend to stay wet.

■ If you do get mold growth around tubs, clean with full strength vinegar and water. A bit of detergent will wet it better. For caulking problems, white silicon bathroom caulk works to help prevent mold re-growth.

## Make a Gas Stove Safer

Natural gas and propane will produce by-products such as formaldehyde, nitrogen oxide, and carbon monoxide, so they need to be properly vented.

■ When using a gas stove, you should have an exhaust fan going to stave off the fumes. The exhaust system should actually be vented to the outside and not be recirculated through the hood and back in the home.

## Check Your Building Materials

■ New paneling and cabinets generally produce formaldehyde outgassing. Formaldehyde is a binder used in interior grade plywood (which is worse than exterior grade from the standpoint of emissions). Particleboard, pressed board, and anything labeled "wood products" tend to have formaldehyde. Buy products that don't contain formaldehyde.

■ Use water-based, low-odor paints if possible. If you already have a coat of oil-based paint, you can't use water-based over it. Therefore, make sure there is adequate ventilation and wait for the paint to dry before a person with allergies enters the room. Some of the newer, oil-based paints with low VOCs will actually give off chemicals for a longer time.

## Tips for Special Situations

**During Pollen Season:**
- Keep house windows closed.
- Use a clothes dryer rather than hanging clothes out to dry.

**In the Car:**
- Don't smoke or allow others to smoke in your car.
- Use a specially designed air filtration system. Car air conditioners and vents can send mold spores and pollens throughout the vehicle.

**While Shopping:**
- Avoid walking through perfume sections, or walk very quickly through them while holding your breath.

- In houses built prior to 1978, which might have lead-based paint, don't sand the paint off and create airborne lead, which you can inhale. Generally, the lead is encapsulated by painting over it with a new paint. Try not to get any chipping or peeling.

### Use Your Fireplace Safely

People with asthma or respiratory problems are discouraged from using fireplaces or wood-burning stoves, as the vapors released can often trigger allergic reactions.

- Don't use scrap woods, newspaper, plastics, or any scrap materials because of toxic by-products, particularly painted lumber. Hard wood is preferred.
- Keep the flue closed when not in use.
- Make sure you have good exhaust and ventilation.

### Keep Your Refrigerator Clean

- Condensate pans should be drained and cleaned more often in humid weather.
- Clean coils at least twice a year. If you have pets, more often.
- Damp-wipe the top of the refrigerator regularly.
- Check door gaskets and make sure they are sealed well so you don't get moisture buildup and mold growth.
- The bottom refrigerator drawers should be kept clean.

# Clean Up Your Body's Environment

Cleaning up your home is a major step in preventing and treating allergies, but that's only half the battle. You also need to deal with toxins in your food, personal-care products, clothes, and dental fillings.

### Use Only Organically Raised Foods

Eat foods that are grown and certified organic. They will be free of the synthetic pesticides and herbicides, hormones, preservatives, dyes, artificial colorings, and antibiotics found in conventionally raised foods. Many health food and grocery stores offer organic produce and meat as do some farmers markets. "Transitional" food products are grown without pesticides, hormones, and other chemicals, but have not met all of the requirements for organic certification. These are safer than conventional foods, but certified organic foods are the best choice.

## Get the Poisons Off Your Produce

Since the U.S. Food and Drug Administration tests only about 1% of produce for pesticide residues, cleaning your food is the only way to ensure that you are not eating agricultural poisons. Even organic foods may have residues of potentially harmful substances. The solution to this problem may be naturally derived produce washes, now available to consumers concerned about preventing food-borne illnesses.

However, people with food allergies, especially to coconuts, yeast, or citrus, should exercise care in using natural produce washes, which contain commonly allergenic ingredients. Common cleansing agents include sodium lauryl sulfate (a chemical made from coconuts, which has other adverse side effects); sugar/fatty acid cleansers derived from yeast; citrus foods, such as lemons; and extracts of bilberry, sugar cane, or sugar maple. Be sure to carefully read the labels.

## Use Natural Hygiene Products, Cosmetics, and Clothing

Personal-care products and dry-clean-only clothes contain many toxic substances that should never touch our skin.

■ Stop using commercial toothpaste and mouthwash. Use fluoride-free natural tooth-care products or baking soda instead.

■ Avoid aerosol hair and deodorant sprays. Use herbal hair products and non-aluminum deodorants; health food markets carry deodorants that contain enzymes, lichen, crystal, baking soda, and other safe alternatives.

■ Use natural, preferably organic, cotton-fiber feminine products that have not been bleached.

■ Avoid cosmetics containing talc, toluene (a petrochemical), or other hazardous substances. Contact the manufacturer for ingredient details.

■ Wear natural-fiber clothing instead of dry-clean-only apparel. If you do continue to wear dry-clean clothes, considering hand-washing them in gentle, safe laundry soap.

## Remove Mercury Dental Amalgams

Allergic people can often expect a marked improvement when their

# Four-Week Mercury Detoxification Program

## FIRST WEEK

***Chlorella***—Helps move mercury out of connective tissue so that substances such as DMPS can then remove it from the body. Begin with only one chlorella capsule daily for the first few weeks after amalgam removal, then gradually increase to three daily.

***Methylsulfonylmethane (MSM)***—This natural supplement, found in some greens and animal products, is high in sulfur, which enables it to bind up (chelate) toxic metals and chemicals, and to work against harmful microbes. Two to three grams of MSM, in crystal or capsule form, per day should be sufficient.

***Silymarin***—Also known as milk thistle seed, it has long been used as a liver-purifying agent. Take one capsule three times daily.

***Vitamin C***—Ascorbic acid has a protective effect against free-radical damage that occurs as heavy metals are being removed and excreted through the kidneys. Take 1,000 mg twice a day.

***Vitamin B complex***—Take 15-20 mg of each B vitamin daily to help replenish nutrients lost when heavy metals are bound up and excreted.

***Essential minerals***—During the detoxification process, some minerals may become depleted. Supplement daily with 15-30 mg of chelated zinc, 2.5-5.0 mg manganese, 450 mg magnesium, and 0.2 mg chromium.

***Homeopathic amalgam drops***—This is a combination of homeopathically prepared elements found in amalgam fillings given for the purpose of enhancing the removal of heavy metals from the body. Beginning one week prior to amalgam removal, take ten drops, three times daily; continue this dosage for one week after amalgam removal.

Once all the amalgams have been removed, begin taking homeopathic mercury (*Mercurius solubilis* 30C) at the rate of 30 drops, two to three times weekly, for the duration of the oral detoxification program or until you feel improved.

## SECOND WEEK

Decrease vitamin C to 1,500 mg daily.

## THIRD WEEK

Decrease vitamin C to 1,000 daily.

## FOURTH WEEK

Decrease vitamin C to 500 mg daily.

---

mercury amalgams are removed. At the 33rd Annual Meeting of the American Academy of Environmental Medicine in 1998, Barbara Solomon, M.D., of Baltimore, Maryland, presented more than ten case studies in which removal of dental amalgams eliminated such symptoms as headache, fatigue, and gastrointestinal distress in patients with allergies.[48] To realize similar results, however, it is imperative that your dentist knows how to properly remove mercury amalgams.

James Hardy, D.M.D., of Winter Park, Florida, and author of *Mercury Free*, says a typical patient in good health can have all mercury amalgams removed in four visits, spaced seven to ten days apart.

Dentists should remove and replace fillings in one quadrant (upper left or right, lower left or right) during each visit. Numerous plastic composite filling alternatives are available and, according to Dr. Hardy, they are durable for at least ten years.

Biological dentist Hal Huggins, D.D.S., of Colorado Springs, Colorado, recommends that people who choose to have their amalgams removed ask their dentists to use a rubber dam, a thin sheet of rubber that slips over the teeth. "Dams prevent over 95% of the mixture of mercury and water produced by the drilling out of old fillings from going down your throat. They also reduce the amount of mercury that you might absorb from your cheeks and under your tongue." Dr. Hardy, however, prefers using a specialized compact device (called Cleanup), which fits snugly over the tooth being worked on and suctions up to 90% of the mercury vapor. This device, says Dr. Hardy, is more effective than rubber dams at preventing mercury from being swallowed during the removal process.

Dr. Huggins suggests that people consider early morning appointments for amalgam removal, rather than later in the day, because the mercury vapor from other patients' sessions can linger in the air for hours and be absorbed by breathing. To avoid this, find a dentist who uses a HEPA mercury-vapor filter system and/or mercury vapor ionizer.

**Mercury Detoxification Program—**While removal of amalgam fillings stops any further source of poisoning from mercury fillings, you still need to detoxify the body to eliminate the residual effect from mercury that remains behind. Even if the fillings are removed, the negative influence of mercury will continue unless it is appropriately detoxified and eliminated from your body. The following guidelines for detoxifying mercury come from Dr. Hardy's clinical practice (see "Four-Week Mercury Detoxification Program," p. 154). Dr. Hardy recommends that patients seek the supervision of a naturopath or other health-care provider during the detoxification and removal process.

On the day of amalgam removal, vitamin C should not be taken until after the procedure; otherwise, it may interfere with the anesthesia.

This four-week detoxification program should begin simultaneously with your amalgam removal sessions. Begin the program with each removal session. Some doctors may advise their patients to supplement with DMSA (2,3-dimercaptosuccinic acid) and DMPS (2,3-dimercaptopropane-1-sulfonate) during the detoxification process. These chemi-

For more tips on **detoxifying your body**, see Chapter 8: Intestinal Detoxification, pp. 212-235.

cals cross the blood-brain barrier to remove the toxic residues from the central nervous system. Consult your physician about these supplements; Dr. Hardy believes they are too strong for some allergy patients suffering from poor health.

Prior to beginning the detoxification and removal process, it's a good idea to build up your body's defense system with antioxidants such as vitamins C and E and beta-carotene. Additionally, clean up your diet before and during the detoxification process. Avoid sugar, carbonated beverages, caffeine, tobacco, alcohol, excessive dairy or meat products, and processed foods. Instead, eat foods high in complex carbohydrates, fiber, vegetables, fruits, and protein sources other than meat. Dr. Hardy recommends eating lightly steamed sulfur-containing vegetables such as asparagus, broccoli, cabbage, garlic, onion, and cilantro, as the sulfur in these foods helps move mercury out of the collagen in tissue so the toxin may be excreted from the body. As with any detoxification process, you may experience a "healing crisis," with flu-like symptoms such as headache, fatigue, and weakness. If so, contact your doctor to see if you should modify your program. The usual length of time required for body elimination of mercury is three to six months.

For **natural fruit and vegetable washes**, contact: Citricidial*, Bio/Chem Research, Inc., (for licensed physicians only); tel: 800-225-4345 or 707-263-1475. Organiclean™, 10877 Wilshire Blvd., Suite 1200, Los Angeles, CA 90024; tel: 888-VEG-WASH or 310-824-2508; website: www.organiclean.com. EarthSafe™, GrowMore, 15600 New Century Drive, Gardena, CA 90248; tel: 310-515-1700; fax: 310-527-9963. VegiWash™, Consumer Health Research, P.O. Box 1884, Bandon, OR 97411; tel: 800-282-WASH; fax: 541-347-7772; website: www.vegiwash.com. For **referrals to dentists trained in mercury amalgam removal**, contact: Holistic Dental Association, Box 5007, Durango, CO 81301; tel: 970-259-1091. American Academy of Biological Dentistry, P.O. Box 859, Carmel Valley, CA 93924.

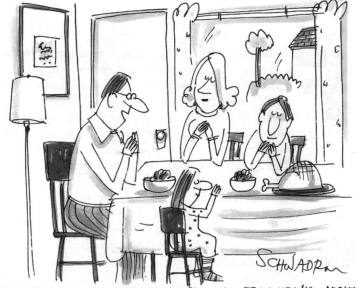

"BLESS THIS FOOD, AND PROTECT US FROM THE PESTICIDES AND ADDITIVES THEREIN."

# CHAPTER

# 6

# Therapeutic Diets

FOODS PLAY A DUAL ROLE in allergies and sensitivities, as both triggers of and contributors to adverse reactions. The problem with food allergies and sensitivities is that 85% of them involve delayed reactions, manifesting up to 72 hours after consumption of the offending food. You may not realize that the wheat bread you ate two days ago is responsible for your headache today. And the symptoms may shape-shift; that is, change over time and with repeated exposure. Further complicating matters is that people tend to experience sensitivity reactions from as little as ten to as many as 50 or more foods; immediate antibody-mediated allergic reactions are usually to a few foods. Even if you realize your headache was caused by a food, it may be hard to determine which of the potentially allergenic foods was the trigger.

For more out about **tests that detect food allergy triggers**, see Chapter 3: Allergy/Sensitivity Testing, pp. 70-105.

The elimination diet, presented here as well as in Chapter 3, is the gold standard for detecting food allergens. It is also a useful therapy in reducing reactions caused by food allergy and sensitivity. This chapter also describes other diet regimens—the rotation, anti-lectin, and anti-*Candida* diets—that minimize reactions. These eating plans, in conjunction with the therapies in Chapter 7: Healing Leaky Gut Syndrome, and Chapter 8: Intestinal Detoxification, will greatly improve intestinal barrier function, not only by treating existing allergies but also by preventing other allergies and associated diseases from occurring.

## In This Chapter

- Are Food Reactions Making You Sick?
- How Diet Leads to Allergy/Sensitivity
- Success Story: Diet Reverses Ulcerative Colitis
- Therapeutic Diets That Minimize Food Reactions

# Are Food Reactions Making You Sick?

Most people realize that food allergy—that is, antibody-mediated reactions to food—can cause health problems, including hives, eczema, and asthma. However, up to 80 different illnesses and disorders have been linked to food allergies and sensitivities. Even cognitive, emotional, and mental problems ("brain allergies") may be responses to offending foods. It's important to note that foods may not be solely responsible for these disorders; biological pollutants, chemicals, and other factors, may also contribute to their development. However, since food sensitivity is often overlooked, it is crucial to emphasize food's association with the health problems described below.

## Ear Infection (Otitis Media)

Ear infections are almost a given during early childhood, accounting for half of all visits to pediatricians. Two-thirds of American children will experience at least one bout of acute (episodic) ear infection and two-thirds of youngsters will experience chronic (recurrent) ear infections by age 6.[2] Acute ear infections usually develop after upper respiratory infections or allergies, but up to 93% of cases of chronic ear infection are caused by allergies to food and/or inhalants.[3] Cow's milk, wheat, egg white, peanuts, soy, corn, tomato, chicken, and apples are the most common triggers of chronic ear infections.[4]

## Types of Food Reactions

Food allergies and sensitivities are hard to detect, not only because of the limitations of conventional allergy tests, but because the symptoms can change, depending on other variables, such as exposure to toxins and digestive dysfunction. Food reactions can manifest in four ways:[1]

■ Fixed Reaction: You always have the same allergic reaction to the food.

■ Cumulative Reaction: You can eat a little of the food, but if it has not passed out of your bloodstream (four to seven days) before you eat more, you may react allergically. This is why a rotation diet is effective in stemming a cumulative allergic reaction.

Another type of cumulative allergic reaction occurs only when your system is overwhelmed by more than one allergen at the same time. For example, you can eat a food in a pristine environment, but if you eat it during hay fever season or when a cat is nearby, you may react.

■ Variable Reaction: You have indigestion after eating the food on one occasion and puffy, watery eyes the next time.

■ Addictive Reaction: You crave the food, consciously or subconsciously, and will experience withdrawal symptoms when it is eliminated from your diet. This is indicative of allergic addiction syndrome.

For more on how **early childhood feeding practices lead to allergy**, see Chapter 4: Prevention of Sensitization, pp. 106-127.

Joining the middle ear and the throat is a passageway called the eustachian tube. It protects the middle ear from bacteria and mucus secretions from the nose and throat, drains fluid, and controls air pressure in the middle ear. During an allergic reaction, chemical mediators inflame the eustachian tube as well as the nasal passageways. When the nasal passages are blocked, swallowing with your mouth closed causes air and mucus secretions to drain into the middle ear. This allows fluid to build up; bacteria can thrive in this environment, leading to infections. If allowed to persist, infections in the ear can travel to the mastoid (bone located behind and under the ear) and into the brain, and can be fatal. Conventional medicine treats ear infections with antibiotics and in many instances, myringotomy tubes—plastic tubes inserted in the middle ear to facilitate drainage. A 1994 report in the *Journal of the American Medical Association* reported that only 42% of the one million myringotomy operations performed each year are useful in minimizing ear infections.[5]

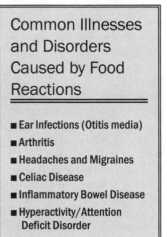

## Common Illnesses and Disorders Caused by Food Reactions

- Ear Infections (Otitis media)
- Arthritis
- Headaches and Migraines
- Celiac Disease
- Inflammatory Bowel Disease
- Hyperactivity/Attention Deficit Disorder
- Enuresis (Bed-wetting)
- Depression, Anxiety, Schizophrenia, and Autism

Bottle-feeding and early introduction of food have been shown to promote chronic ear infections, while breastfeeding prevents them.[6] Eliminating food allergens from the diet also prevents ear infections from recurring. In one study, 81 children with chronic ear infections were put on elimination diets (free of milk, wheat, peanuts, and corn) for 11 weeks; 70 (78%) experienced a significant improvement. Reintroducing the allergenic foods caused a relapse in 66 children (94%).[7]

### Arthritis

Both rheumatoid arthritis and the inflammation in osteoarthritis are caused to some degree by food sensitivities.[8] High levels of circulating immune complexes (SEE QUICK DEFINITION) have been found in both the blood serum and the fluid around the joints of arthritis patients.[9]

Evidence is gradually mounting that strongly links arthritis and allergies. One study tracked the medical history and progress of a 52-year-old woman who had suffered from inflammatory arthritis for 11 years to see if her symptoms were linked with food sensitivities. The researchers were especially concerned to study her reactions to milk, meat, and beans. First, they evaluated her while on her regular diet, then while fasting, and then while being "challenged" with foods known to provoke allergies. When she was given eight ounces of milk four times a day, this produced 30 minutes of morning stiffness, 14 tender joints, and four swollen joints 24-48 hours later. She also experienced morning stiffness during her normal diet period. In contrast, when the woman fasted for three days, she had no morning stiffness, no swollen joints, and only one tender joint. This study clearly showed that food sensitivities were associated with arthritic symptoms in this patient.[10]

Researchers at the Asthma and Allergy Research Center at Sahlgren's University Hospital in Göteborg, Sweden, also reported strong correlations between milk consumption and arthritis. Of 58 patients who came to the hospital with food-related gastrointestinal symptoms, 41% (24 patients) had joint swelling and 71% (41 patients) had joint pain (arthralgia).[11] In another study, researchers at the All India Institute of Medical Sciences examined 14 patients with rheumatoid arthritis. These patients abstained from grains, cereals, milk, and non-vegetarian protein foods for two weeks; 71% showed "significant clinical improvement" as a result of eliminating these foods from their daily intake. The researchers concluded that dietary factors may influence inflammatory response in rheumatoid arthritis.[12]

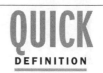

**DEFINITION**

Circulating immune complexes (CICs) form in the body when poor digestion results in undigested food proteins "leaking" through the intestinal wall and into the bloodstream. The immune system treats these foreign substances or antigens as invaders, causing antibodies to form and couple with them. This antigen and antibody combination is known as a CIC. In a healthy person, CICs are neutralized, but in someone with a compromised immune system, they tend to accumulate in the blood where they burden the detoxification pathways or initiate an allergic reaction. If too many CICs accumulate, the kidneys and liver cannot excrete enough of them via the urine or stool. The CICs are then deposited in soft tissues, causing inflammation and bringing stress to the immune system. The overload can lead to a variety of chronic health conditions.

To learn more about **allergies and arthritis**, see *Arthritis: An Alternative Medicine Definitive Guide* (AlternativeMedicine. com, 1999; ISBN 1-887299-15-7); to order, call 800-333-HEAL.

## Headaches and Migraines

Adverse reactions to food, whether mediated by antibodies or other immunological processes, can cause headaches. The inflammatory chemicals released during allergy and sensitivity responses simultaneously constrict blood vessels and initiate blood clotting, causing localized pain and throbbing, often in the head. Migraine headaches, severe head pains accompanied by visual disturbances, fatigue, disorientation, nausea, and even vomiting, are often triggered by eating an offending food and, to a lesser degree, food additives and environmental sub-

For more on the **allergy-headache connection**, see *Alternative Medicine Definitive Guide to Headaches* (Future Medicine Publishing, 1997; ISBN 1-887299-03-3); to order, call 800-333-HEAL.

stances. Although the percentage is disputed, researchers suggest that between 20% and 90% of all migraines are related to allergy/sensitivity factors.

A groundbreaking study conducted by Joseph Egger of the Hospital for Sick Children in London, suggests that the percentage may be even higher. In a carefully controlled study, Egger showed that it was possible to eliminate the incidence of migraine in 93% of the study's 88 migraine sufferers when sensitivity-causing foods were eliminated from their diet. Most of the participants in the study were found to be intolerant to more than one type of food, and as is often the case with food sensitivities and allergies, the offending foods were also the foods they craved or ate most frequently. A double-blind placebo test was included as a control, and it was proven that when the offending foods were introduced back into the diet, the migraine pain would return.[13] The foods most often implicated as a cause of headaches were cow's milk (in 30% of patients), eggs (27%), chocolate (25%), oranges (24%), wheat (24%), cheese (15%), and tomatoes (15%).

## Celiac Disease

Wheat is among the most common triggers of food allergy and sensitivity. People suffering from reactions to wheat or its constituent proteins gluten and gliadin often suffer from diarrhea, stomach pain, and other gastrointestinal discomforts. A condition called celiac disease is also characterized by intolerance to gluten and gliadin, found in wheat, rye, barley, oats; similar proteins are also found in buckwheat (a grass seed) and millet. Not all people experiencing reactions to wheat and other gluten/gliadin foods have celiac disease. Patients with celiac disease experience diarrhea, foul-smelling, greasy stools, and weight loss, due to multiple vitamin and nutrient deficiencies. They also have damaged small intestine tissue folds (known as jejunoileal fold pattern reversal) caused by exposure to wheat proteins. The liver is also damaged in celiac disease.[14] A recent report in the *Journal of Pediatrics* states that one out of every 33 children in the United States may have this disease.[15]

Despite some diagnostic differences, celiac disease appears to share many of the causes of other food allergies, including genetic susceptibility (particularly to people from northern and central Europe and northwest India),[16] enzyme deficiency, and intestinal permeability. Children who are not breast-fed and who are introduced to cow's milk early are at higher risk than other children for developing celiac disease.[17] Additionally, celiac patients also tend to become lactose deficient, leading to lactose intolerance;[18] they also frequently develop multiple food allergies, due to leaky gut.

Celiac disease has also been linked to Type I (insulin-dependent) diabetes mellitus,[19] schizophrenia, thyroid problems, and hives.[20] Women with celiac disease are at a higher risk for experiencing reproductive problems, including infertility, miscarriage, and low-weight-infant births.[21] Celiac disease is also implicated in bone loss and osteoporosis. In one recent study, 86 newly diagnosed celiac disease patients were placed on a gluten-free diet for one year. These patients, including postmenopausal women, showed a significant improvement in bone mineral density and bone metabolism compared to the control group that did not undergo the elimination diet.[22]

## Inflammatory Bowel Disease
## (Crohn's Disease and Ulcerative Colitis)

Inflammatory bowel disease (IBD) is the generic term for several chronic disorders in which gastrointestinal organs become inflamed and often permanently damaged by exposure to food antigens. The two most common IBDs are Crohn's disease and ulcerative colitis. Researchers believe that both diseases develop as part of a genetic susceptibility to lactase (enzyme that breaks down milk sugar) deficiency. However, bacterial overgrowth and prolonged fecal transit time (time it takes for bowels to eliminate waste after eating) also appear to impair the health of the gastrointestinal system.[23] In addition to dairy foods, chocolate, fats, and artificial sweeteners often trigger both types of inflammatory bowel disease.[24]

Named after U.S. gastroenterologist Burril Crohn (1884-1983), Crohn's disease is also called enteritis or regional ileitis. It is caused by a T cell–mediated (type IV) reaction, usually to milk sugars as a result of lactase deficiency. A chronic, recurrent problem often affecting young adults (age 20 to 40), it involves an inflammation mainly of the intestines, particularly of segments of the small intestine, such as the ileum or ileocecal valve. As the ileocecal valve is located on the right side of the intestines, Crohn's is sometimes called "right-sided disease." When similar lesions occur in the large intestine, the condition is called colitis. Symptoms may include abdominal pain, weakness and fatigue, cramps, diarrhea, rectal bleeding, 24- to 48-hour fever, weight loss, canker sores in the mouth, and a thickening of the gastrointestinal lining.

Ulcerative colitis, another T cell–mediated food allergy, shares many of the characteristics of Crohn's disease. It likewise afflicts

To understand what happens in **inflammatory bowel disease and other T cell–mediated allergic reactions**, see Chapter 1: Understanding Allergy and Sensitivity pp. 14-37.

younger adults but is approximately twice as prevalent as Crohn's disease.[25] The symptoms of this disease may resemble those of Crohn's disease but can include blood diarrhea with cramps in the lower abdomen, as well as some abdominal tenderness, weight loss, and fever. Unlike Crohn's disease, however, the colon, not the small intestine, is inflamed in patients with ulcerative colitis. Also unlike Crohn's disease, ulcerative colitis is an autoimmune disease. The immune system makes antibodies to its own bowel tissue—an allergy to self. If left untreated, ulcerative colitis can lead to colorectal cancer.[26]

### Hyperactivity/Attention Deficit Hyperactivity Disorder

Healthy children are expected to be full of energy, but hyperactive youngsters suffer from numerous emotional, mental, and behavioral problems, most notably excessive restlessness, aggressiveness, stubbornness, and temper tantrums. Hyperactive children can't seem to sit still or concentrate for even short periods or time and are easily distracted. They may also experience anxiety, fright, migraines, and loose bowel movements.

Hyperactivity is a childhood epidemic. It's estimated that 3% to 5% of U.S. children between the ages of 6 and 12 have been clinically diagnosed with attention deficit hyperactivity disorder (ADHD), a severe form of hyperactivity, with 8% to 10% of children showing symptoms of ADHD.[28] Two and a half million children with hyperactivity problems are currently taking the prescription drug Ritalin, a mild form of amphetamine called methylphenidate, to manage symptoms.[29] Pharmaceutical treatment of ADHD is on the increase; for instance, between 1991 and 1995, Ritalin use almost tripled in children ages two to four years.[30] Ritalin is rife with potentially dangerous side effects: it can stunt growth, induce seizures in epileptic children, and cause extreme anxiety and insomnia, as well as skin rashes, nausea, headaches, drowsiness, joint pain, chest pain, weight loss, anemia, and hair loss, among other symptoms.[31]

Often parents and teachers notice that hyperactivity increases after snacks or lunchtime, indicating that food is the culprit. And, indeed, research has found that some hyperactive and ADHD children are intolerant to foods and food additives (especially food dyes and preservatives). It appears that offending foods and additives abnormally impact the brain, provoking mood and behavioral problems. In 1997, a group of Australian researchers measured the brain activity of 15 children with food-induced ADHD. The researchers found that brain activity in the

## Is Food Intolerance All in Your Head?

As with chemical sensitivity, mainstream medicine tends to look at claims of food intolerance with a great deal of skepticism. The absence of antibodies in food-sensitivity reactions not only makes these conditions difficult to diagnose, it also leads conventional doctors to dismiss the health complaints of food-intolerant patients. In fact, researchers have conducted studies to determine the psychosomatic nature of patients with perceived food intolerance.

In a study published in 1999 in the *Journal of Psychosomatic Research*, researchers at the University of Birmingham (U.K.) School of Psychology surveyed more than 500 subjects, including those who perceived themselves to be food intolerant. They asked the subjects to fill out two questionnaires, one on general health and the other on personality/psychological states. The researchers found that women with perceived food intolerance showed more symptoms of neurosis, anxiety, insomnia, and severe depression than controls.[27] However, the researchers emphasize that the prevalence of psychiatric disorders in perceived food-intolerant women and men was comparable to that of control groups in previously conducted studies.

Although some conventional doctors may use these findings to confirm the view that food sensitivity is psychosomatic, this study also illustrates that people with food intolerance suffer more symptoms than gastrointestinal distress. It appears that adverse reactions to food does indeed correlate with "brain allergies"—cognitive, emotional, and mental health problems caused by food sensitivity.

fronto-temporal areas of the brain increased in all children during consumption of the offending foods, while it returned to normal when the children avoided the same foods.[32] Diets in which reactive foods and additives were eliminated have been shown to reverse ADHD.[33]

## Enuresis (Bed-wetting)

Bed-wetting (nocturnal enuresis) is a common occurrence in toddlers and is only recognized as a disorder after the age of five. It's estimated that 3% of youths between the ages of 12 and 18 suffer from chronic sleep enuresis.[34] Some children also experience diurnal enuresis, or daytime incontinence. Less than 1% of nocturnal enuresis cases is attributed to emotional problems.[35] Physiological abnormalities and disorders, including a small bladder, metabolic or hormonal imbalances, urethral stricture, bladder infections, and obstructive sleep apnea are associated with the development of this disorder. Food allergies and sensitivities are also implicated.

Research has found that enuresis is significantly more common in children with ADHD than in other children. In fact, 6-year-olds with

ADHD are 2.7 times more likely to have nocturnal enuresis and 4.5 times more likely to suffer from diurnal enuresis than non-ADHD children.[36] Like ADHD, enuresis is often induced by food and can be reversed by eliminating the offending foods. In one study, 21 children who suffered from enuresis as well as ADHD and/or migraines were placed on an elimination diet. Of those, 12 children were soon able to control their bladders, while another four experienced significant improvements in their enuresis. The hyperactivity and migraines also subsided on the elimination diet. When allergenic foods were reintroduced, symptoms of incontinence, hyperactivity, and migraines recurred.[37]

## Mental Disorders: Depression, Anxiety, Schizophrenia, and Autism

Research indicates that some cases of mental and behavioral disorders, including depression, anxiety, schizophrenia, and autism, are caused by food allergies. Studies have shown that asthmatic children[38] and people who suffer from allergic rhinitis,[39] conditions often triggered by biological pollutants but also by food, are more likely than others to suffer from anxiety, depression, schizophrenia, and other psychiatric disorders. Another report showed that 71% of people clinically diagnosed with depression had a history of IgE-mediated allergies including hives, eczema, allergic rhinitis, and asthma.[40]

Researchers suggest that one of the ways in which allergy may trigger psychological disorders is that chemical mediators released during an allergic response travel to the brain. There, they appear to interact and disrupt the function of neurotransmitters (brain chemicals) that regulate mood and mental stability. In clinical ecology, this reaction is called a "brain allergy." Interestingly, histamine can also act as a neurotransmitter, further disrupting the normal biochemical processes in the brain.

Brain allergies to food and other substances may also be implicated in the development of schizophrenia and autism. Research suggests that at least some cases of schizophrenia are induced by adverse reactions to foods, especially to wheat and gluten. In one study, two of 24 schizophrenics experienced remission of their disorder when fed a gluten-free diet for 14 weeks; they relapsed when gluten was reintroduced.[41] In a 1995 study, 36 autistic patients tested positive for food allergies, most frequently to cow's milk. Researchers placed the patients on a diet that excluded the allergenic foods for eight weeks, by which time all patients experienced a marked improvement in symptoms. The researchers concluded food allergens have toxic effects on the central nervous system in some people, causing autism.[42]

# Food Allergies: The Mental Illness Link

Abram Hoffer, M.D, an orthomolecular psychiatrist based in Victoria, British Columbia, has found that the majority of his psychiatric patients experience a quick reversal of their problems after removing allergenic foods. Below, he relates his experiences with the four-day water fast as a diagnostic tool for identifying food triggers in persons with mental disorders:

"Allergies play a major role in both physical and psychiatric illnesses. I became interested in them when Dr. Alan Kant, a New York psychiatrist, came back from Russia where he had studied the Russians' use of a 30-day fast for treating chronic schizophrenia. I had a few patients who were not getting better, so I placed one of my patients on a 30-day water fast. She had never responded to anything else, but, to my amazement, four days after she went into her fast, she was fine.

"Then, when I put her back on food, she became psychotic again. I asked her once more if she would go on another fast, but this time I only ran it for five days. She became normal once again. Convinced she must have food allergies, I began to put back one item per meal into her diet. What I discovered was that she was allergic to all meats and when she avoided them she remained normal.

"One case doesn't prove much so, over the next few years, I fasted 200 of my schizophrenic patients who had not responded particularly well to previous treatments. Most of them did it at home. They drank only water for four days and, on the fifth day, I began reintroducing one food at a time. I would ask them to drink only milk or eat only porridge. And, if they became sick again within a matter of hours, this would be the positive response to the challenge. With many foods it was just a matter of hours before they experienced their symptoms again; with some of the grains, it might take days. I had many cases where milk, for example, became a hallucinogen.

"As it turned out, 60% of my 200 patients did respond to the fast, and when I placed them on diets that eliminated the allergenic foods, they continued to make improvement towards recovery."

Other conditions sometimes triggered by brain allergies to food include memory impairment, spaciness, insomnia, irritability, and fatigue.

**Other Disorders**—Numerous disease states have been linked to food allergy and sensitivity in clinical studies. Among them are childhood epilepsy (often to milk),[43] gallbladder disease and gallstones (especially to eggs),[44] peptic ulcers (especially to milk),[45] and low back pain.[46] Other common symptoms of food reactions are edema (tissue swelling), muscle soreness, diarrhea, stomach pain, bloating, belching, and gas.

# How Diet Leads to Allergy/Sensitivity

Nutritionist Lindsey Berkson, M.A., D.C., of Santa Fe, New Mexico, sees today's typical American diet as containing too few foods. "Unfortunately, most Americans tend to avoid variety and commit the dietary sin of monotony," she says, "eating the same foods meal after meal, only disguised by different names." They also consume food not according to what is best for them but according to what tastes best to them.

According to Dr. Berkson, the American menu is actually made of various combinations of the same foods, usually wheat, beef, eggs, potatoes, and milk products. For example, she points out, a breakfast of eggs, sausage, white toast, and hash browns is the same as a lunch of a hamburger, white bun, and fries, which is the same as a dinner of steak and potatoes or white pasta. James Braly, M.D., medical director of Immuno Laboratories and author of *Dr. Braly's Food Allergy & Nutrition Revolution*, concurs with Dr. Berkson's perspective. He reports that Americans typically get 80% of their calories from 11 types of foods, and that among these foods are the most highly allergenic: milk, eggs, wheat, rye, nuts, and soy.[47] What's the connection? A leaky gut.

If you suffer from intestinal permeability and constantly eat the same foods over and over again, undigested molecules from these foods will frequently leak into the bloodstream, activating an allergic response. "A repetitive diet can contribute greatly to the development of allergies," says Marshall Mandell, M.D., medical director for the New England Foundation for Allergies and Environmental Diseases. "If someone eats bread every day, for instance, he could easily develop a wheat allergy due to the immune system's continuous exposure to it."

For more on **alternative therapies for leaky gut**, see Chapter 7: Healing Leaky Gut Syndrome, pp. 184-211.

A main step in eliminating allergies is to vary your diet. If you are no longer triggering allergic reactions and sending your immune system into chaos, you can begin the process of healing your leaky gut and immune function. The rotation diet is a good way to change your repetitive, allergy-inducing eating habits.

## Allergic Addiction Syndrome

Do you ever crave a particular food? Can't imagine going through the day without bread or cheese or chocolate? You may believe that these urges are good, that your body is signaling you that it needs these foods to remain healthy. However, these cravings often mean the exact opposite—that your body is being assaulted by these foods. This is called the allergic addiction syndrome.

Allergy to addictive foods develops as any other allergy does—with a leaky gut and improper digestion. One day you eat cheese; for some reason, your gastrointestinal system is unable to fully break down the cheese molecules. Some undigested molecules escape through the intestinal barrier and enter your bloodstream, leading to sensitization. When you consume cheese again and macromolecules again leak through the gut wall, an antibody-mediated allergic reaction ensues. Among the chemicals released during this immune process are narcotic-like substances called opioids, which help the body deal with ("mask") the discomfort caused by the allergic reaction. These opioids are like tranquilizers with a boost; they give you an immediate physical and emotional high. After a while, the inflammatory response subsides, and so does the opioid high. Your spirits and energy levels flag.

## Commonly Reactive Foods

If you were to ask ten doctors to name their patients' top offending foods and food additives, chances are their lists would look similar to this one, compiled from patient tests in my practice. Testing was done with electrodermal screening. Note that these foods and additives are found, in varying combinations, in most processed foods.

| Item Tested | Testing Positive |
| --- | --- |
| Wheat | 73% |
| Egg | 70% |
| BHA (preservative) | 70% |
| BHT (preservative) | 70% |
| Fluoride | 70% |
| Corn | 68% |
| Peanut | 68% |
| Cow's Milk | 68% |
| Soy | 68% |
| Red Dye | 68% |
| Monosodium Glutamate (MSG) | 68% |
| Nitrates | 65% |
| Nitrites | 65% |
| Sulfite | 65% |
| Yellow Dye (tartrazine) | 62% |
| Blue Dye | 62% |
| Sorbic Acid | 62% |
| Sulfur Dioxide | 62% |
| Violet Dye | 57% |
| Chicken | 57% |
| Turkey | 57% |
| Hydrolyzed Vegetable Protein | 54% |
| Beef | 51% |
| Nutrasweet™ | 49% |
| Chocolate | 46% |
| Bacon | 46% |
| Tuna | 43% |
| Tabasco Sauce | 43% |
| Pork | 41% |
| Cane Sugar | 41% |

As with any addiction, you will begin to crave this opioid lift—and the food that triggered it. The more you eat the allergenic food, however, the more damage it does to your body. The type III (arthus) allergic reactions that occur during allergic addiction damage cells. Additionally, the constant release of opioid chemicals and accompanying stress hormones (such as cortisol, which also provides an energy boost) exhausts the adrenal glands and the nervous system. Without the food, you will begin to feel withdrawal symptoms, including nervousness, shakiness, fatigue, weakness, perhaps headaches. But you need to eat larger quantities of the allergenic food for your brain to release greater amounts of feel-good chemicals to fight the withdrawal symptoms. Over time, you will truly be addicted to the offending food, bingeing on it, while your body deteriorates as a result of the allergic inflammation.

## Dietary Lectins

If you've ever read the diet book *Eat Right 4 Your Type* by Peter D'Adamo, N.D., you're familiar with the concept of lectins, types of proteins found in beans, grains, and soy, as well as in pollens, bacteria, and viruses. These proteins are able to bind with specific sugars on the surface of all cells of the body. This feature enables lectins to clump cells together for various biochemical functions, some of which are beneficial. Lectins found on cells in the liver's bile duct bind with bacteria and parasites, clumping them together, and facilitating their elimination from the body. Lectins can also perform pathogenic roles; for example, lectins on bacteria and viruses stick like Velcro® to mucosal linings in our body, causing irritation and infection. Dietary lectins are particularly damaging to the gastrointestinal linings. One study found that dietary lectins, especially those found in lentils, induced a significantly large release of histamine, causing tissue inflammation.[48] Soybean and wheat lectins can produce an increase in permeability in the cells they bind to, often leading to cell death. Further, lectins can cause the intestinal villi (the fingerlike projections that give the intestine its absorptive surface area) to atrophy.

Some lectins also cause illness in individuals with certain blood types, while promoting health in those with different blood types. Blood is classified into four blood types or groups according to the presence of type A and type B antigens on the surface of red blood cells. These antigens are also called agglutinogens and pertain to the blood cells' ability to agglutinate, or clump together. Blood type A contains antibodies to type B, and vice versa. Blood type O carries antibodies for both type A and type B. Blood type AB has no antibodies to any blood type. Blood type is considered relevant to food allergy because agglutination also occurs in the body in response to lectins.

Lectins are found in 30% of the foods we eat; they have characteristics similar to blood antigens and can thus sometimes become an "enemy" when they enter the body. Nutritionist Ann Louise Gittleman, M.S., C.N.S., author of *Your Body Knows Best*, notes that there are 65 different lectins known to have an agglutination reaction in the body, leading to intestinal damage, disrupted digestion and absorption, and food allergy, among other health problems.[49] Milk lectins are similar to type B blood cells. If someone with type A blood consumes milk, anti-B antibodies will be mobilized, causing an allergic reaction. However, milk is generally well tolerated in people with type B blood. Gluten, a lectin found in wheat and other grains, counteracts strongly with type O blood and tends to cause gastrointestinal inflammation. Tomatoes provoke strong reactions in type A and B blood types, but are often properly absorbed by types O and AB.[50]

In general, our immune systems protect all of us—regardless of blood type—from lectins entering the bloodstream. However, according to Dr. D'Adamo, approximately 5% of dietary lectins do enter our blood,[51] likely due to intestinal permeability.

## Lectins and Cross-Reactivity

Over the years, physicians have noticed that some patients who are allergic to certain pollens are also allergic to certain foods. For example, people with ragweed pollen allergy often are allergic to foods in the *Curcubitaceae* family (watermelon, melon, and cucumber) as well as banana. Why is this so? It appears that lectins are partly responsible for this cross-reactivity—edible plant foods contain lectins also found in common pollens.[52] This may also be the reason that people with allergies to latex also experience banana allergy.[53] Here are some other common instances of cross-reactivity that may be due to shared lectin content:

- Birch pollen—apple, carrot, potato, kiwis, and hazelnut
- Mugwort pollen—carrot, celery, nuts, mustard greens, and legumes
- Grass pollen—tomato, potato, green peas, peanut, watermelon, melon, apple, orange, and kiwi
- Plantain pollen—melon

### The Candidiasis Connection

There are more than 400 species of bacteria living in the human body and the majority of these bacteria reside in the gastrointestinal tract. Under conditions of intestinal health, "friendly" bacteria (such as *Lactobacillus acidophilus* and *Bifidobacterium bifidum*) predominate and contribute to digestion and the overall health of the body. But, increasingly, the shift observed today is towards a predominance of pathogenic bacteria, a condition of intestinal imbalance called dysbiosis. The unfriendly or pathogenic bacteria that dominate the intestines impair digestion, the absorption of nutrients, and the normal elimination cycle. They also provoke allergic reactions to food and contribute to the erosion of the intestinal mucosa and the infiltration of inappropriate substances into the bloodstream—a condition referred to as "leaky gut syndrome."

Dysbiosis is considered a primary cause or major cofactor in the development of many health problems, such as rheumatoid arthritis, acne, chronic fatigue, depression, digestive disorders, bloating, PMS, cancer, and food allergies. Of the pathogenic organisms most significantly implicated in food allergy is the yeast *Candida albicans*; its overgrowth is called candidiasis.

The modern North American way of eating is largely responsible for dysbiosis. The foods we eat are not pure and, to an extent, full of poisons. The typical diet is replete with meat products, which contain large amounts of chemical residues from the pesticides and herbicides used in livestock feed, and hormones and antibiotics used to make the animals grow larger and more rapidly. Ingestion of antibiotics, either through food products or prescribed medications, severely alters the intestinal flora by killing off bacteria, including beneficial microorganisms. As the bacterial communities repopulate after prolonged use of antibiotics, the colonic environment favors the growth of disease-causing organisms in lieu of the healthier bacteria.

We also tend to eat too many of the nutritionally wrong foods. Consider the huge amount of sugar and refined carbohydrates found in what's called the Standard American Diet (SAD). It is a sad diet indeed, for it has led to a nation with a staggering number of obese individuals and has caused chronic aberrations in the digestive flora. The SAD decreases the amount of intestinal secretions that aid in the proper breakdown of foods and this favors the overgrowth of pathogenic microorganisms.

# Success Story:
# Diet Reverses Ulcerative Colitis

For years, Claudia, 39, suffered from bloating, cramps, and other digestive disturbances shortly after eating even a very simple meal. She also experienced chronic sinus and ear problems, muscle and joint pains, mood swings, and hyperactivity, but accepted these physical and psychological problems as a fact of life.

One day, Claudia took some conventional cold medicine with orange juice and, soon after, she began to bleed from her rectum. Her doctor diagnosed ulcerative colitis and prescribed anti-inflammatory drugs that only exacerbated the problem. Soon Claudia started having esophageal reflux, in which stomach acids leak upward into the esophagus, producing an intense sensation of heartburn. Her reflux was so bad, she occasionally regurgitated fecal matter and the reverse movement of her stomach acids, which could potentially digest membranes lining the esophagus, soon produced mouth blisters.

Claudia consulted numerous specialists, none of whom was able to improve her condition or even ferret out its causes. One doctor told her she would have to learn to live with it. Another recommended that she have her intestines removed and move her bowels by way of a colostomy (a feces collection unit). Claudia refused the surgical procedure and instead began researching the possible causes of her condition. She discovered that food allergies were probably involved, but she was unable to accurately correlate specific allergic reactions with foods she ate. Frustrated, she decided to adopt a vegetarian diet, hoping a non-meat, non-dairy diet would be the solution.

After three months on this new diet, Claudia had gained 12 pounds, was excessively bloated all the time, and had developed a painful foot sore that prevented her from wearing any shoes but sandals. None of her other symptoms improved. Claudia then sought the help of Dr. Braly, of Immuno Laboratories in Fort Lauderdale, Florida.

Dr. Braly ran an IgG ELISA blood test called the Immuno 1 Bloodprint to determine if Claudia was suffering from delayed food allergies. He determined that Claudia had significant food allergies to 17 foods, or 16.6% of the 102 foods tested, including bananas, chili peppers, clams, eggs, oysters, green peppers, pineapples, scallops, spinach, sugar cane, wheat, yeast (baker's and brewer's), and green, kidney, and yellow wax beans. Some of these foods, particularly wheat and its constituent proteins gluten and gliadin, formed the basis for Claudia's vegetarian diet, and explained why her symptoms worsened when she adopted vegetarianism. The blood test also disclosed that Claudia had candidiasis, an infestation of *Candida albicans*, a yeast that often overgrows in the intestines as a result of a faulty diet, such as one high in sugar and yeasted foods, or excessive use of antibiotics or steroids.

Dr. Braly immediately recommended that Claudia not eat any of the 17 allergenic foods so as to avoid any symptomatic flare-ups. Additionally, he suggested that she avoid all foods and beverages containing yeasts, including buttermilk, cereals, cheeses, mushrooms,

For more about the **ELISA test**, see Chapter 3: Allergy/Sensitivity Testing, pp. 70-105.

olives, wine, soy sauce, pickles, and even certain vitamins. This prevented the proliferation of the *Candida* fungus. He further advised that Claudia follow a rotation diet, in which she avoided all allergenic foods and did not eat the same non-allergenic foods two days in a row. This ensured that she wouldn't develop new food allergies while her digestive tract healed.

Claudia had excellent results from these dietary changes. Over the next few months, she lost 22 pounds, her bowel bleeding stopped, and the rest of her symptoms cleared up. When Claudia's specialist performed a follow-up colonoscopy (an examination of her bowel), he was surprised at how healthy it had become. Not only did Claudia's physical symptoms resolve, but her state of mind improved as well. She no longer felt tense, domineering, hyperactive, or argumentative, and found a new sense of peace.

# Therapeutic Diets to Minimize Reactions

The following diets, which focus on varying the foods you eat, help the digestive and immune systems heal. In many cases, if a food is totally eliminated for a period of up to eight weeks or more, the body should be able to repair its intestinal membrane and replenish its enzyme store. Thus, the offending food may be tolerated when it is reintroduced. However, there is no guarantee that you will be able to safely resume eating allergenic foods, particularly in the case of antibody-mediated allergy. But the following diets, along with adjunct therapies in chapters 7 and 8, increase your chances of permanent recovery.

## Therapeutic Diets

- Elimination Diet
- Rotation Diet
- Stone Age Diet
- Proper Food Combining
- Anti-Lectin Diets
- Anti-*Candida* Diet

## Elimination Diet

Once you have identified the foods you are allergic to (see Chapter 3: Allergy/Sensitivity Testing), the next step is to eliminate them from your diet. Initially, you should completely refrain from eating all allergenic foods for 60 to 90 days. After this period, you can begin to slowly reintroduce them into your diet. You should also vary the foods that you eat on a daily basis to avoid developing new allergies (see "Rotation Diet" below). In most cases, this diet allows the body to repair intestinal barrier function, enabling patients to reintroduce the reactive foods into their diets. Dr. Braly estimates that only about 5% of delayed food allergies will not subside using the elimination and rotation diets, necessitating the use of other alternative therapies.

Remember that eliminating an allergenic food can cause withdrawal reactions. "The majority of people who give up foods they're allergic to go through a mild to moderate withdrawal phase, lasting one to five days, while the body detoxifies itself," says Dr. Braly. Allergic symptoms may get worse during this period and cravings can be intense. If the allergy foods were also your comfort foods, you may experience emotional feelings of loss and distress. Dr. Braly explains that "once the withdrawal phase has passed, the cravings also abate, and the allergy sufferer is free of dependence on that food, free of both the physiological and psychological desire to consume it so frequently, and in such great quantities."[54] In my clinical experience, I've found most cravings that accompany

To learn how to use the **elimination diet to detect food allergens**, see Chapter 3: Allergy/Sensitivity Testing, pp. 70-105.

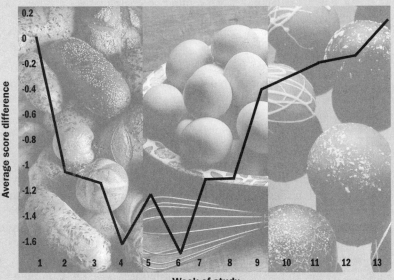

**Week of study**

**HOW TO STOP YOUR FOOD ALLERGIES FAST**—The graph shows the rapid decline in reactions to suspected allergenic foods when patients completely avoided them for about two months, in a study sponsored by Immuno Laboratories. Maximum freedom from food allergy–related symptoms was achieved between the third and sixth weeks. Among foods most commonly identified as allergenic are wheat, eggs, and chocolate (pictured above), as well as milk and corn.

allergic addiction syndrome resolve after 14 days of complete abstention from offending foods.

**The Trouble with GEOs**—When you're following the elimination diet, you have to carefully read the labels to commercial products to screen out allergenic substances. But in the past decade, the introduction of genetically engineered organisms (GEOs, also called genetically modified organisms) into foods has complicated this process. In order to accelerate crop growth and enable crops to tolerate more pesticides, the genetic codes of food plants are combined with genes from other food sources. This crossbreeding procedure is called horizontal gene transfer, whereby scientists take a gene from one organism (chicken, for example) and force it into the DNA code of another organism (potato). This procedure is radically different from traditional plant crossbreeding, which works within species, not across species boundaries.

You may think you are eating "safe," nonallergenic foods, but often they contain components of foods that can, and do, trigger allergic reactions. Brett Kettlehut, M.D., committee chair of the Adverse Food Reactions Committee at the American Academy of Allergy, Asthma & Immunology in Milwaukee, Wisconsin, warns that a person who has food allergies should be concerned about the possible allergenicity of genetically engineered foods.[55] And research supports his alarm. For instance, a 1996 study reported that eight of nine people allergic to Brazil nuts also showed an allergic response to genetically engineered soybeans containing the Brazil nut protein 2S albumin.[56]

Additionally, people allergic to antibiotics may also experience adverse reactions to genetically engineered foods. According to Joe Cummins, Ph.D., a retired genetics professor at the University of Western Ontario, in Canada, most GEO crops produce an enzyme that creates antibiotics intended to make plants resistant to harmful bacteria. The GEO antibiotics contain a similar molecular structure to antibiotics manufactured for human use. In a person who has allergies to antibiotics, the immune system confuses GEO antibiotics with the allergenic type. "Thus, most genetically engineered crops are likely to be allergenic to people sensitive to antibiotics," says Dr. Cummins.

Presently, the altered substances are not listed on food labels in the U.S. In May 2000, the federal government rejected a proposal that would require that food labels disclose GEO ingredients. (However, the Food and Drug Administration stated it would develop voluntary labeling procedures and further examine the safety of GEO crops.) Industry estimates tell us that many packaged foods, especially those containing corn or soy, contain genetically engineered organisms.

Numerous public opinion polls in North America and
Europe demonstrate strong opposition to genetically engineered foods and some European countries have begun
labeling one or more food items containing GEOs, generally soy. France now requires the labeling of all GEOs, and
Italy has actually banned the production of GEO corn.
Currently, in the U.S., the only certain way to avoid GEOs
is by eating organically grown foods.

## Rotation Diet

Another way of minimizing the risk of exposure to allergenic foods is to increase the variety of foods eaten and
rotate them so that they aren't eaten too frequently. This is
known as a rotation diet. This diet facilitates the rejuvena-
tion of the intestinal membrane and reversal of leaky gut
syndrome and the resultant food allergies. Some alternative
medicine practitioners only use the rotation diet if a patient
has difficulty staying desensitized to a food item, as a result
of chronic digestive barrier function default.

To follow the rotation diet, vary your foods every four
days. "You might be able to have the same food more than
once a day, but then you would not have it again until four days
later," explains Dr. Braly. This requires some attention to food and beverage components. For instance, if you eat eggs on a Friday, they cannot
be ingredients in your meals on Saturday. Likewise, you should check the
ingredients of your nutrient supplements to ensure that they do not contain binders, fillers, or other food products that you are avoiding or rotating. Also note that you should avoid eating foods in the same family (e.g.,
broccoli and cabbage) two days in a row (see "Food Family Chart,"
p. 179).

## Stone Age Diet

The "Stone Age diet" is another potentially useful diet plan for allergy sufferers. The theory behind this diet is that our bodies are not
genetically adapted to the synthetic, processed foods that constitute
much of our modern eating practices. Therefore, we are unable to
digest many foods properly and they become allergenic as our body
tries to defend against them.

According to Dr. Hoffer, due to the slow course of evolution, our
digestive apparatus has remained the same for 10,000 years. Thus, we
are best suited for the foods prevalent during the Paleolithic era—

For information about **consumer action ini-
tiatives against GEOs**, contact: Alliance for Bio-Integrity, 406 West Depot Avenue, Fairfield, IA 52556; tel: 515-472-5554; web-site: http://www.bio-integrity.org. For **feder-al regulations and information on GEOs**, visit the Food and Drug Administration's web-site at www.fda.com., or the USDA's biotech-nology website at www.aphis.usda.gov/biotechnology. For **rotation and other therapeutic diet plans**, contact: Immuno Laboratories, Inc., 1620 West Oakland Park Blvd., Fort Lauderdale, FL 33311; tel: 800-231-9197 or 954-486-4500; fax: 954-739-6563; website: www.immunolabs.com.

# Sample Rotation Diet

The following sample of a four-day rotation plan was created by Immuno Laboratories. Your own rotation diet may differ since it should contain foods to which you are not allergic. It is advisable to eat a variety of foods every day. You may move a food from one day to another (for example, if you like peas and rice together), but be careful not to repeat the same food two days in a row. Reading food labels is important, and it is recommended that you consult your physician or health practitioner for further guidance.

| DAY ONE | DAY TWO | DAY THREE | DAY FOUR |
|---|---|---|---|
| **Protein:** | | | |
| Beef/Veal | Chicken | Cod | Crab |
| Haddock | Flounder | Lamb | Halibut |
| Salmon | Scallops | Lobster | Pork |
| Sole | Trout | Shrimp | Snapper |
| | Whitefish | Tuna | Turkey |
| **Vegetables:** | | | |
| Asparagus | Acorn Squash | Eggplant | Endive |
| Broccoli | Carrot | Mushroom | Green Pepper |
| Brussels Sprouts | Cucumber | Potato (White, Sweet) | Radish |
| Cabbage | Green Bean | Spinach | Yam |
| Cauliflower | Parsley | Tomato | |
| Celery | Yellow Squash | | |
| Lettuce | Yellow Wax Bean | | |
| Onion | Zucchini | | |
| **Beans/Grains/Legumes:** | | | |
| Alfalfa | Pea | Mung Bean | Corn |
| Pinto Bean | Soybean | Kidney Bean | |
| **Fruits and Nuts:** | | | |
| (Plus beverages derived from these foods) | | | |
| Almond | Cantaloupe | Apple | Cherry |
| Blueberry | Orange | Apricot | Grapefruit |
| Peach | Pear | Grape | Plum |
| Strawberry | Tangerine | Peanut | Sunflower |
| | | Watermelon | |
| **Condiments:** | | | |
| Black Pepper | Chili Pepper | Lemon | Cinnamon |
| Garlic | Ginger | Lime | Clove |
| Mustard | Nutmeg | Olive | Cocoa |
| Safflower | Sage | Chocolate | |
| White Pepper | Sesame | | |
| | Vanilla | | |

**Beverages:**

Beverages should also be rotated.

©1997 Immuno Laboratories Inc.

# Food Family Chart

**Meat:** beef, cow's milk, goat's milk, pork, lamb

**Fowl:** chicken, turkey, duck, goose, eggs,

**Freshwater fish:** bass, perch, pike, salmon, trout

**Saltwater fish:** anchovy, cod, eel, herring, mackerel, mullet, sardine, sole, tuna

**Crustacean:** crab, lobster, shrimp

**Mollusks:** clams, mussels, oyster, scallop

**Grass:** barley, corn, kamut, malt, millet, oat, quinoa, rice, rye, spelt, wheat, wild rice

**Legumes:** beans, lentil, peanut, peas, soybean, tamarind, alfalfa sprouts, licorice, carob

**Mustard greens:** broccoli, Brussels sprout, cabbage, cauliflower, horseradish, kale, kohlrabi, mustard greens, mustard seed, radish, turnip, watercress

**Parsley:** anise, caraway, carrot, celery, celeriac, chervil, coriander, cumin, dill, lovage, parsley, parsnip

**Potato:** cayenne, chili pepper, eggplant, paprika, peppers, potatoes, white potatoes, tobacco

**Lily:** asparagus, chive, garlic, leek, onion

**Sunflower (aster):** artichoke, chicory, endive, Jerusalem artichoke, dandelion, tarragon, chamomile, sunflower, safflower, yarrow

**Beet:** beet, chard, spinach, sugar beet

**Buckwheat:** buckwheat, rhubarb, sorrel

**Laurel:** avocado, camphor, cinnamon, bay leaf

**Melon:** cantaloupe, cucumber, honeydew, pumpkin, squash, zucchini

**Plum:** almond, apricot, cherry, nectarine, peach, plum

**Citrus:** citron, grapefruit, lemon, lime, orange, tangerine

**Banana:** arrowroot, banana, plantain

**Palm:** coconut, date, date sugar

**Grape:** grape, raisin, cream of tartar

**Rose:** blackberry, loganberry, raspberry, rosehip, strawberry

**Apple:** apple, loquat, pear, quince

**Blueberry:** blueberry, cranberry, huckleberry

**Cashew:** cashew, mango, pistachio

**Nuts:** Brazil nut, pecan, walnut

**Beech:** beechnut, chestnut

**Birch:** filbert, hazelnut

**Walnut:** butternut, hickory nut, pecan, walnut

meat, fish, vegetables, fruit, and a few seeds. "You ate different foods in the spring, summer, fall, and winter and never had too much. You also did not load up on any one item," says Dr. Hoffer. However, modern agriculture and processing advances now allow us to eat an abundance of the same foods, especially grains, every day of the year. "Today, you may find 100 cereals in the supermarket, but they're all made from corn, wheat, rice, sugar, and artificial color," explains Dr.

Hoffer. "If you overload the gut with one particular item, for instance bread three times a day, then eventually the body breaks down." Malnourishment and a leaky gut are elements of this breakdown.

Leon Chaitow, N.D., D.O., of London, England, speculates that the change away from a caveman-type diet over the centuries is associated with the increase in allergies worldwide. Lending weight to this theory is the fact that it is precisely those foods our cave-dwelling ancestors did not eat—cereal grains, dairy products, and modern processed foods—that most frequently provoke allergic reactions

The Stone Age diet requires eating only seasonal produce as well as protein foods, such as meat, fish, and seeds, and few grains and processed foods. No food chemicals or additives are allowed. Dr. Chaitow reports that patients following the Stone Age diet report impressive results. "In the majority of cases, most allergy problems vanish after a few weeks of eating this way. And with many patients, a gradual reintroduction of the offending foods is possible on a rotating basis."

### Proper Food Combining

If your food allergies/sensitivities are caused by poor digestion, which allows food molecules to escape the gut barrier, proper food combining may help restore healthy digestion. The general rule, according to Patrick Donovan, N.D., of Cancer Centers of America, in Seattle, Washington, is that proteins and carbohydrates are never eaten at the same time (rice is an exception). Proteins may be eaten with non-starchy vegetables; carbohydrates (grains, starchy vegetables) may be eaten with all vegetables as well as legumes. Fruits must be eaten alone, usually as a snack; the same is true with dairy products.

"The rational for this approach is the difference in digestion time for various food groups," Dr. Donovan explains. "Digestion is optimal if foods eaten together have roughly the same digestion time." Many alternative medicine practitioners have found that food combining helps patients avoid gas, belching, and bloating, which is often caused when sugars (carbohydrates) ferment in the gut because the stomach is busy processing fats. However, some studies have shown that food combining isn't necessarily effective—certain foods may still not be properly absorbed, even if you follow the combining rules. Once again, the efficacy of this diet depends on individual response and various biochemical factors. Your doctor can help you decide whether this may be an effective therapy for your condition.

### Anti-Lectin Diets

This diet is based on Dr. Peter D'Adamo's recommendations in *Eat Right*

*4 Your Type*. Blood types A and B should both avoid tomatoes, which is called a panhemaglutinan because it contains lectins that can agglutinate every blood type. However, blood types O and AB can generally tolerate tomatoes. Even people who do not have allergic symptoms experience health-promoting improvements on the anti-lectin diet. For instance, I have a patient who runs marathons and claims a 29-minute decrease in his marathon time that he attributes to the anti-lectin diet alone.

**Diet for Blood Type A**—Avoid the following foods and products containing these foods, because they harbor lectins that can be confused for type B blood antigens:

■ Whole cow's milk and dairy products, including most cheeses, cream cheese, butter, and buttermilk, which contain sugars called D-galactosamine, a primary building block of type B antigen. Fermented low-fat or nonfat milk products are usually tolerable, including goat's milk and yogurt, cow's milk yogurt, kefir, nonfat sour cream, and cultured dairy products (mozzarella, ricotta, string cheese). Soy milk and soy cheeses are well tolerated.

■ Corn, cottonseed, peanut, sesame, and safflower oils
■ Kidney, lima, navy, and garbanzo beans
■ Whole-wheat and wheat products (sprouted wheats and grains are allowed)
■ Tomatoes, potatoes, sweet potatoes, yams, cabbage, and olives (olive oil is permitted)

**Diet for Blood Type B**—Avoid the following foods and products containing these foods, because they harbor lectins that can be confused for type A blood antigens:

■ Chicken (eggs are allowed because the damaging lectin is found in muscle tissue), shellfish (crab, lobster, shrimp, mussels, etc.)
■ Peanuts, sesame seeds, and sunflower seeds
■ Lentils, garbanzo beans, pinto beans, and black-eyed peas
■ Wheat (sprouted is excepted), rye, corn, and buckwheat
■ Tomatoes, olives (olive oil is permitted)
■ Coconut, persimmons, pomegranates, prickly pears, rhubarb, starfruit
■ White and black pepper

**Diet for Blood Type AB**—On the whole, individuals with type AB blood can tolerate most foods, because they do not possess antibodies to any blood antigens. However, this blood type is still susceptible to damage caused by some dietary lectins. Dairy products usually are acceptable,

For **bloods test that can help you identify allergenic lectins**, contact: Peter D'Adamo, N.D., Blood Type Test (available to public), P.O. Box 2106, Norwalk, CT 06852-2106. Meridian Valley Laboratory, 515 West Harrison, Suite 9, Kent, WA 98042; tel: 253-859-8700; fax: 253-859-1135; website: www.meridianvalleylab.com.

but if you experience signs of respiratory problems, sinus attacks, or ear infections, this may be due to intolerances or allergy to milk products. In that case, reduce your consumption of these foods. Avoid the following foods and products that contain these foods:

- Chicken (eggs are allowed), sole, and flounder
- Filbert nuts, poppy seeds, pumpkin seeds, sesame seeds, and sunflower seeds
- Kidney, lima, and garbanzo beans, and black-eyed peas
- Buckwheat and corn
- Banana and tropical fruits (except for pineapple)

**Diet for Blood Type O**—Avoid the following foods and products containing these foods, because they harbor lectins that can be confused for either type A and type B blood antigens:

- Wheat, rye, oat, and all gluten-containing foods (sprouted grains are permitted)
- Cabbage, Brussels sprouts, cauliflower, mustard greens, eggplant, potato, corn, alfalfa sprouts, mushrooms, and olives
- Blackberries and coconut

### Anti-*Candida* Diet

Although alternative medicine physicians sometimes include conventional or natural antifungal medications in severe cases of candidiasis, diet is always an important part of the cure. While diet does not get rid of yeast, it does make it harder for the unfriendly bacteria to thrive.

Traditionally, anti-*Candida* diets are based on avoidance of all sugar products since yeast thrives on sugar, alcohol (composed of fermented and refined sugar), white flour, fermented and aged food products, and anything containing yeast. As meat, poultry, and milk products may contain traces of the antibiotics routinely fed to conventionally raised farm animals, the consumption of organic meat and poultry (without antibiotics or hormones) is recommended. For allergy sufferers, it is prudent to avoid foods with yeast-stimulating molds (cheeses, grapes, fermented foods, and mushrooms), as well as environmental molds to which you may now be more susceptible.

Brad Rachman, D.C., of Fort Myers, Florida, has found the following program useful for treating candidiasis and easier for patients to follow than some of the more restrictive diets.

**Beneficial Foods**—Chicken, turkey, lamb, cold-water fish such as salmon, halibut, and mackerel; all types of beans, lentils, and dried peas; unsweetened live-culture yogurt, milk substitutes such as rice milk, nut milk, and soy beverages; white potatoes, sweet potatoes; brown rice, tapioca, buckwheat, gluten-free products made with millet, corn, soy, and arrowroot; unsweetened fresh or frozen fruits, canned fruits packed in water; almonds, cashews, pecans, and walnuts and butters made from these nuts; pumpkin, sesame, sunflower, and squash seeds and spreads made from these seeds; expeller-pressed, unrefined canola, flaxseed, and olive oils; all vegetables, and freshly prepared vegetable juices.

For more **therapies that fight *Candida* overgrowth**, see Chapter 7: Healing Leaky Gut Syndrome, pp. 184-211, and Chapter 8: Intestinal Detoxification, pp. 212-235.

**Foods to Avoid**—Beef, pork, cold cuts, frankfurters, sausage, canned meats; eggs; milk, cream, cheese, ice cream, nondairy creamers; all products made with wheat, wheat gluten, wheat flour, oats, spelt, kamut, rye, barley, amaranth, quinoa; coffee, black teas, cocoa, Postum, soda, alcoholic beverages, citrus juices, sweetened fruit juices; strawberries, dried fruit, citrus fruits; peanuts; margarine, shortening, refined oils; bottled salad dressings and spreads, butter (unless clarified); canned or creamed soups and vegetables; and fried foods.

**Herbal Adjuncts**—Also helpful for removing yeast is a formula called Candacin, containing grapefruit seed extract, black walnut, goldenseal, and bear berry leaf. Chlorophyll tablets can chemically create an internal environment that is not conducive to *Candida* growth. The herb pau d'arco has also proven helpful in fighting *Candida*, as have aloe vera and biotin, a B vitamin (take with the other B-complex vitamins).

Dr. Braly gives his candidiasis patients caprylic acid, a fatty acid found in coconut oil, before relying on conventional antifungal medications. However, many alternative medicine physicians find that pharmaceuticals such as Diflucan are the best treatment for primary *Candida* overgrowth. If you are taking antifungal drugs, supplementing with the probiotics *Lactobacillus acidophilus* and *Bifidobacterium bifidum* cultures is recommended.

**Brad Rachman, D.C.**: Healthy Living Enterprises, Inc. 12734 Kenwood Lane, Suite 77, Fort Myers, FL 33907; tel: 941-275-3575 or 888-333-5935; fax: 941-275-8694. For **Candacin**, contact: Metagenics, Inc., 971 Calle Negocio, San Clemente, CA 92673; tel: 800-692-9400 or 949-366-0818; website: www.metagenics.com. For **supergreen concentrates**, contact: Nutricology, Inc., Allergy Research Group, 30806 Santana Street, Hayward, CA 94544; tel: 800-545-9960 (info), 800-782-4272 (orders), or 510-487-8526; website: www.nutricology.com. New Spirit Naturals, Inc. P.O. Box 3300, San Dimas, CA 91773; tel: 800-922-2766; fax: 909-599-4035. For **organic, low-fat meats**, contact: Laura's Lean Beef, 2285 Executive Drive, Suite 202, Lexington, KY 40505; tel: 800-ITS-LEAN (487-5326) or 606-299-7707; fax: 606-299-6822; website: www.laurasleanbeef.com.

# Healing Leaky Gut Syndrome

**A** HEALTHY INTESTINAL TRACT is a dual-functioning system: it must allow nutrients to pass unhindered into the body with maximum absorption while simultaneously insuring that the toxins within the tract are not absorbed and allowed to contaminate tissues, glands, and organs. But when the structural integrity of the intestines breaks down, a condition known as intestinal permeability or "leaky gut syndrome" develops, which allows undigested food proteins and other toxins to enter the bloodstream. The immune system recognizes these undigested proteins as foreign substances, and sends antibodies to attack these "invaders" and neutralize them. In leaky gut, an endless supply of toxins escape into the blood, overwhelming the immune system, sparking allergic reactions, and accumulating in soft tissues, in joints, and elsewhere.

Inflammatory bowel disease, such as Crohn's disease and ulcerative colitis, and arthritis are among the many inflammatory conditions caused by these allergic reactions.

Restoring gut barrier function involves three components: healing the gut, improving digestion, and detoxifying the digestive tract. This chapter will present therapies that help repair intestinal permeability, with a focus on restoring the balance of intestinal microflora and replenishing the supply of digestive enzymes and hydrochloric acid. Chapter 8: Intestinal Detoxification focuses on therapies that further support your intestinal barrier function and immune function by eliminating parasites and toxins from your intestinal system.

## In This Chapter

- Success Story: Throwing Away the Ritalin
- Restoring Intestinal Integrity
- Hypothyroidism and Malabsorption
- Hypochlorhydria and Maldigestion
- Enzyme Deficiency and Leaky Gut
- Illuminating the *Candida* Connection
- Ridding the Body of *Candida* Overgrowth

# Success Story: Throwing Away the Ritalin

Caroline was a six-year-old girl who couldn't sit still at school. Caroline's mastery of speech was delayed, she had a chronically runny nose, and she was on Ritalin for her hyperactivity. By the time her parents sought help from Constantine A. Kotsanis, M.D., medical director of the MindBody Health Center International in Grapevine, Texas, her doctors were on the verge of clinically diagnosing her with attention deficit disorder (ADD). Furthermore, her teacher recommended that she find another school to attend.

Dr. Kotsanis doesn't like putting medically convenient labels, such as ADD, on children because it can stigmatize the child and often it obscures the real causes of the heightened or uncontrolled activity. Many times one of those real causes is an undiagnosed allergy, as it turned out to be with Caroline.

Her parents first noticed she had a problem at age seven months, when she had a high fever accompanied by a seizure. This continued intermittently until she was 18 months old. When she was four years old, Caroline had frequent urinary infections and was diagnosed with hyperactivity and borderline ("high function") autism. At this point, she was put on Ritalin. By the time her parents found Dr. Kotsanis, two years later, they were eager to get their child off the drug.

In studying Caroline's face, Dr. Kotsanis saw many familiar signs of unresolved allergies. The nasal drip, for example, was indicative of mold and food allergies, says Dr. Kotsanis. A skin prick test for IgE and IgG antibodies confirmed that Caroline had allergies to several foods, tree pollens, and glycerin.

Dr. Kotsanis took Caroline off all sugar products, both natural and synthetic, and had her avoid all milk products, food dyes, white flour, gluten, and canned and processed foods. Dr. Kotsanis also asked Caroline's parents to feed her exclusively at home using organically raised produce. In consultation with Jay Apte, a specialist in Ayurvedic (SEE QUICK DEFINITION) nutrition on the MindBody Health Center's staff, Dr. Kotsanis also decided to have Caroline avoid all cold foods and any foods that would

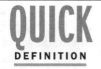

**DEFINITION**

**Ayurveda** is the traditional medicine of India, based on many centuries of empirical use. Its name means "end of the Vedas" (which were India's sacred scripts), implying that a holistic medicine may be founded on spiritual principles. Ayurveda describes three metabolic, constitutional, and body types (*doshas*), in association with the basic elements of Nature in combination. These are *vata* (air and ether, rooted in intestines), *pitta* (fire and water/stomach), and *kapha* (water and earth/lungs). Ayurvedic physicians use these categories (which also have psychological aspects) as the basis for prescribing individualized formulas of herbs, diet, massage, breathing, meditation, exercise and yoga postures, and detoxification techniques.

create mucus in the body, such as dairy and "junk" foods.

To get a more detailed understanding of Caroline's digestive system and nutrient absorption, Dr. Kotsanis ordered a comprehensive stool analysis. This gave him the information he needed to prescribe specialized nutrients to correct the digestive underpinnings of Caroline's symptoms. The analysis showed that Caroline had a malabsorption problem and an overgrowth of the yeast *Candida albicans*.

For more on **digestive stool analysis and other tests**, see Chapter 3: Allergy/Sensitivity Testing, pp. 70-105. For more on **homeopathic antigens**, see Chapter 13: Desensitizing the Immune System, pp. 328-347.

To address the *Candida*, Dr. Kotsanis started Caroline on a short-term dose of Nystatin, a conventional drug for fungal infections, which she took in capsule form two times daily for four weeks. He also gave her a series of four injections, at two-month intervals, containing homeopathic remedies to desensitize her against food, inhalant, mold, and dander allergens. Typically, a patient receives 11 shots during a three-year period, then goes on to a maintenance schedule of occasional injections. The homeopathic remedies (also called homeopathic antigens because they're made from the allergens themselves) are low potency and "piggy-backed" onto shark cartilage as a carrier.

Next, he gave her Permeability Factors, ¹/₂ capsule, three times daily between meals for six weeks, followed by the same dosage for one week per month for one year. This is a "nutritional stabilizing formula" containing amino acids, oils, and vitamins derived from marine sources, borage and rice bran oils, and lecithin. Its purpose is to regulate the lining and activity of the gastrointestinal tract, especially the intestines, where food allergies often begin.

Dr. Kotsanis also put Caroline on UltraFlora Plus, ¹/₄ teaspoon, two times daily in four ounces of warm water for six weeks, then up to ¹/₂ teaspoon, two times daily for six weeks. The purpose of this formula is to replenish beneficial bacteria (such as *Lactobacillus acidophilus*) in the intestines and thereby improve the absorption of nutrients made possible by these bacteria, says Dr. Kotsanis.

To enhance digestion in the stomach and small intestine, Dr. Kotsanis started Caroline on Vital Zymes, an enzyme mixture, taken once daily just before lunch. A nutrient formula called Super Nu-Thera®, specifically developed for hyperactive children and containing vitamin B6 (and other B vitamins), magnesium, and additional key nutrients, was next on Dr. Kotsanis' program for Caroline. Super Nu-Thera #200 Nutrient Powder was given at the rate of ¹/₈ teaspoon once daily, building to twice daily, then to ¹/₂ teaspoon daily for at least six weeks.

Research reported by Bernard Rimland, Ph.D., of the Autism Research Institute in San Diego, California, indicates that 30% to

40% of autistic children (out of a test group of 200) responded favorably to high-dose vitamin B6 in combination with magnesium, two nutrients often found to benefit allergic conditions. Improvements included better eye contact, fewer tantrums, more interest in the outer world, and more normal behavior in general.

Over the years, Dr. Kotsanis has perceived similarities between symptoms and causes of such seemingly different problems as autism, hyperactivity, attention deficit disorder, and learning impairments. He construes these conditions as part of a larger category of sensory developmental disorders that he calls Sensory Deficit Syndrome. "We do not medicate symptoms to cover them up," says Dr. Kotsanis. "We address the root cause of the breakdown." These include food/environmental sensitivities and allergies, nutritional deficiencies, bowel dysfunction, sensory hypersensitivity, and metabolic anomalies. "The therapies we prescribe for this are holistic and natural, and address digestive, immune, endocrine, and neurological system integrity."

For best results, timing is crucial, emphasizes Dr. Kotsanis. "Nutrition is the first step, then allergy elimination and immune stabilization, followed by gross-sensory integration, visual prism lenses, and finally, auditory training." As part of her sensory integration training, Dr. Kotsanis had Caroline brush her skin (torso and extremities, but not head or genitals) in a circular fashion every two hours using a dry stiff brush. Ideally, she was to do the brushing while performing a balancing exercise or walking in a straight line. This stimulates multiple senses simultaneously.

In autism, Dr. Kostsanis explains, the brain is underaroused. "The brain needs to be stimulated to balance out the hyperactivity of the muscles. Ritalin is routinely given to wake up the brain, but it doesn't accomplish anything useful in the long run. For long-term success, you must replace what is missing in the child's body. Correct the physiology and the body chemistry and give the right nutrients in the right proportions—but don't forget the physics. This is why we give filtered sound therapy."

**Constantine A. Kotsanis, M.D.:** MindBody Health Center International, Baylor Medical Plaza, 1600 W. College St., Suite 260, Grapevine, TX 76051; tel: 817-481-3131; fax: 817-488-8903. For **Permeability Factors**, contact: Tyler Encapsulations, 2204-8 N.W. Birdsale, Gresham, OR 97030; tel: 800-869-9705 or 503-661-5401; fax: 503-666-4913. For **Vital Zymes**, contact: Klaire Labs, Inc., 1573 W. Seminole, San Marco, CA 92069; tel: 800-533-7255 or 619-744-9680; fax: 619-744-9364. For **Super Nu-Thera® #200 Nutrient Powder**, contact: Family Resource Services, 231 Columbia 61, P.O. Box 1146, Magnolia, AR 71753; tel: 800-501-0139; fax: 501-234-9021. For **UltraFlora Plus**, contact: Metagenics West, Inc., 12445 East 39th Avenue, Suite 402, Denver, CO 80239; tel: 303-371-6848 or 800-321-6382; fax: 303-371-9303; website: www.metagenics.com.

Using this audio enhancement technique, which involves music, Dr. Kotsanis has a special device that filters out certain frequencies to which the patient is hypersensitive. After a while, the patient's hearing normalizes on these frequencies. "Patients like Caroline are usually hypersensitive to loud noises; this technique helps to retrain them to listen more selectively, and it teaches their auditory system to communicate with the environment," says Dr. Kotsanis. He has used this process to transform nonverbal children into speaking ones. Often, they emerge with better socialization skills as well as eating and sleeping patterns, he adds.

Dr. Kotsanis' multifaceted program for Caroline yielded successful results. By the time of her second homeopathic antigen injection (about one month after beginning treatment), she was stable and calm enough to be taken off the Ritalin, which she had been receiving at 10 mg daily. Caroline's school behavior, which formerly her teachers had rated as "terrible," now quickly improved to "good" and her teachers began remarking "how well she was doing," recalls Dr. Kotsanis.

Caroline's mother reported that her daughter's speech abilities grew quickly and, after about five months on the program, expanded from one or two words at a time to full sentences. Caroline was also able to sit still for up to 2$^1/_2$ hours of special education classes, whereas formerly the most she could manage before fidgeting was ten minutes. She sleeps much better at night and can fall asleep now without the presence of a parent. Caroline no longer needs diapers and is able to play with other children, where before she could not.

# Restoring Intestinal Integrity

Naturopathic physicians and other holistically oriented doctors use various approaches to strengthen the digestive functions of the intestines.

### Dietary Tips to Reduce Leaky Gut Syndrome

Here are two key dietary adjustments that can make a significant difference to the operation of your intestines:

■ Avoid alcohol, foods containing antibiotic residues (animal proteins, including dairy products, except those designated organic and free-range) and artificial substances (which can irritate the intestinal lining), foods known to be allergenic to you, sources of dietary lectins, sugars, and refined foods. Instead, use organically grown foods whenever possible. While completely abstaining from alcohol and sugar may seem unrealistically austere, even a substantial reduction of these substances in your diet will produce beneficial results.

■ Eat with awareness. Eat and chew slowly, chew thoroughly until the food is liquified, and try to be conscious of the fact you are consuming foods. Begin the digestive process in a state of calm with appreciation of the sensory qualities of the foods. Consider using chopsticks instead of a knife and fork; the chopsticks will slow you down and induce a more contemplative approach to eating. If you eat with your right hand, switch to your left. Put down your fork between bites and take smaller bites. When you're eating, do nothing else—don't watch TV, don't read the newspaper—eat with purpose to heal yourself. Drink only a small volume of liquid with meals, because large amounts of liquid dilutes digestive juices, rendering digestion less effective.

**Low-Salt Water**—In a 1999 study published in *Dermatology*, 12 patients with atopic dermatitis and leaky gut syndrome drank and topically applied low-salt water for 18 days. At the end of this time, all patients had improved intestinal function, as evidenced by the lactulose and mannitol test. Lactulose levels in urine are a good indicator of intestinal permeability. In people with a healthy gut, this sugar is excreted in feces, while in people with a leaky gut, lactulose is excreted in the urine. In this study, all 12 patients had an average 55% decrease in lactulose in their urine, indicating reduced intestinal permeability.[1] Exactly why this is effective is unknown. However, we do know that hypotonic (low-salt) solutions cause tissues to swell in order to equilibrate with the salt concentration of the water being applied. It appears that this would result in moisturizing the bowel, helping to repair the gut membrane.

### Herbs and Botanicals to Decrease Leaky Gut

**Ginkgo biloba**—The ginkgo tree is one of the oldest living trees on earth. Its leaves contain biochemical compounds responsible for ginkgo's healing properties.[2] Clinical and laboratory tests have shown that standardized *Ginkgo biloba* extract has significant benefit in the treatment of increased intestinal permeability, as well as many other health problems associated with inadequate blood supply. Ginkgo protects the intestine by reducing the oxidative damage in the intestinal lining due to free-radical (SEE QUICK DEFINITION) activity. Recommended dosage: 300 mg, two times daily.

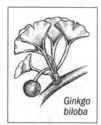

Ginkgo
biloba

# QUICK

## DEFINITION

A **free radical** is an unstable molecule of oxygen that destroys healthy molecules. The process develops when molecules within cells react with oxygen, or oxidize. Free radicals then begin to break down cells, especially the cell membranes, and can harmfully alter proteins, enzymes, and even DNA.

The **arachidonic acid cascade** is a chemical reaction occuring in cell membranes that results in the production of molecules such as prostaglandins and leukotrienes that cause many negative physiological reactions. These include bronchial constriction (in asthmatics), intestinal permeability or leakiness, water retention and swelling, allergies, inflammation, and, ultimately, tissue destruction. Arachidonic acid is a fatty acid found primarily in animal foods such as meat, poultry, and dairy products. When the diet is abundant with arachidonic acids, these are stored in cell membranes; an enzyme transforms these stored fatty acids into chemical messengers called prostaglandins and leukotrienes that instigate inflammation.

## CAUTION

Because licorice root mimics some of the adrenal hormones so closely, it can cause retention of sodium and water and thus raise blood pressure. This is not normally a concern, but if you tend to have a blood pressure problem, it is best to use a type of deglycyrrhizinated licorice (DGL), which will help in the regeneration of stomach and intestinal cells, without the increase in water retention.

**Khella (*Ammi visnaga*)**—Khella is an under-utilized herb in the treatment of leaky gut syndrome. The use of khella was part of the Bedouin folk medicine for centuries. Khellin, the chief active component, inhibits the release of histamine, which otherwise induces an inflammatory response, and also has anti-spasmodic properties.[3] The allopathic antihistamine drug Intal® is based on this ancient remedy.

**Chinese Skullcap or Scute (*Scutellaria baicalensis*)**—Japanese research has yielded new information that Chinese skullcap has significant anti-allergenic and antioxidant properties.[4] The active ingredient, baicalin, is responsible for its anti-inflammatory action. Chinese skullcap has been shown to block highly inflammatory end products of the arachidonic acid cascade (SEE QUICK DEFINITION).

**Licorice Root (*Glycyrrhiza glabra*)**—Licorice is a traditional herbal remedy with an ancient history. Modern research has shown that it has beneficial effects on the endocrine system, adrenal glands, and liver; it is also a systemic anti-inflammatory.[5] The anti-irritant effect on the gastrointestinal system is thought to be due to flavonoid derivatives of licorice called steroidal saponin glycosides, which exert a protective effect. Licorice root is used internationally for its anti-ulcer and healing effects on the gastrointestinal system.[6]

### Demulcent Herbs and Foods

*Demulcent* is a term used by herbalists to describe an herb that has a protective effect on the mucous membranes. Most of the herbs that contain demulcents have large amounts of mucilaginous materials—gummy, slimy chemicals that have a direct action on the lining of the intestines, soothing irritations. In general, all mucilage-containing demulcents minimize irritation down the whole length of the bowel, reducing the sensitivity of the digestive system to gastric acids, relaxing painful spasms, and decreasing leaky gut and digestive inflammation and ulceration.[7]

**Marshmallow (*Althea officinalis*)—**Marshmallow root contains 25% to 35% mucilage. The root of the plant is used by herbalists for any inflammation of the gastrointestinal system. It is usually taken as a tea: take several teaspoons of the root or leaves, cover it with boiling water, and steep for 20-30 minutes to extract all the medicinal components. Six cups of this tea a day can be useful in severe cases of leaky gut.

**Slippery Elm Bark (*Ulmus fulva*)—**Slippery elm bark has traditionally been used in the treatment of ulcers, colitis, irritable bowel, infections, and diarrhea.[8] Slippery elm is available as tinctures or capsules, or a decoction can be made where the bark is very gently simmered, one part of the bark to eight quarts of water; bring to a boil and let it simmer for 20-30 minutes; drink 2-3 cups a day.

**Cabbage Juice—**Raw, green, organic cabbage juice contains high amounts of glutamine, an essential amino acid that aids in the metabolism of gastrointestinal cells. Cabbage juice can be made in combination with other vegetables that are effective in reconstructing a healthy gut mucosa, such as chickweed and plantain banana. Four to eight ounces a day is generally advisable.

**Fenugreek—**Crushed fenugreek seeds contain 28% mucilin and makes an excellent demulcent. Fenugreek seeds can be steeped as a tea or used in capsules. To make tea, use one teaspoon of fenugreek to one cup of water. In capsule form, typically take one capsule (250 mg) 2-3 times daily with hot water.

## Anti-Inflammatory and Astringent Herbs
Anti-inflammatory herbs help to reduce localized tissue swelling and inflammation in the gut. Astringent herbs tighten and tonify tissues, thus sealing the permeable intestines.

**Meadowsweet (*Filipendulia ulmaria*)—**Meadowsweet contains anti-inflammatory glycosides, tannins, mucilage, and flavonoids. The anti-inflammatory properties in combination with other effects makes meadowsweet one of the prime herbs in the treatment of ulcers or other problems with the gastrointestinal system. Its astringent properties allow this herb to strengthen the connective tissue bonds between the cells of the gastrointestinal tract, thus solidifying the protective barrier, which helps to decrease leaky gut. Meadowsweet is a powerful astringent and can actually help stop bleeding in the digestive tract. Typical recommended dosage: 250 mg, twice daily.

**Chamomile (*Matricaria chamomilia*)**—The flower of the chamomile plant produces a calming effect, easing anxiety and reducing tension. It can be helpful with overall anxiety, sleep disorders, and muscle tension, and its calming properties have a beneficial effect on the gastrointestinal system as well. In addition, it stimulates digestive secretions, so it can improve digestive function. In Europe, chamomile is

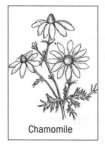
Chamomile

recognized as a digestive aid, a mild sedative, and an anti-inflammatory, notably in antibacterial oral hygiene and skin preparations.[9] Its anti-inflammatory properties also reduce allergic responses. In Germany, chamomile is licensed as an over-the-counter drug for internal use against gastrointestinal spasms and inflammatory diseases of the intestinal tract. Chamomile's Latin name, *Matricaria chamomilia*, means "mother of the gut." Typical dosage: 250 mg, 2-3 times daily.

**Goldenseal (*Hydrastis canadensis*)**—One of the most widely used American herbs, goldenseal is considered to be a tonic remedy that stimulates immune response and is a germ destroyer as well. In addition, because of its astringent effects, goldenseal can help in many digestive problems, from peptic ulcers to colitis.[10] It promotes the production and secretion of digestive juices. Goldenseal's germ-fighting properties are due to berberine. Berberine is effective against bacteria, protozoa, and fungi, including *Staphylococcus*, *Streptococcus*, *Candida*, and *Giardia lamblia*.[11] Berberine has also been shown to increase immune function by activating the white blood cells that digest cell debris and other waste matter in the blood.[12] Physicians often recommend the use of berberine-rich substitutes for goldenseal (such as barberry), because over-harvesting is a major problem with this herb. Goldenseal also contains alkaloids and tannins that support the intestinal barrier and is considered a major herb for treating chronic gastrointestinal inflammatory conditions. Goldenseal also stimulates epithelial surfaces to make new cells. Typical recommended dosage: 250 mg, 2-3 times daily.

### Other Nutrients for Leaky Gut
**Quercetin**—Quercetin is a naturally occurring bioflavonoid (vitamin C helper) found in many species of plants, including oak, onion, and blue-green algae. As a bioflavonoid, it has powerful antioxidant and

## Chinese Herbal Combinations for Leaky Gut

A good herbal remedy for leaky gut is to combine ginkgo, quercetin, scutellaria, khella, and okra with any of the Chinese patent medicines mentioned below. These formulas work well in combination with herbs; especially good pre-formulated combinations including Gastro Guard from Nature's Answer and Robert's Formula from Phyto-Pharmica or Naturopathic Formulations (available at health food stores). In Chinese medicine, there are several excellent patent formulas that have a soothing effect on the digestive system:

**Pill Curing Formula**—Pill Curing Formula helps cramping, abdominal pain, diarrhea, irritation, and mucusy stools. Some physicians call it the alternative to Pepto Bismal. It is made up of many ingredients, including coix seed, atractylodes, chrysanthemum flowers, and citrus peel.

**Chinese patent medicines** are available in most Chinese pharmacies. For information about the patent medicines mentioned here, contact: Lin's Sister, 4 Bowery Street, New York, NY 10013; tel: 212-962-5417. For **Gastro Guard**, contact: Nature's Answer, 320 Oser Avenue, Hauppauge, NY 11788; tel: 800-439-2324 or 516-231-7492; fax: 516-231-8391. For **Robert's Formula**, contact: Phyto-Pharmica, P.O. Box 1745, Green Bay, WI 54305; tel: 800-558-7372 or 920-469-9099; fax: 920-469-4418.

**Shenling Baizhupian**— Shenling Baizhupian is a classic patent medicine formula for digestion, erratic loose stools, and symptoms of irritable bowel. It includes codonopsis, wild yam root, citrus peel, and licorice root.

**Yunnan Paiyao**—Yunnan Paiyao is a valuable first-aid remedy for internal and external bleeding; studies indicate that it can cause blood to clot 33% faster. The main ingredient is pseudo ginseng root. When taken internally, Yunnan Paiyao has been shown to stop internal bleeding in the gastrointestinal system and is used for the treatment of gastrointestinal inflammation.

anti-inflammatory properties and has been used by alternative practitioners for many years in the treatment of arthritis, autoimmune diseases, asthma, and cataracts. Quercetin blocks inflammation that can otherwise lead to leaky gut syndrome. Quercetin has an excellent affinity for the gut and, in the treatment of leaky gut syndrome, it represents one of nature's most perfect medicines. By decreasing the rapid opening of mast cells and basophils—white blood cells that release histamines—quercetin stabilizes the gut and decreases permeability. Typical dosage: 200 mg, 2-3 times daily between meals.

**Glutamine**—The amino acid glutamine is an important nutrient for the intestinal mucosa. An increase in the diet of L-glutamine has been shown to support gastrointestinal mucus integrity.[13] Glutamine reduces unwanted movement of bacterial forms through the permeable intestinal wall and into general circulation, where they can often instigate inflammatory conditions or bowel disease.[14] Glutamine is used in the synthesis of an important nutrient known as N-acetyl-D-glucosamine (NAG), which is fundamental to the production of the protective mucus lining the digestive and respiratory tracts and the first line of defense against leaky gut syndrome. Glutamine supplementation also enhances glutathione, an important antioxidant.[15] Typical recommended dosage for patients with leaky gut syndrome: 3,000-10,000 mg per day, in divided doses between meals.

**Glutathione—**Glutathione is a small protein consisting of three amino acids that functions as a principle antioxidant, scavenging free radicals and toxins that would otherwise damage and destroy cells. Further, glutathione regulates the activities of other antioxidants, such as vitamins A, C, and E. Vitamin C can also help increase glutathione levels.[16] When the body is overrun by free radicals, supplies of glutathione become depleted. This condition—known as oxidative stress—negatively affects the musculoskeletal, nervous, immune, and endocrine systems and may underlie many of the symptoms associated with allergy. Glutathione exerts another protective and scavenging role in concert with the liver, the body's primary organ of detoxification. In the liver, glutathione quenches free radicals as a way of neutralizing them and securing their elimination from the body. In addition, glutathione must be present for white blood cells to perform their function of immune regulation. Some studies have shown that the absorption of oral glutathione supplements is limited.[17] However, several studies refute this conclusion, finding that oral glutathione is indeed absorbed by the body.[18] Glutathione is best absorbed orally when combined with anthocyanidins (bioflavonoids found in such fruits as berries)—in fact, it increases its oral activity by more than 100 times. You can also increase the availability of glutathione by increasing the precursors that the body needs to manufacture it, including foods in the cabbage family as well as onions and garlic.

For more about **glutathione**, see Chapter 10: Supporting the Respiratory System, pp. 260-277.

For **glutathione supplements combined with anthocyanidins**, contact: Tyler Encapsulations, 2204-8 N.W. Birdsale, Gresham, OR 97030; tel: 800-869-9705 or 503-661-5401; fax: 503-666-4913.

**N-Acetyl-D-Glucosamine—**N-acetyl-D-glucosamine (NAG) is a sugar that is important to the formation of a type of mucus, glycocalyx, that protects the delicate intestinal tissues and acts as a first line of defense against bacteria, fungi, and viruses. These disease-causing microorganisms attempt to adhere to the cell surface and invade the intestinal walls. NAG also functions as a decoy sugar, attracting and binding dietary lectins, which prevents them from attaching to the gut and damaging it. Patients with a compromised gastrointestinal lining are more likely to experience the irritation caused by food allergies, dietary lectins, and bacterial, fungal, and viral organisms. Also, they are more susceptible to the damage due to aspirin, NSAIDs, and the contents of their own intestines, such as bile acid.[19] Again, elevated levels of circulating immune complexes are the end result, which cause inflammation and create serious problems for allergy sufferers. NAG promotes the growth of friendly bacteria and is quickly digested by healthy intestinal bacteria. Typical dosage: 500 mg, three times daily on an empty stomach.

**Vitamins and Minerals—**The nutrients zinc, selenium, ascorbic acid, vitamin E, beta carotene, and vitamin A, the enzymes superoxide dismutase (SOD) and catalase, and the amino acid N-acetyl-cysteine have been shown to quench various types of free radicals. Some intestinal lining damage is due to free radicals, so neutralizing free radicals is beneficial. Not only do the antioxidants help the gut in preventing intestinal damage due to oxidation, but these antioxidants systemically decrease inflammation.

# Hypothyroidism and Malabsorption

The thyroid gland plays a key role in digestion, as it controls the body's metabolic rate. When this gland isn't working properly, due to toxic overload, poor diet, medication use, yeast infections, or stress, it can lead to a sluggish digestive system. Symptoms of hypothyroidism (SEE QUICK DEFINITION) include a number of gastrointestinal problems, including constipation, gas and bloating, abdominal pain, and decreased absorption of nutrients. Decreased digestive efficiency may lead to leaky gut syndrome.

## Alternative Therapies for a Healthy Thyroid
Alternative medicine practitioners generally treat hypothyroidism by strengthening intestinal health and digestion. Proper nutrition and exercise help restore a weakened thyroid. Thyroid glandular

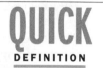

**QUICK DEFINITION**

**Hypothyroidism** is a condition of low or underactive thyroid gland function that can produce numerous symptoms. Among the 47 clinically recognized symptoms: fatigue, depression, lethargy, weakness, weight gain, low body temperature, chills, cold extremities, general inappropriate sensation of cold, infertility, rheumatic pain, menstrual disorders (excessive flow, cramps), repeated infections, colds, upper respiratory infections, skin problems (itching, eczema, psoriasis, acne, dry, coarse, or scaly skin, skin pallor), memory disturbances, concentration difficulties, paranoia, migraines, oversleep, "laziness," muscle aches and weakness, hearing disturbances, burning/prickling sensations, anemia, slow reaction time and mental sluggishness, swelling of the eyelids, constipation, labored or difficult breathing, hoarseness, brittle nails, and poor vision. A resting body temperature (measured in the armpit) below 97.8° F may indicate hypothyroidism. Menstruating women should take the underarm temperature only on the second and third days of menstruation.

therapy and thyroid hormone therapy are two other options available to return the thyroid to normal functioning.

**Dietary Recommendations**—Goitrogens are foods that reduce the release of thyroid hormone. Examples include walnuts, sorghum, cassava, almonds, peanuts, soy flour, millet, and apples. These foods should be avoided by anyone suffering from hypothyroidism. Mustard greens, kale, cabbage, spinach, Brussels sprouts, cauliflower, broccoli, and turnips also have a mild antithyroid effect and should be avoided until the condition is normalized or stabilized.[20]

Thyrotrophs are foods that stimulate thyroid hormone production. Examples include seaweeds (bladderwrack, laminaria, kelp, and dulse), garlic, radishes, watercress, seafood, egg yolks, wheat germ, brewer's yeast, and mushrooms. Fruits and fruit juices (especially tropical varieties), watermelon, and coconut oil are also thyroid-stimulating. A two- to four-week diet of only raw foods, with heavy emphasis on raw greens, seaweed, nuts, sprouted beans and seeds, and freshly extracted juices, is an excellent way to improve thyroid function.

**Vitamins**—A deficiency of vitamin E will reduce iodine absorption by the thyroid by 95%. Iodine is required for optimal thyroid function. Vitamin E deficiency commonly occurs in women during pregnancy and menopause, which may help explain why thyroid disorders are so often triggered by these conditions. A typical recommended dosage is 800-1,200 IU of vitamin E per day.

Hypothyroid patients do not effectively convert beta carotene—the natural form of vitamin A found in yellow and green fruits and vegetables—to a biologically usable form. Vitamin A is necessary for the thyroid to absorb iodine.[21] Most vitamin A supplements are sold in the beta carotene form. As a typical recommendation, patients with impaired thyroid function should take 10,000-20,000 IU of vitamin A daily. Unless closely supervised by a physician, your intake of pure vitamin A should never exceed 20,000 IU per day.

Daily supplementation with vitamins C (3-5 g) and B complex (100-150 mg) can help strengthen the thyroid. Vitamin C deficiency will make capillaries in the thyroid bleed and normal cells in the gland will begin to multiply abnormally, a condition called hyperplasia;[22] B complex is important for keeping all cells, including those of the thyroid, in good health.

**Iodine**—Iodine is essential in the production of thyroid hormones that keep the gland balanced and functioning properly. The best food supplements for iodine are kelp and cod liver oil.[23] Kelp, a type of sea-weed, is best taken in tablet form. Lobster, shrimp, crab, and saltwater fish such as haddock, cod, halibut, and herring, are also good sources of iodine. The recommended daily allowance for iodine is 100 mcg for women and 120 mcg for men. Don't take more than this amount, as too much iodine can suppress the formation of a necessary thyroid hormone (T3). Also, don't use too much table salt, a source of iodine that is also frequently high in sodium. Too much salt can alter the rel-ative concentrations of sodium and potassium in the body, which, in turn, can result in serious disorders, such as heart disease, high blood pressure, and obesity.

**Minerals—**Zinc helps in the conversion of thyroid hormones and increases the sensitivity of cell membranes to these hormones; a typi-cal dose is 25 mg per day along with 3 mg of copper (because zinc tends to deplete copper reserves). With medical supervision, the dosage of zinc can be increased, if necessary; however, dosages should be increased with caution, as too much zinc can interfere with the functioning of the immune system.

Selenium also plays an important role in the conversion of thyroid hormones; the generally recommended dose is 200 mcg per day. In addition, a diet low in iron will cause anemia, which has been found to lead to low thyroid function; typical dose is 100 mcg per day.[24]

**Tyrosine—**The amino acid tyrosine is an important building block of thyroid hormones. Tyrosine is found in soybeans, beef, chicken, fish, carob, bean sprouts, oats, spinach, sesame seeds, and butternut squash. L-tyrosine can also be taken as a nutritional supplement; typical recommended dose is 250-750 mg per day, taken between meals.

**Herbal Therapy—**Gugulipid, an Ayurvedic herb that has been used in India for more than 2,500 years, is helpful for supporting the thyroid. It is derived from the resin of a small myrrh tree native to Asia and is traditionally used for a number of health conditions, including rheumatoid arthritis and high cholesterol. Studies have shown that gugulipid stimulates thyroid function.[25]

*Coleus forskohlii*, a member of the mint family, is another Ayurvedic herb for stimulating the thyroid. Research has shown that the prima-ry active ingredient, forskolin, increases the production of thyroid hormones and stimulates their release.[26]

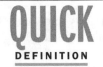

**QUICK**
**DEFINITION**

A **glandular extract** is a purified nutritional and therapeutic product derived from one of several animal glands including the adrenal, thymus, thyroid, ovaries, testes, pancreas, pineal, and pituitary. It is prescribed by a physician for a person whose corresponding gland is underfunctioning and not producing enough of its own hormone.

**Thyroid Glandular Therapy**—While good nutrition is important, some patients require additional help to restore thyroid function, particularly second-generation hypothyroids—patients whose parents also had the disease. In such cases, doctors prescribe desiccated thyroid glandular extract (SEE QUICK DEFINITION) rather than synthetic hormones. Thyroid glandular is usually derived from calves or pigs and contains both types of thyroid hormones (T4 and T3). Thyroid therapy is best undertaken with the guidance of a qualified health-care practitioner.

# Hypochlorhydria and Maldigestion

Many allergy patients, especially those suffering from food sensitivities, are deficient in hydrochloric acid (a conditon known as hypochlorhydria), a stomach acid needed to adequately break down food so that cells can absorb important nutrients. When digestion is incomplete or inadequate, large food molecules can be inappropriately absorbed into the bloodstream, contributing to the onset of allergies and sensitivities. Inside the stomach, a very low pH (acid level) is needed to break down food. To maintain the optimal pH (around 2, which is very acidic), the stomach secretes hydrochloric acid (HCl). With age, HCl levels tend to decline, leading to impaired digestion.

A combination of physical symptoms can indicate low levels of hydrochloric acid or a deficiency in digestive and pancreatic enzymes. If you answer "yes" to at least three of the questions below, your body may not be producing enough HCl or digestive enzymes for optimal digestion.

After eating, do you suffer from:
gas? _____
bloating? _____
abdominal discomfort? _____
undigested food in stool? _____

## Therapies for Insufficient Stomach Acid

If insufficient hydrochloric acid is a factor in your poor digestive function, there are a number of steps you can take to remedy this situation. First, thoroughly chew your food and reduce your stress level at meal times. Take care to avoid excessive amounts of fat and sugar in your diet. Have yourself tested for potential underlying problems, such as adrenal stress, hypothyroidism, or *Helicobacter pylori* infection. You may also want to take bitter herbs to promote the secretion of digestive juices.

For **testing for hydrochloric acid levels**, see Chapter 3: Allergy/Sensitivity Testing, pp. 70-105.

**Bitter Herbs**—Chemicals present in bitter-tasting herbs stimulate the central nervous system (via nerves in the tongue); a message is then sent to the gut to activate a powerful digestive hormone, gastrin.[27] Bitters stimulate the production of hydrochloric acid, increase the liver's production of bile, and stimulate the appetite. Bitters can also promote saliva and gastric juices and accelerate the emptying of the stomach, thus triggering the pancreas to begin to release digestive enzymes. Bitters are useful for sluggish digestion, heartburn, dyspepsia, bowel tension, flatulence, and bloating.

While bitters have been used for thousands of years as a digestive tonic in many traditional cultures, most Americans shun them and have not, like many Europeans and Asians, become accustomed to their taste. We suggest an excellent, pleasant-tasting bitters formula: brew one teaspoon each of gentian, dandelion, goldenseal, rue, artemesia, and prickly ash in six cups of boiling water to make a tea. Add a few drops of peppermint oil. Bitters need to be sipped and tasted, because they work through the slow stimulation of the tongue.

A bitters salad can be made with dandelion leaves, escarole, endive, and other bitter salad greens. These can be combined with romaine, green leaf and red leaf lettuce, and some olive oil, flaxseed oil, spices, and lemon juice. This salad triggers the entire digestive system to function more effectively. Bitters are available commercially as "Swedish Bitters" in health food stores and as Italian Fernet Brancha in any liquor store. Be aware that Swedish Bitters contains camphor, which can sabotage the effectiveness of homeopathic remedies.

People who are taking nonsteroidal, anti-inflammatory drugs (like cortisone or aspirin) should not take additional betaine hydrochloride, as it could cause ulcers. Hydrochloric acid supplementation should be done under medical supervision, as it is possible to take too much betaine hydrochloride without any immediately evident symptoms, which could lead to ulcers or serious bleeding in the stomach.

**HCl Supplements**—If these measures prove ineffective, you may want to consider (in consultation with a health-care provider) taking hydrochloric acid supplements. The most common form of supplement is betaine hydrochloride (an edible compound that forms hydrochloric acid in the stomach), available at most health food stores or pharmacies. Typically, physicians recommend taking one capsule (usually 5-10 grains) at the beginning of each meal. If after three days, this does not cause any adverse symptoms (heartburn, abdominal pain, nausea), the dose can be increased to two capsules, then three capsules, per meal. If symptoms do occur, reduce your dosage. (You can quickly neutralize any adverse effect by drinking milk, eating yogurt, or taking a bicarbonate like baking soda.)[28]

# Enzyme Deficiency and Leaky Gut

Like hypochlorhydria, enzyme deficiency may be responsible for maldigestion. Inadequate amounts of digestive enzymes (for example of lactase, which breaks down milk sugars), means certain foods cannot be broken down into molecules small enough to be used by the body's cells. In addition, enzyme deficiency can cause gastrointestinal problems, such as diarrhea and bloating, which are not symptoms of allergy but of intolerance.

Patients with allergy and leaky gut syndrome need the digestive tonification enabled by digestive enzymes. Tonifying the digestive system breaks down large food molecules, decreases the amount of food allergies, inactivates dietary lectins, stimulates digestion, and halts or alters the growth of dysbiotic microorganisms in the gut. In essence, it arrests the processes responsible for allergy.

Our bodies manufacture enzymes and we also derive some from our foods. With the modern diet of highly processed, devitalized convenience foods, many people no longer obtain enough enzymes from their diet. At the same time, environmental toxins, prescription drugs, and physical or emotional stress diminish the body's ability to manufacture its natural enzymes and we must supplement them. This is particularly true for allergy and sensitivity sufferers.

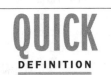

## DEFINITION

**Amino acids** are the building blocks of the 40,000 different proteins in the body, including enzymes, hormones, and the brain chemical messengers called neurotransmitters. Eight amino acids cannot be made by the body and must be obtained through the diet; others are produced in the body but not always in sufficient amounts. The body's main "amino acid pool" consists of: alanine, arginine, aspargine, aspartic acid, carnitine, citrulline, cysteine, cystine, GABA, glutamic acid, glutamine, glycine, histidine, isoleucine, leucine, lysine, methionine, ornithine, phenylalanine, proline, serine, taurine, threonine, tryptophan, tyrosine, and valine.

### Treating Allergies with Digestive Enzymes

In this section, Lita Lee, Ph.D., an enzyme therapist from Lowell, Oregon, and author of *The Enzyme Cure*, discusses the primary digestive enzymes: protease, amylase, and disaccharidase, along with some of the allergy-related deficiency symptoms associated with each.

**Protease**—Protease digests protein into smaller units called amino acids (SEE QUICK DEFINITION), but not only protein from food, but other organisms that are composed of proteins. These include the protein coating on some viruses, toxic debris

## Enzyme Sources and Functions

The enzymes we need for digestion are manufactured in the pancreas but they are also available in food sources. Other types of enzymes are metabolic enzymes, which activate all the biochemical processes that sustain your body. Antioxidant enzymes (glutathione peroxidase and superoxide dismutase), a subset of metabolic enzymes, destroy free radicals (which break down cells) and convert them into neutral oxygen and water.

**Pancreatic Enzymes**—The pancreas, located behind the stomach, secretes 22 kinds of enzymes that function mainly in the intestines and the blood. Their primary purpose is to aid in digestion. These enzymes include protease (digests protein), amylase (digests carbohydrates, or starches), disaccharidase (digests sugar), and lipase (digests fats). Pancreatic enzymes, when deficient, can be obtained from supplements.

**Plant or Food Enzymes**—Raw foods (but not cooked) have living enzymes embedded within their structure. These enzymes function in the stomach, predigesting the food even before hydrochloric acid accumulates in the stomach to begin the next stage of digestion. This phenomenon was first proposed by Edward Howell, M.D., a pioneer in the field of enzyme therapy in the United States. He stated, "If the stomach is performing its proper role, and we are eating our foods uncooked, a large portion of the intake will be partially digested before reacting with the stronger digestive juices found there. Moreover, fewer of your body's internal digestive enzymes will be called upon to perform the digestive function." It is this easing of the body enzymes' workload that is thought to contribute substantially to the healing effects of enzyme therapy.[29]

Enzyme supplements need to be taken on an empty stomach. To digest food and prevent food allergens and toxins from migrating from the colon to the bloodstream, enzymes should be taken on a full stomach.

from dead bacteria and other organisms, and certain harmful substances produced at sites of injury or inflammation. Protease enzymes are particularly helpful for allergy sufferers, as partially undigested protein molecules are often responsible for food sensitization.

Lita Lee, Ph.D.: P.O. Box 516, Lowell, OR 97452; tel: 541-937-1123; fax: 541-937-1132.

Protease is especially effective during inflammatory processes due to its ability to control swelling, redness, heat, fever and pain. Enzyme therapist Howard Loomis, M.D., refers to protease as the first line of immune defense among food enzymes. He compares it to the neutrophils (54%-65% of the white blood cells), whose principle activity is to digest harmful bacteria and fungi. In fact, immune system disorders such as allergies are among the most common symptoms of protease deficiency, as are bacterial and viral infections.

To learn more about **enzyme therapy**, see *The Enzyme Cure* (Future Medicine Publishing, 1998; ISBN 1-887299-22-X); to order, call 800-333-HEAL.

For more about **enzyme testing**, see Chapter 3: Allergy/Sensitivity Testing for Allergies, pp. 70-105.

Toxic colon syndrome, also called indicanuria or intestinal toxemia, is another result of protease deficiency. Here, undigested proteins decompose at the intestinal level. The products of this putrefication (called indican) leak into the bloodstream from the intestines (where they may be treated as allergens). Elevated levels of indican in the urine reflects poor protein digestion only and, since it is a bowel toxin, some information about toxic load. It can be identified by a simple 24-hour urine analysis.

Papain from papaya and bromelain from pineapples are effective proteases when taken along with food. These same enzymes can be used for their anti-inflammatory action when taken without food. Pancreatic enzymes from animal sources are also extremely useful. Pancreatic enzyme supplements aid in the production of pancreatic enzymes and strengthen the gland. The pancreas can recycle and recirculate pancreatic enzyme extracts, so not only do they support digestion while it's occurring in the small intestine, but they also support future digestion and tonify the pancreas and small intestine.

Possible allergy-related deficiency symptoms: weakened immunity, frequent bacterial or viral infections, fluid in the ears, chronic constipation, toxic buildup in the large intestine.

**Amylase**—Amylase digests carbohydrates (polysaccharides), breaking them down into smaller units that are later converted into monosaccharides (simple sugars) such as glucose and disaccharides such as fructose. People who can't digest fats often eat large amounts of sugar and carbohydrates to make up for the lack of fat in their diet. If their diet is excessive in carbohydrates, they can develop an amylase deficiency.

Amylase possesses antihistamine properties and can relieve many kinds of skin problems, such as hives and rashes, contact dermatitis, allergic reactions to bee stings, bug bites, and poison oak or ivy. Amylase, in conjunction with lung-healing herbs, helps alleviate the wheezing of asthmatics who are intolerant to sugar. The combination also acts as a lung expectorant.

Possible allergy-related deficiency symptoms: hives, eczema, allergies to bee stings and insect bites, muscle pain and joint stiffness.

**Disaccharidase**—Since disaccharidase digests sugars, the inability to digest complex sugars (sucrose, lactose, fructose and maltose) and convert them into simple sugars (glucose) lowers the blood sugar level and deprives the

# Natural Enzyme Supplements

Two enzymes from pineapples and papayas have proven valuable in improving digestion and relieving allergic inflammation.

**Bromelain**—According to clinical research, bromelain helps break down fibrin, a substance that accumulates in an inflamed area and blocks off blood and lymph fluid, causing swelling.[30] Bromelain also interferes with the production of prostaglandins (see quick definition) and other substances that contribute to inflammation and increases the production of prostaglandins that decrease inflammation. Bromelain can also act along with other pancreatic enzymes to help clear the blood of allergens, which can contribute to or trigger inflammation. As a digestive aid, bromelain is usually used in combination with ox bile and hydrochloric acid.[31]

For anti-inflammatory effects, take bromelain on an empty stomach; taken with food, it helps improve digestion.[32] Juicing an organic non-irradiated pineapple along with half of an organic lemon, and a quarter- or half-inch piece of fresh ginger root, is an excellent way to get high amounts of bromelain. For consistent therapeutic value, bromelain supplements should be used. Typical therapeutic dose: 500-2,000 mg, three times daily. Precautions: Bromelain can cause sensitivity in people who are allergic to bee stings, olive tree pollen, or pineapple.[33] Those with a history of heart palpitations are advised to limit the dose of bromelain to 460 mg per day.[34]

**Papaya**—A tropical fruit, papaya contains the digestive enzyme papain, which has the power of digesting 300 times its own volume in protein. The skin of the fruit, especially when it is still green, has been used to treat ulcers and infectious wounds.[35] As with all digestive enzymes, papain helps to break down immune complexes, which aggravate inflammatory allergic conditions. Papain is included in many digestive enzyme combinations, often along with bromelain and hydrochloric acid. Typical therapeutic dose: 250-500 mg daily.

## QUICK DEFINITION

**Prostaglandins** are hormone-like, complex fatty acids which affect smooth muscle function, inflammatory processes, and constriction and dilation of blood vessels. Essential fatty acids in the diet (omega-6 and omega-3) provide the raw material for prostaglandin production; once ingested, these essential fatty acids can be converted to prostaglandins by nearly any cell in the body. Omega-6-derived prostaglandins can have either pro-inflammatory or anti-inflammatory properties, while most prostaglandins converted from omega-3 sources help reduce pain and inflammation. For proper body function, an appropriate balance of both types of prostaglandins must be maintained.

brain of nourishment. People who are intolerant of sugar or disaccharides (such as lactose) tend to compensate by eating more protein, as proteins can be converted to glucose as needed. The major cause of sugar intolerance is probably excessive consumption of refined sugars.

Possible allergy-related deficiency symptoms: asthma, environmental illness, dizziness, hyperactivity/attention deficit hyperactivity disorder (ADHD).

# Illuminating the *Candida* Connection

While there are many species of microorganisms that can overgrow in the body and cause an increase in intestinal permeability, of prime concern here is *Candida albicans*. This is a yeast-like fungus found widely in nature, in the soil, on vegetables and fruits, and in the human body. It is frequently present in small quantities in the intestines and in the vagina. *Candida* overgrowth, a condition called candidiasis, can become pathogenic and cause allergic reactions throughout the body. These reactions can lead to a wide range of symptoms, including depression, fatigue, weight gain, anxiety, rashes, headaches, and muscle cramping.

Predisposing factors for candidiasis include: the use of steroid hormone medications such as cortisone or corticosteroids, which are often prescribed for skin and respiratory allergies; prolonged or repeated use of antibiotics; oral contraceptive use; estrogen therapy; and a diet high in sugar, both natural and refined. Certain illnesses, such as AIDS, cancer, and diabetes, which are accompanied by extreme immune suppression, can also increase susceptibility to *Candida* overgrowth.

This organism changes form as it develops, and sends hyphae (microscopic "root-like" filaments) through the intestinal wall, similar to the way English ivy grows up a wall and adheres to the bricks. This analogy is helpful in understanding how *Candida* produces illness. The ivy's rootlets infiltrate the mortar between the bricks and severely damage it. Similarly, *Candida*'s root-like filaments become attached to the intestinal wall and loosen the intracellular "cement" (the connective tissue between cells), create holes through the cell membranes, and release toxic waste products (*Candida* toxin) that circulate throughout the system, causing an increase in toxemia in the body.

Yeasts like *Candida* contain decarboxylases, enzymes that convert (and putrefy) amino acids into vasoactive amines (such as putricine from arginine, ornithine and indican from tryptophan), which cause alterations in the permeability of blood vessels and other tissues and affect how easily materials permeate the walls of cells. Vasoactive amines can cause leaky gut syndrome and dissolve the intestinal membrane.

*Candida albicans* can also produce more than 400 mycotoxins, any of which can cause systemic illness. A mycotoxin is a fungal poison; more specifically, it is a toxic chemical released into the blood as a byproduct of the yeast's metabolism or from cell fragments from dead yeast cells. Some of these mycotoxins, like acetylaldehyde and alcohol, can produce the feelings of being "hung over" that many patients affected with *Candida* tend to experience. One mycotoxin in particular, gliotoxin, has been shown to suppress the immune system, particularly the ability of the white blood cells to engulf foreign material. It suppresses the thymus gland, the lymph nodes, the spleen, and the bone marrow in the production of white blood cells. Gliotoxin also interferes with normal glutathione metabolism; the depletion of glutathione not only robs the *Candida* patient of this important antioxidant, but it contributes to other systemic illnesses associated with low levels of glutathione, such as sensitivity, allergies, and symptoms of chemical sensitivity.[36]

## *Candida*'s Role in Allergy

*Candida* not only damages the intestinal membrane, it can also trigger allergic reactions. *Candida* is particularly implicated in sparking outbreaks of atopic dermatitis. In one study, 15 patients with atopic dermatitis and seven controls were exposed to extracts of *Candida*. IgE levels were significantly higher in all of the eczema sufferers, and cytokine chemical mediators were released for up to 96 hours after *Candida* exposure—a delayed allergic response.[37] Other studies have shown that *Candida* triggers immediate reactions in atopic dermatitis patients[38] and that treating the *Candida* overgrowth with various antifungal medications improves eczema symptoms in between 28% to 60% of patients.[39]

Research also shows that recurrent vaginal candidiasis is often associated with allergic rhinitis. For 28 months, Brazilian researchers studied 95 women with recurrent yeast infections and 100 controls, and found that 64 (71%) of the yeast-infected women also suffered from allergic rhinitis, compared to only 42% of the controls.[40] The yeast-infected women also had a higher incidence of family history of allergies (73% compared to 61%). The researchers concluded that atopic (susceptible to allergies) women tend to experience recurrent vaginal candidiasis.

## Do You Have Candidiasis? A Self-Test

William Crook, M.D., author of *The Yeast Connection*, popularized the idea that *Candida* can create numerous health problems. During the course of his research, Dr. Crook developed a reliable patient questionnaire for assessing potential *Candida* involvement in a patient's health picture. Among the questions are the following:

■ Have you taken repeated courses of antibiotics or steroids (e.g. cortisone)?

- Have you used birth-control pills?
- Have you had repeated fungal infections ("jock itch," athlete's foot, ringworm)?
- Do you regularly have any of these symptoms—bloating, headaches, depression, fatigue, memory problems, impotence or lack of interest in sex, muscle aches with no apparent cause, brain fogginess?
- Do you experience symptoms of PMS (pre-menstrual syndrome)?
- Do you have cravings for sweets, products containing white flour, or alcoholic beverages?
- Do you repeatedly experience any of these health difficulties— inappropriate drowsiness, mood swings, rashes, bad breath, dry mouth, post-nasal drip or nasal congestion, heartburn, urinary frequency or urgency?[41]

A study conducted at Bastyr University showed the degree of *Candida albicans* growth in stool cultures correlated well with the symptomatic scores for the same patients on Dr. Crook's *Candida* questionnaire.[42] In another study, out of 854 patients considered, the predominant fungal species isolated were *Candida albicans* (64.5%), followed by *Candida tropicalis* (23.3%) and *Candida krusei* (6.9%).[43] Other fungal species, such as trichosporon, geotrichum, rhodotorula, and conida, are lesser-known fungi that can also contribute to yeast overgrowth.

# Ridding the Body of *Candida* Overgrowth

Successful treatment of candidiasis requires the reduction of factors that predispose a patient to *Candida* overgrowth and the strengthening of the patient's immune function. Diet, nutritional supplements, herbal and Ayurvedic remedies, acupuncture, and enzyme therapy are some of the choices often employed to help people accomplish these ends. Recovery from chronic candidiasis seldom takes less than three months and it may take much longer. However, many experience relief from some symptoms after only one week. Note that many alternative medicine practitioners will use conventional antifungal medications such as Diflucan or Nystatin to fight severe yeast infections.

### Probiotics
High doses of probiotics, "friendly" bacteria such as *Bifidobacterium bifidum* and *Lactobacillus acidophilus*, *bulgaricus*, *plantarum*, and *salvarius*, are available as nutritional supplements. Treatment may last from

eight to 12 weeks. Leon Chaitow, N.D., a British naturopath, reports an 80% success rate using this method in cases of seriously ill people afflicted with yeast overgrowth and parasites. Recolonizing the intestines with friendly bacteria can help prevent illness by depriving the pathogenic (disease-causing) bacteria of the opportunity to over-grow and flourish.

Probiotic supplementation has been clinically proven to reverse eczema and other conditions caused by food allergy. In study of 14 infants with atopic dermatitis fed a hydrolyzed whey formula and 13 fed a whey formula with *Lactobacillus*, researchers noticed a significant improvement after one month in the *Lactobacillus* group.[44] It appears that probiotics help repair and preserve the integrity of the intestinal mucosa.[45]

**How to Take Probiotics**—Dr. Chaitow advises that "to be effective, pro-biotic supplements should be freeze-dried, contain only the declared and desirable strains of the species, and have concentrations of the friendly bacteria of about one billion parts per gram. They should also be kept refrigerated."

Patients with food allergies and sensitivities are advised to avoid yogurt because of its high lactose (milk sugar) content and allergenic-ity, despite its high concentration of *Lactobacilli*. Freeze-dried, nondairy-derived acidophilus supplements in capsule form are more effective in reducing bacteria than unsweetened raw yogurt. Below are some of the more common friendly bacteria.

■ *Lactobacillus acidophilus* is the predominant friendly bacteria in the upper intestinal tract. *Lactobacillus* is the general (genus) name of the bacteria, *acidophilus* is the particular strain (species). *L. acidophilus* is involved in the production of B vit-amins (niacin, folic acid, and pyridoxine) during the diges-tive process.

Dietary recommenda-tions for eliminating *Candida* overgrowth are discussed in Chapter 6: Therapeutic Diets, pp. 158-183.

■ *Bifidobacterium bifidum* and *B. longum* are the primary friendly bacteria in the large intestine. Note that these bac-teria only competes with the yeast for space and food source; they don't kill it or create a barrier to it. These probiotics also manu-facture B vitamins.

■ *Streptococcus thermophilus* and *L. bulgaricus* are most commonly found in yogurt and exist only transiently in the human digestive tract. They produce lactic acid, which encourages the growth of other friendly bacteria, and they also synthesize bacteriocidins (natural antibiotic-like substances) that kill harmful bacteria.

## Why Friendly Bacteria are Essential to Your Health

A study of 154 newborns found that *L. acidophilus* given shortly after birth encouraged the growth of normal intestinal flora and reduced the number of opportunistic infections and inflammatory diseases in those infants. Another study demonstrated that *L. acidophilus* prevents the attachment of harmful bacteria to human intestinal cells, thus providing a barrier against these bacteria in the digestive system. The pathogenic bacteria affected included *E. coli*, *Salmonella typhimurium*, and *Yersinia pseudotuberculosis*, *L. acidophilus* is also effective against *Campylobacter pylori*, common bacteria that cause acid-peptic disease.

One of the common side effects of treatment with antibiotics (especially the broad-spectrum type) is that levels of both friendly and pathogenic bacteria are killed off, opening the door to yeast infestation and gastrointestinal distress, particularly diarrhea. Steroids, such as cortisone, and birth control pills can contribute to probiotic damage as well.

Supplementing with *Lactobacilli* and other probiotics can restore the normal intestinal microflora damaged by antibiotics. In one double-blind study, 98 patients taking the antibiotic ampicillin were divided into two groups, one receiving a *Lactobacilli* supplement while the other group received a placebo. There were no cases of ampicillin-induced diarrhea in the group receiving *Lactobacilli*, while 14% of the placebo group had diarrhea as a result of the antibiotics. Another study involved 27 patients with ear, sinus, or throat infections who were given the antibiotic amoxicillin/clavulanate; some of the patients were also given *L. acidophilus*. According to the researchers, there was "a significant decrease in patient complaints of gastrointestinal side effects and yeast superinfection" in the group given *L. acidophilus* supplements.[46]

■ *Lactobacilli*, *Bifidobacteria*, and *Streptococci* are the bacteria most commonly found in probiotic supplements. Other beneficial species that may be included are *L. casei*, *L. plantarum*, *L. sporogenes*, *L. brevis*, and *Saccharomyces boulardii*.

### Ayurvedic Anti-Fungal Therapies

Ayurvedic medicine considers candidiasis to be a condition caused by *ama*, the improper digestion of foods, according to Virender Sodhi, N.D., M.D. (Ayurveda), of Bellevue, Washington. As do other alternative physicians, Dr. Sodhi attributes this malfunction, and thus candidiasis, to the widespread use of antibiotics, birth control pills, and hormones, environmental stress, and society's addiction to sugar in the diet. "Ayurvedic medicine believes that these stresses on the system cause carbohydrates to be digested improperly," he says. "Furthermore, the immune system in the gut becomes worn down."

Dr. Sodhi's candidiasis protocol involves strengthening the immune system and improving digestion through stimulation of secretory IgA, the immunoglobulin, or antibody, found in the mucoid lining of the intestines and lungs; it may help prevent invasion of those surfaces by disease-producing bacteria and viruses.

Dr. Sodhi uses grapefruit seed oil and tannic acid, which act as antifungals and antibiotics, and *acidophilus*, which helps restore the balance of friendly bacteria in the intestines. Long pepper, ginger, cayenne, and the Ayurvedic herbs trikatu and neem taken 30 minutes before meals increase immunoglobulin and digestive functions. He further recommends that his patients cleanse toxins from their systems using the *pancha karma* program, which involves herbs and dietary modification. With Dr. Sodhi's approach, candidiasis can usually be eliminated in four to six months.

### Herbal Remedies

Herbs are often used to kill harmful yeasts and to shore up immune function. Herbs containing berberine (an alkaloid) have proven to be particularly useful for *Candida*. These include goldenseal, Oregon grape root, and barberry. Berberine acts as a natural antibiotic against *Candida* overgrowth, normalizes intestinal flora, helps digestive problems, and stimulates the immune system.[47] Other herbs helpful for candidiasis include artemisia, quassia bark, red clover, and pau d' arco. The commercial formula PlantiBiotic (which contains barberry, berberine, citrus seed extract, thyme oil, oregano oil, tea tree oil, garlic, and other herbs) is also helpful in treating *Candida* infections.

### Nutritional Supplements

Enzyme therapist Dr. Lita Lee has three recommendations for treating candidiasis. First, Citricidal (grapefruit seed and pulp extract) which is a nontoxic antibacterial, anti-parasitic, antifungal, and antiviral; it kills 11 fungi, including *Candida albicans*. Typical dosage: 1-2 tablets (each tablet contains four drops), three times daily.

Second, Dr. Lee recommends soil-based organisms (SEE QUICK DEFINITION). This is an intestinal formula of beneficial bacteria, which kill pathological microbes and help prevent prolifera-

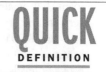

**DEFINITION**

**Soil-based organisms (SBOs)** are beneficial microbes, or probiotics, found in soil. Before chemical farming, the earth was rich in these organisms which naturally destroyed molds, yeast, fungi, and viruses in the soil. Transmitted to humans in the food supply, SBOs performed the same function in the human body, working with the "friendly" bacteria inhabiting the gastrointestinal tract to maintain balance in the intestinal flora and thus ensure a healthy digestive system. Since soil has become depleted of SBOs, the ratio of good to bad bacteria in the intestines has become skewed and a host of health problems, including allergies, candidiasis, and Crohn's disease among other gastrointestinal conditions, are the result.

For **Citricidal** (available to health practitioners only), contact: Nutribiotic, P.O. Box 238, Lakeport, CA 95453; tel: 800-255-435 or 707-263-0411; fax: 707-263-7844. The equivalent for consumers is Nutribiotic's Standardized Extract of Grapefruit, available in health food stores. For **soil-based organisms**, contact: GanEden Ltd., 15355 72nd Drive North, Palm Beach Gardens, FL 33418; tel: 800-622-8986 or 561-748-2478; fax: 561-575-5488. Life Sciences, 321 North Mall Drive, Building F-201, St. George, UT 84790; tel: 801-628-4111; fax: 801-628-6114. For **Thera-zyme Sml** (for health-care professionals only), contact: 21st Century Nutrition, 6421 Enterprise Lane, Madison, WI 53719; tel: 800-662-2630 or 608-273-8100. For **PlantiBiotic**, contact: Nature's Answer, 320 Oser Avenue, Hauppauge, NY 11788; tel: 800-439-2324 or 516-231-7492; fax: 516-231-8391; website: www.naturesanswer.com. For other **anti-*Candida* remedies**, contact: Environmental Detoxification Consultants, 413 Grassy Hill Road, Woodbury, CT 06798; tel: 203-263-2970.

tion of toxins in the intestines. Typical dosage: one capsule daily, increasing by one capsule per week up to six capsules daily in divided doses.

Third, Dr. Lee advises taking a multiple digestive enzyme formula, determined by urinalysis, to address the foods the person has difficulty digesting or eats in excess. She also recommends a product called Thera-zyme SmI, which contains a form of cellulase (the enzyme that digests plant fiber) that breaks down pathogenic yeast. The formula also contains *L. acidophilus* and *B. bifidum*, which reestablish friendly bowel flora, thus lessening the likelihood of yeast overgrowth in the future.

**Caprylic Acid—**This is a fatty substance found in coconut oil that is an effective antifungal agent. Caprylic acid is readily absorbed into the body and should be taken in coated tablets or in a sustained-release form that ensures release in the small intestine rather than the stomach. In one study, 16 patients were given 1,800 mg daily of caprylic acid for 16 days, three patients were given 2,700 mg daily, and six received 3,600 mg per day. The results were a 30%-90% reduction in *Candida* levels among those with the 1,800 mg dosage; a 70%-100% reduction in the three patients taking 2,700 mg; and complete elimination in two weeks in all of those taking 3,600 mg.[48]

However, doctors have seen (through darkfield blood analysis) an increase in the fragility of red blood cells in patients who stay on caprylic acid for more than two months; perhaps the same factors that attack *Candida* also begin to attack blood cell membranes. Many alternative medicine practitioners use caprylic acid only for short-term intervention and rely on dietary and lifestyle changes for a long-term cure. Typical dosage: 1,800 mg to 3,500 mg per day.

**Garlic—**It was Louis Pasteur, the 19th-century formulator of modern germ theory, who first recognized the antibiotic properties of garlic. Although now eclipsed by penicillin and other antibiotics, garlic often is more effective and more versatile in treating fungal, bacterial, and viral infections.[49] In treating the overgrowth of *Candida albicans*, researchers in the U.S. and Europe found that an injection of fresh raw garlic extract into *Candida*-infected cells inhibited growth of the fungus by 70%. Allicin, the active antifungal component in garlic, attacks the surface of the *Candida* cells, alters its fat content, and oxidizes a group of its essential enzymes.[50] Garlic has the added benefit of stimulating the immune system rather than depressing it. Recommended dosage: two fresh cloves daily.

**Oregano Oil**—Oil of oregano is used to treat topical and internal candidiasis. Its powerful antimicrobial properties come from a combination of carvacrol, a naturally occurring antiseptic, and thymol, a compound similar to that found in thyme. Carvacrol is a phenol that rivals in strength the synthetic phenol known as carbolic acid, once used to sterilize medical instruments. For internal *Candida* infections, a relatively small amount of oil of oregano is needed to kill the overgrown fungi. But while this amber-colored liquid may look mild, it has a strong and almost spicy flavor, so it is recommended that you mix it with vegetable juice. Oil of oregano is also a safe alternative to commercially produced anti-inflammatory drugs, such as aspirin, Motrin, and Indocin.[51] Typical dosage: a few drops sublingually two or three times a day for two weeks.

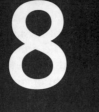

CHAPTER

# 8

# Intestinal Detoxification

**A**S OUR ENVIRONMENT and food are increasingly saturated with pollutants and chemicals, the body's mechanisms for elimination of toxins cannot keep up with the chemical deluge. All organs involved in detoxification, which include the intestines, liver, skin, and respiratory system, can become overloaded. The constant circulation of toxins in the body taxes the immune system, which must continually strive to destroy or eliminate them. Toxic overload is a major contributor to a hyperactive immune system.

It is advisable to take measures to support these detoxification organs and to remove toxins stored in the body. In this chapter, we cover steps on detoxifying the intestines and liver. Chapter 9: Supporting the Skin features skin detoxification therapies, and Chapter 10: Supporting the Respiratory System discusses detoxification tips for the respiratory system.

## Success Story: Detoxification Helps Reverse Asthma

Brad, 54, had asthma for many years and suffered with frequent attacks, requiring that he use his inhaler three times a day as well as two to three doses of Allegra®, a conventional antihistamine. He also complained of extreme fatigue, digestive problems (gas, diarrhea, and abdominal pain), swollen lower extremities and feet, lower back pain and bone pain, and excessive joint mobility causing frequent ankle sprains. At 260 pounds, Brad was also too fat for his 5'11½" frame.

Brad finally sought the help of Kevin Davison, N.D., of Haiku, Hawaii. "He had exhausted all other possibilities in terms of getting control of his asthma," says Dr. Davison. As part of his diagnostic procedure, Dr. Davison assessed Brad's thyroid function. He had Brad measure his basal (resting) body temperature, which involves taking underarm temperatures on consecutive mornings. Brad's average on his temperature test was 96.5° F, indicating depressed thyroid function (a normal average would be 97.8° F or higher). A blood test revealed that Brad's cholesterol level (223) and triglycerides (101) were both elevated.

Because he felt food allergies were a factor in both Brad's asthma and obesity, Dr. Davison started Brad on a modified elimination diet, which excluded yeast-derived products, caffeine, dairy, gluten-containing grains such as wheat, refined carbohydrates, and food additives. He also recommended a macromineral supplement to help rebalance Brad's acid levels. Because of the depressed thyroid function, Dr. Davison recommended Metabolic Enhancer (two capsules, three times daily), a formula containing thyroid glandulars and nutrients to support the production of thyroid hormones, which helps increase the metabolic rate.

Dr. Davison then started Brad on a liver detoxification program. He recommended a product called UltraClear, manufactured by Metagenics. UltraClear is a "medical food" based on rice protein to provide necessary nutrients to the body during the detoxification process. Brad was put on a diet of low-carbohydrate fruits and vegetables, large quantities of water, essential fatty acids (EFAs; sources include flaxseeds, pumpkin seeds, and walnuts), and protein from fresh ocean fish, free-range poultry, or legumes.

After four days, Dr. Davison moved Brad into the intensive clearing phase. He increased Brad's dose of UltraClear to five times per day, with a tablespoon of ground flaxseeds for EFAs. Brad's diet was to consist exclusively of a broth containing natural minerals to promote his body's alkalinity. The broth was made from equal amounts of celery, green beans, zucchini, spinach, and parsley, steamed, then blended with the water to form a puree (to be eaten at least twice per day). The combination of UltraClear and the diet "are very good for cleaning out the hardware of the system and all the bile channels of the liver," explains Dr. Davison.

For **Metabolic Enhancer** (available to licensed health-care practitioners only), contact: Professional Health Products, 211 Overlook Drive, Suite 6, Sewickley, PA 15143; tel: 800-929-4133 or 412-741-6351; fax: 412-741-6372. For **UltraClear and UltraClear Sustain** (available to licensed health-care practitioners only), contact: Metagenics, Inc., 971 Calle Negocio, San Clemente, CA 92673; tel: 800-692-9400; fax: 949-366-0818; website: www.metagenics.com.

He had Brad take a buffered vitamin C supplement as well, to help reduce any detoxification symptoms. After one week, the swelling in Brad's feet and ankles had reduced by 70%, his bowel movements normalized, and he was able to reduce his asthma medication by 80%.

Two months later, Dr. Davison put on UltraClear Sustain, a formula to help rebuild his intestinal lining, and started reintroducing foods into his diet, noting any allergic responses that arose. Brad took a multivitamin/mineral formula for nutritional support and Dr. Davison also used acupuncture treatments to increase liver circulation and bile flow.

After five months, Brad's weight was down to 195 and his cholesterol levels were healthier. Most importantly, Brad felt great and he was completely off his asthma medication.

# The Congested Intestines

Most of the digestion and absorption of nutrients that happens in the body occurs along the 25-foot-long passageway that comprises the small and large intestines. Your intestines, which make up 80% of your immune system, are key players in keeping you free from allergies. When they perform properly, they break down food particles and keep large molecules from entering your bloodstream. If, on the other hand, your intestines can't handle your toxic load, large molecules from poorly digested food or foreign substances may leak through the intestinal wall into the bloodstream. There, they are treated as foreign invaders and can trigger an allergic response. It has been estimated that 2% of ingested protein is absorbed undigested in normal adults. Keeping your intestinal barriers intact with a normal pH and alive with healthy digestive microbes is vital to maintaining an allergy-free life.

Digestion begins in the mouth with proper chewing and digestive enzymes secreted by the salivary glands. From the mouth, food travels to the stomach where hydrochloric acid activates pepsin to break down proteins into absorbable molecular components. The partially digested food then moves to the upper part of the small intestine (duodenum), where digestion continues with enzymes (produced by the pancreas) and bile, from the liver and gallbladder. In the next section of the intestine (jejunum), the majority of nutrients from food are absorbed into the blood. The metabolic end-products, insoluble fiber, and any toxic residues are then solidified by the extraction (reabsorption) of water (about a liter a day) as the stool bolus passes through the large intestine.

Around 1900, most people in the United States had a brief intestinal transit time—meaning that it took 15-20 hours from the time food entered the mouth until it was excreted as feces. Today, many have a seriously delayed transit time of 50-70 hours. Constipation and sluggish transit time allows for the stool to putrefy, harmful microorganisms to flourish, and toxins to be reabsorbed by tissues and lymph vessels, triggering inflammation throughout the body. In addition, undigested proteins that pass into the small and large intestines without being broken down into their constituent amino acids (due to inadequate levels of hydrochloric acid) produce toxins that further poison the intestines and can escape into the blood or lymph fluids. Inadequate digestion of dietary protein often results in insufficient production of amino acids, hormones, digestive enzymes, and other substances important for proper immune function and allergy-free health. Long transit time also increases colon cancer risk due to reabsorption of toxins.

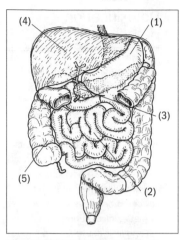

THE DIGESTIVE SYSTEM. Digestion begins in the mouth, then food travels to the stomach (1), where it is further broken down by gastric juices. Next, the partially digested food goes to the small intestine (2) where enzymes from the pancreas (3) and bile produced by the liver (4) act upon the food to extract nutrients for absorption into the blood and lymph cells. The unusable food materials are sent tot the large intestine (5) for evacuation from the body.

# Intestinal Detoxification Therapies

Cleansing the intestines of this toxic buildup is vital for allergy sufferers in order to modulate the immune system and stop the chronic inflammatory response that often accompanies an overburdened detoxification system. Repopulating the intestines with friendly bacteria is also important for maintaining healthy digestive functioning.

## Colon Hydrotherapy
Colon hydrotherapy (colonics or colonic irrigation) helps to normalize a sluggish intestinal tract, scour the crevices of the

CAUTION

People with severe heart disease, appendicitis, aneurysm, gastrointestinal hemorrhage, severe hemorrhoids, colon cancer, intestinal wall herniation, pregnancy, severe colitis, and intestinal blockages should not undergo colon hydrotherapy.

In my practice, I encourage allergy/sensitivity patients to detoxify all barrier functions—intestines, skin, and respiratory system. Enemas, dry skin brushing, and nutritional supplements are important steps in the detoxification process. I advise that patients also take UltraClear, a powdered beverage mix developed by Metagenics, during the intestinal and liver detoxification period. UltraClear contains a specific blend of vitamins, minerals, amino acids, and other nutrients that support Phase I and II liver detoxification processes, protects against free-radical damage, and provides overall nourishment for the intestines. UltraClear contains the antioxidants beta carotene, L-glutathione, N-acetyl-cysteine, selenium, and vitamins C and E, as well as a host of other nutrients that are beneficial for allergy/sensitivity sufferers. This formula is available from your doctor.

intestinal membrane for pathogens, and prevent inflammation (which allows toxins to escape through the intestinal walls). Colon hydrotherapy is a safe and minimally uncomfortable procedure that involves the gentle infusion of warm, filtered water into the colon. It is unsurpassed in its ability to detoxify the colon, correct disordered intestinal bacteria (dysbiosis), and treat intestinal permeability (leaky gut syndrome). It also tones the muscles of the colon and stimulates the wave-like contractions of the intestines to propel food through the digestive tract and prevent the reabsorption of toxins.

Two to three bowel movements a day, at regular times, soon after the consumption of a meal, are the ideal goal. The average American eliminates less than once per day, which means that most people are actually constipated. With constipation, the stool is hard and dry and hardened fecal stones (fecoliths) get caught in the folds of the colon, contributing to toxic buildup. In third-world countries, where five to ten times more fiber is eaten than in the standard American diet, the stool is typically larger, softer, and more frequent. There is a corresponding lower incidence of colon cancer and other gastrointestinal diseases.

**The Colonic Procedure**—Colonic hydrotherapy begins with the insertion of a small, rectal tube (speculum) into the patient by the therapist, nurse, or physician. The colon hydrotherapy machine is a closed system. Water, oxygenated water, food-grade hydrogen peroxide, ozone, botanical anti-microbials, nutritional supplements, or an "implant" of friendly intestinal flora (probiotics) is gently infused into and out of the intestines. The temperature, water pressure, and flow are continuously monitored throughout the treatment. The colonic machine is self-sanitizing, featuring a built-in check valve that prevents wastewater from returning and contaminating the water source. All instruments used in the treatment are sterile and disposable, eliminating any possible contamination to the patient.

The water pressure used during the colonic treatment is a safe and gentle five pounds per square inch. The treatment usually lasts for approximately one hour, which includes time for evacuating the bowels after a treatment. A series of 3-12 colonic treatments is often prescribed, depending on the diagnosis. The medications or therapeutic substances are changed often so as to expose the disease-causing microorganisms found in the colon to the widest spectrum of disease fighters, guaranteeing maximum eradication. Using healthy bacteria during colon hydrotherapy (at the end of the treatment) is recommended, because it is much more effective than taking oral supplements.

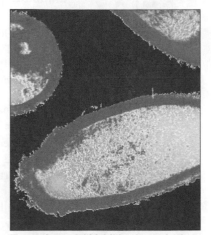

The estimated 100 trillion bacteria that live in the human intestines do so in a delicate balance. Certain bacteria such as *Lactobacillus acidophilus* and *Bifidobacterium bifidum*, are "friendly" bacteria that support numerous vital physiological processes. They help insure that bowel movements are regular and frequent and they also oppose the overgrowth of yeasts and parasites. Other bacteria, such as *Citrobacter*, *Klebsiella*, and *Clostridium*, are also present, but are considered "unfriendly" because they produce a variety of toxic substances. A healthy proportion of microorganisms in the colon is 85% friendly bacteria to no more than 15% unfriendly bacteria. Unfortunately, in most people, the proportions are the exact opposite. A number of factors can throw off the balance of intestinal flora, including stress, the use of antibiotics and other drugs, and processed foods.

## Enemas

Enemas can easily be done at home and adding medicinal herbs or the friendly bacteria *L. acidophilus* makes an enema even more effective. A coffee enema causes bile (SEE QUICK DEFINITION) dumping, which clears the biliary tree (intestinal passageways where bile flows) and causes biliary and intestinal peristalsis (movement by alimentary organs to push out its contents). The enema is prepared by brewing organic caffeinated coffee through a natural brown filter (white filters often contain toxic compounds), letting it cool to body temperature, and delivering it via an enema bag.

# QUICK

### DEFINITION

**Bile**, secreted by the liver, stored in the gallbladder, and pumped into the small intestine as needed through the bile ducts, is a yellowish brown, orange, or green fluid meant to alkalinize (make less acidic) and emulsify the intestinal contents to support fat digestion. Bile also increases peristalsis and prevents putrefaction of intestinal contents. Its chief components are bile salts, which are combinations of bile acids with amino acids, such as glycine or taurine, formed in the liver and secreted in the bile to break down fat globules enabling them to be digested. Bile acids are derived from cholesterol, made either in the liver or intestines; bile acids are regularly returned to the liver.

## Eliminating Constipation

The following are gentle intestinal cleansers to restore proper bowel function; thereby avoiding the buildup of toxins that can be reabsorbed into the bloodstream and intensify the chance of an allergic reaction.

**Anti-Constipation Bars**—Combine the following ingredients: 1 cup of aloe vera liquid, 4 tbsp unsweetened black cherry concentrate, ⅓ cup flaxseeds, 2 tsp slippery elm, ½ cup agar flakes, and 1 quart water (add some psyllium seed for blood sugar and bulk).

Place all ingredients in a saucepan; bring to a boil, then immediately lower to a simmer. Continue to simmer until consistency is like a thick gravy. Allow it to cool. Place in a container and chill until firm. Cut into one-inch squares. Take two one-inch squares daily until constipation is relieved. Will keep three to four weeks in the refrigerator.

**CAUTION**

Avoid chronic use of stimulant laxative herbs like *Cascara sagrada* or senna. They are too irritating to the intestine and chronic use may increase risk of colon cancer.

For more about **vitamin C, magnesium, and allergies**, see Chapter 10: Supporting the Respiratory System, pp. 260-277, and Chapter 11: Supplements for Symptom Control, pp. 278-303. For more on **probiotics**, see Chapter 7: Healing Leaky Gut Syndrome, pp. 184-211.

## More Easy Constipation Remedies—

■ Sprinkle 1-2 tablespoons of flaxseed powder on breakfast cereal or other foods once or twice a day (1 teaspoon only for children under 12).

■ Drink ½ cup aloe vera juice three times daily.

■ Increase intake of magnesium and vitamin C, both of which assist food in passing through the intestines. They also have a laxative effect. As an extra benefit, vitamin C helps in the formation of cortisone by the adrenal glands, which helps check the allergic response.[1]

## Probiotics

—Whenever you undergo any form of intestinal cleansing, all of the bacteria, both friendly and unfriendly, are washed out. It is therefore important to repopulate your intestine with friendly bacteria, particularly *Lactobacillus acidophilus* and *Bifidobacterium bifidum*. Cabbage is one of the best food sources of friendly bacteria; eat it raw daily or juice it. Other foods that can help revitalize the colon and encourage the growth of normal bacteria include rice protein, chicory, onions, garlic, asparagus, and bananas. Friendly bacteria are also found in yogurt and kefir (a fer-

## How to Administer a Coffee Enema

Here is the regimen generally recommended by health researcher Etienne Callebout, M.D., of London, England, for administering the coffee enema:

1) Add three tablespoons of ground organic coffee (not instant or decaffeinated) to two pints of distilled water. Boil for five minutes (uncovered) to burn off oils; then cover, lower heat, and simmer for an additional 15 minutes.

2) Strain and cool to body temperature. Lubricate rectal enema tube with K-Y Jelly or other lubricant. Hang enema bag above you, but not more than two feet from your body; the best level is approximately six inches above the intestines (hang it on the bathroom doorknob). Lying on your right side, draw both legs close to the abdomen.

3) Insert the tube several inches into rectum. Open the stopcock and allow fluid to run in very slowly to avoid cramping. Breathe deeply and try to relax. Retain the solution for 12-15 minutes. If you have trouble retaining or taking the full amount, lower the bag; if you feel spasms, lower the bag to the floor to relieve the pressure. After about 20 seconds, slowly start raising the bag toward the original level. You can also pinch the tube to control the flow.

4) With symptoms of toxicity, such as headaches, fever, nausea, intestinal spasm, and drowsiness, one may increase the frequency of enemas. Take in one to two pints each time for these conditions.

5) Upon waking the next morning, if you experience headaches and drowsiness, an additional enema is recommended that night. Eat a piece of fruit before the first coffee enema of the day to activate the upper digestive tract. Keep all equipment clean.

---

mented milk drink). Another way to repopulate the intestines with friendly bacteria is to take a probiotic supplement. Use non-dairy sources if you have been diagnosed with dairy allergies/sensitivities.

# The Overburdened Liver

The liver, located beneath the right lower part of the rib cage, is one of the most complicated organs in the body, rivaled only by the brain. The liver collects and removes foreign particles and chemicals from the blood and detoxifies these poisons through three systems: (1) the Kupffer cells; (2) Phase I and Phase II systems, involving more than 75 enzymes; and (3) the production of bile. Each system feeds into the other, and all three need to be operating at full efficiency for proper detoxification.

Approximately 1,500 milliliters of blood pass through the liver each minute for filtering. The major players in this filtering project are the Kupffer cells, a type of stationary white blood cell that engulfs foreign matter in the blood before it passes through the rest of the liver. When the liver is damaged, toxic, congested, or sluggish, the Kupffer cells become overburdened and the filtration system slows down, allowing increased levels of antigens, foreign proteins, bowel microorganisms, and dietary waste products to pass through the liver and enter the general circulatory system. Inflammatory agents called cytokines are also released, contributing to the development of inflammatory allergic conditions.

The most complex of the liver's detoxification mechanisms are referred to as Phase I and Phase II biotransformation systems. When a toxic chemical such as alcohol enters the liver, reactions begin that attempt to break these chemicals down into harmless substances. There are two phases to this complex breakdown process. Phase I is the oxidation phase, in which enzymes "burn" or oxidize chemicals into intermediate substances. Phase II enzymes act to combine these decomposed substances with other molecules (such as sulfur, glutathione, and glycine) to make them more water-soluble and easier for the body to excrete.[2] Bile (excreted by the liver, stored in the gallbladder, and pumped into the small intestine as needed) is a yellowish-brown, orange, or green fluid meant to make intestinal contents less acidic and to emulsify or digest fat; bile prevents putrefaction of intestinal contents and speeds up peristalsis. The goal of all the liver's detoxification systems is to convert toxins into a water-soluble form for easy elimination from the body via the stool.

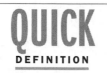

**DEFINITION**

A **free radical** is an unstable molecule of oxygen with an unpaired electron that steals an electron from another molecule and produces harmful effects. Free radicals are formed when molecules within cells react with oxygen (oxidize) as part of normal metabolic processes. Free radicals then begin to break down cells, especially the cell membranes, often in a matter of minutes to an hour. Their work is enhanced if there are not enough free-radical quenching nutrients, such as vitamins C and E, in the cell. While free radicals are normal products of metabolism, uncontrolled free-radical production plays a major role in aging and the development of most degenerative diseases, including cancer and heart disease. Free radicals harmfully alter important molecules, such as proteins, enzymes, fats, even DNA. Other sources of free radicals include pesticides, industrial pollutants, smoking, alcohol, viruses, most infections, allergies, stress, even certain foods and excessive exercise.

## Causes of Defective Detoxification

Defects in the body's ability to activate these detoxification pathways will create an accumulation of toxins in the system or a slowed excretion rate, causing damage to sensitive physiological systems. Over-activation of Phase I causes excessive production of free radicals (SEE QUICK DEFINITION) and toxic by-products. In addition, if Phase II is sluggish, it causes a buildup of damaging molecules in the body.

Allergic people tend to have poorly functioning livers. Joseph Pizzorno, N.D., co-author of *Encyclopedia of Natural Medicine*, points out that NSAIDs (nonsteroidal, anti-inflammatory drugs), which are routinely used in the treatment of allergic conditions, are proven inhibitors of the liver's Phase II detoxification enzymes. Other inhibitors include aspirin and acetaminophen. Nutrient deficiencies in folic acid, vitamins B12, B complex, and C, and the amino acids glutathione (as caused by mercury toxicity), cysteine, or methionine stop these detoxification reactions.

For more about **tests that determine the efficiency of your liver processes**, see Chapter 3: Allergy/Sensitivity Testing, pp. 70-105. For more on **how free radicals contribute to allergy**, see Chapter 10: Supporting the Respiratory System, pp. 260-277.

# Liver Detoxification Therapies

Balancing the Phase I and Phase II processes of the liver is extremely important for people with allergies and sensitivities. Techniques that can help cleanse, tone, and repair damaged liver cells include a coffee enema, castor oil packs, and specific herbs, plants, and foods for liver support.

### Coffee Enema
Coffee contains choleretics, substances that increase the flow of bile from the gallbladder.[3] Early research by Max Gerson, M.D., founder of the Gerson Institute, in Bonita, California, and originator of the Gerson Diet Therapy, established that a coffee enema is effective in stimulating the complex system of liver detoxification.[4] (See "How to Administer a Coffee Enema," p. 219).

### Castor Oil Packs
Castor oil comes from the bean of the castor plant, *Oleum ricini*. The plant itself is quite poisonous, but the oil pressed out of the bean is safe to use, since the toxic constituents remain in the seeds. The Egyptians used castor oil as a laxative for cleansing the bowels and as a scalp rub to make hair grow and shine. Castor oil packs have been used for many conditions, including liver problems, constipation, and other ailments involving elimination, as well as non-malignant ovarian fibroid cysts and headaches.[5] Castor oil, when heated on flannel, acts as a "counter-irritant." It irritates the skin surface, causing dilation of the vessels and recruitment of immune cells to the area under the pack. Deeper tissues receive the benefit of the additional circulation and immune stimulation. (The same technique was used for lung infections using mustard for the famous "mustard plaster.")

### Dietary Recommendations to Support the Liver
Foods that help the liver include the cabbage family and cruciferous vegetables (Brussels sprouts, cauliflower, and broccoli), which aid the

## Castor Oil Pack Instructions

1) Fold a flannel sheet into three sections to fit over your whole abdomen.
2) Cut a piece of plastic one to two inches larger than flannel sheet.
3) Soak flannel sheet in gently heated castor oil. Fold it over and squeeze until some of the liquid oozes out. Unfold.
4) Prepare the surface where you will be lying. Place a large plastic sheet and an old towel over the surface to prevent staining.
5) Lie down on the towel and place the oil-soaked flannel sheet over your abdomen. Place fitted plastic piece over the flannel sheet. Apply a hot water bottle over the area.
6) Wrap towel under and around your torso.
7) Rest for one to two hours.
8) Wash your body with a solution of three tablespoons baking soda to one quart water to rinse off the oil, or you will get a rash.
9) Repeat as instructed by a physician.

liver in both Phase I and Phase II detoxification. Brussels sprouts are the best of the cruciferous vegetables for the liver, according to the late John Bastyr, N.D., the namesake of Bastyr University of Naturopathic Medicine, in Seattle, Washington. Other helpful sulfur-containing foods include onions, garlic, leeks, and chives.

Beets contain high levels of betaine, a powerful lipotropic agent (increases the flow of bile). Black radish and artichokes contain cynarin, which has liver-protective properties similar to milk thistle. Olive oil promotes the production of bile in the liver as well as protecting it from microorganisms. Many aromatic cooking spices also aid the liver in its detoxification process. Outstanding among them is rosemary, which assists the production and movement of bile through the liver and gallbladder. Dill, caraway, and fennel aid in Phase II detoxification. Be careful with volatile plants like rosemary and sage; although few people have food intolerances to them, airborne allergies to the plants are possible.

### Therapeutic Herbs for the Liver

■ Silymarin (Milk Thistle)—For centuries, European herbalists have used the bioflavonoids in silymarin for restoring liver function. Bioflavonoids are plant pigments with beneficial properties: they protect against damage from destructive free radicals in the body and enhance the activity of vitamin C. Silymarin accelerates the process of regenerating damaged liver tissue, thereby freeing the organ to carry out its key functions. It has even been proven effective against certain types of mushroom and petrochemical solvent poisoning. The usual dose is 2-3 capsules (420 mg) daily of milk thistle standardized to 70%-80% silymarin content.

■ *Picrorrhiza kurroa* (Katuka)—Picrorrhiza is a tiny plant that grows in the Himalayas at an altitude of 9,000-15,000 feet. Its active ingredient has been found to be comparable or superior to that of silymarin. Typical recommended dose: 500 mg, twice daily.

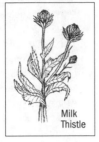

Milk Thistle

■ Dandelion (*Taraxacum officinale*)—As a liver and digestive tonic as well as blood cleanser and diuretic (urine-increasing agent), dandelion aids in detoxification of the body. As testimony to dandelion's powerful influence on the liver, severe hepatitis has been reversed by dandelion tea along with dietary restrictions in as short a period as a week.[6] Given that chemical or heavy metal toxicity is frequently involved in allergies/sensitivities, dandelion can help cleanse the body and support the liver in its own elimination functions. As a digestive tonic, dandelion may also help with the gastrointestinal complaints associated with allergy/sensitivity. Typical recommended dose: 4-10 g of dried root or three cups of fresh dandelion tea, once daily.

■ Other Phytonutrients—Several other phytonutrients ("phyto" meaning plant) have demonstrated anti-inflammatory activity on the liver through various mechanisms. Catechins (a bioflavonoid) are used by European naturopaths and medical doctors to treat chemical hepatitis, cirrhosis, and other environmental and viral forms of liver disease.[7] Catechins can be taken as a nutritional supplement; typical dose is 250 mg, twice daily. Green tea (2-3 cups a day) is also a good source of catechins. Certain botanicals act as Kupffer-cell stimulants, including burdock root, goldenseal, baptisia, smilax, Oregon grape root, and echinacea.

## Parasites in the Intestines

A parasite is an organism that lives off the life and nutrients of another organism, to the host's detriment. Specifically, parasites are the protozoa (single-cell organisms), arthropods (insects), and worms that infect the body and cause serious damage to tissues and organs. Parasites tend to reside in the intestines, but they can also migrate to the blood, lymph, heart, liver, gallbladder, pancreas, spleen, eyes and brain, as well as inside the joints.

It is estimated that more than 300 kinds of parasites can live in the human body, where they often reside as what microbiologists call the

# How Chinese Medicine Views the Liver and Allergies

TCM stresses that an allergy-free and healthy body often depends on a balanced liver. The liver, a yin organ, controls tendons, keeps the qi moving throughout the body, and stores blood. Its yang partner is the gallbladder, which stores and excretes bile, protects the nervous system from overreaction, and helps stabilize emotions.[8] When the liver is congested (made more yang) from eating yang (heating) foods or overloading the body with toxins, the gallbladder's function is likewise impeded, and symptoms of allergies may manifest.

One day, on a hike, Stan, a 39-year-old computer engineer, inadvertently came in contact with poison ivy. He was unaware of the fact until, two days later, when he broke out in a rash, accompanied by uncomfortable itching (allergic contact dermatitis).

Stan tried to relieve the symptoms by taking an over-the-counter antihistamine, Benadryl. This lessened the itching, but the rash continued to get worse. By the time he consulted acupuncturist Ira J. Golchehreh, L.Ac., O.M.D., of San Rafael, California, six days after exposure, he had large, red, raised blisters all over his body, particularly on his abdomen, thighs, and groin.

Dr. Golchehreh discovered that Stan had a history of severe allergies as well as signs of a liver imbalance, which manifested on an emotional level as occasional angry outbursts. According to TCM, this indicates a "hyperactivity of liver yang," explains Dr. Golchehreh, or a liver whose energy, or "fire," is so overreactive (yang) that it creates problems throughout the body and mind. Poison ivy, too, is a manifestation of too much heat, says Dr. Golchehreh, "and the boils are considered an infection of poison in the organs."

The first order of business was to remove the heat from Stan's system so that the toxic manifestation would be eliminated. Dr. Golchehreh used acupuncture to redirect *qi* imbalances and allow the poisons to drain from his system. Additionally, he gave Stan the Chinese herbs *Bupleurum schizonepeta* (commonly used to treat hives) and *Gypsum fibrosum* (calcium sulfate) to help disperse the heat and remove the toxins from his system. Stan also moistened the *Gypsum fibrosum* powder with water to make a paste and applied it topically to cool the lesions. Another remedy in TCM that rebalances the liver is a combination of the herbs Tang-Kuei and Gardenia (3 g, three times a day, between meals).

"I recommended that Stan drink cooling drinks and eat ice cream to cool down his body temperature," Dr. Golchehreh says. "When you have blisters that have become inflamed, it indicates too much heat on the surface of the body and the best thing is to cool down the system with something cold." Applying ice to the skin can also be beneficial for poison ivy symptoms.

Since poison ivy often lingers for weeks, Stan was greatly relieved to find that 48 hours after his visit to Dr. Golchehreh, all traces of his allergic contact dermatitis had disappeared.

Ira J. Golchehreh, L.Ac., O.M.D.: Bay Park Business Center, 2175 Francisco Blvd., Suite D, San Rafael, CA 94901; tel: 415-485-4411.

"great masqueraders." They generate numerous symptoms that are mistakenly associated with other illnesses by conventional medicine, while a parasitic infestation is overlooked. For example, if you have parasites, you may have headaches, back pain, energy loss, spaciness, vomiting, weight loss, colitis, gas, uncontrolled appetite, acne, and many other symptoms. You could easily wander through a labyrinth of unsuccessful treatments for each of the symptoms as the attending physicians never suspect—and therefore never treat—a parasite involvement.

In the U.S., the most common parasites, apart from head lice, are microscopic protozoans. These include *Giardia lamblia*, a virulent form found in the contaminated waters of lakes, streams, and oceans, and a common cause of traveler's diarrhea;[9] *Entamoeba histolytica*, which can cause dysentery and injure the liver and lungs; *Blastocystis hominus*, which is increasingly linked to acute and chronic illnesses; *Dientamoeba fragilis*, associated with diarrhea, abdominal pain, anal itching, and loose stools; and *Cryptosporidia*, which is particularly dangerous to those with compromised immune function. Arthropod parasites, which include mites, fleas, and ticks, can carry smaller parasites that are also infectious to humans. Larger parasites include pinworms, tapeworms, roundworms, hookworms, filaria (thread-like worms that inhabit the blood and tissue) and flukes (which invade the liver).

In case you think it's necessary to travel abroad in undeveloped countries to pick up internal parasites, you are quite mistaken. Many authorities in the field of parasitology now confirm that humans are the vessels of many unreported parasites. In a recent study done at Johns Hopkins Hospital in Baltimore, Maryland, 18% of a random selection of blood samples showed a past or present infection of the parasite *Giardia lamblia*. Parasites can easily evade detection by sophisticated testing; they also have life-cycle phases in which they leave the gastrointestinal system (the site of most parasite testing) and enter the liver, lungs, eyes, kidneys, lymphatic system, or the joints.

## The Link Between Parasites and Allergy
Parasites appear to play two roles in allergy. First, they are highly allergenic; that is, they frequently trigger allergic reactions. In fact, parasitic reactions can be mistaken for food allergy, as is often the case with gastroallergic anisakiasis, a condition in which ingesting raw or undercooked fish containing the parasite *Anisakis simplex* causes a delayed immunoglobulin E allergic reaction. In a recent report, a group of Spanish researchers examined 40 patients who made emergency hos-

pital visits for apparent food allergy symptoms—hives, bronchospasm, anaphylaxis, as well as abdominal pain, vomiting, and diarrhea. Of these, 20 had eaten fish within the past 26 hours. These patients also tested positive for the *Anisakis* parasite and were found to have elevated levels of IgE antibodies, indicating that their bodies were responding allergically to the parasitic invasion.[10]

Parasites also increase intestinal permeability. *Giardia lamblia* is especially implicated in the development of allergy due to leaky gut. In a 1998 study, researchers evaluated a group of Venezuelan children for giardiasis (*Giardia* infestation) and allergy. Seventy percent of the children infected with *Giardia* also manifested symptoms of IgE-mediated food allergy, compared to 43% of non-parasitized children.[11] The researchers concluded that *Giardia* parasites had damaged the children's intestinal mucous membranes and caused sensitization to foods. Another study suggests that parasitic infestation disrupts the regulation of IgE synthesis and causes hypersensitive helper T cell responses, leading to asthma and atopic dermatitis.[12]

# Natural Parasite Elimination Techniques

A period of general body detoxification (elimination, cleansing, and toning) is recommended prior to starting a parasite removal program. This enables the body to handle the destruction of the parasites and the liberation of toxic substances from them. If these toxins are absorbed through the body, they can lead to an unpleasant die-off (Herxheimer) reaction. This means that while, technically, your health is improving because you have destroyed and are removing toxic organisms, you feel terrible during the process, as if your illness were getting worse. Typically, the die-off symptoms may include joint pains, malaise, fever, coated tongue, gastrointestinal disturbances, and diarrhea.

Parasites can be difficult to eradicate, because they can form spores or eggs that are deposited in the body tissues. An anti-parasitic program should be undertaken with the knowledge of the typical life cycle of parasites. The eggs of many of the worms hatch every 2-3 weeks.

For more about **parasitology tests**, see Chapter 3: Allergy/Sensitivity Testing, pp. 70-105.

The length of treatment is critical for successful elimination of parasites—if your program is too short, it may fail to destroy parasites at an advanced stage in their life cycle. Typically, enemas should be performed two to three times weekly for a period of four weeks, followed by an ova (egg) and parasite test, then repeat enemas and other oral anti-parasitic substances, if needed.

According to Dr. Pizzorno, it is essential that you repeat your anti-parasitic program every 2-4 weeks accompanied by a parasitology test (offered by Great Smokies Diagnostic Laboratory). The ova and parasite material, collected from the patient for the test, must be derived from a purged sample or rectal swab in which a saline or other laxative is administered and the purged stool is collected. This should be repeated every two months; do not consider yourself clear of parasites until you have three clearly negative results. Although self-treatment is possible, we advise you to have a knowledgeable health-care practitioner follow your progress; be sure this practitioner is familiar with parasite life cycles, testing, and cleansing procedures. Few local labs, even in large cities, are successful in culturing parasites out of the stool. Great Smokies has a much higher rate of identifying organisms because they do ELISA antibody screens on the stool to detect your antibodies to these organisms.

## Eliminating Parasites with Colon-Cleansing Programs

Colon cleansing is commonly recommended by natural health practitioners as an effective method for eliminating parasites. There are a number of colon-cleansing programs available to help you scrub microorganisms and other toxic materials from the intestines. Colonic irrigations and enemas are highly recommended.

Parasites tend to embed themselves in the intestinal wall, but over the course of several weeks, you can flush them out by using some of these natural substances (preferably in combination): psyllium husks, agar-agar, citrus pectin, papaya extract, pumpkin seeds, flaxseeds, comfrey root, beet root, and bentonite clay (take bentonite only in combination with another substance, such as psyllium). You might also take extra amounts of vitamin C (minimum 2 g daily, but higher amounts up to individual bowel tolerance are more useful) to help flush out your intestine. Note, however, that vitamin C taken at the same time as wormwood (an anti-parasitic herb) makes wormwood ineffective.

Food-grade hydrogen peroxide can be added to an enema (done at home) as an anti-parasitic agent. Add ¼ cup of peroxide per two liters of fluid. Use food-grade hydrogen peroxide because typically drug store brands contain impurities not appropriate for internal consumption. Ozonated water (SEE QUICK DEFINITION) is another safe and effective

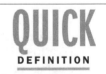

**DEFINITION**

**Ozone** ($O_3$) is a less stable, more reactive form of oxygen, containing three oxygen atoms. This extra atom enables ozone to more readily oxidize other chemicals. In oxidation, the extra oxygen atom breaks off, leaving ordinary oxygen ($O_2$), thereby favorably increasing the oxygen content of body tissues or blood. Medical-grade ozone is used as part of oxygen therapy to increase local oxygen supply to lesions, speed wound healing, reduce infections, and stimulate metabolic processes. Ozone may be administered intravenously or by injection, or applied topically in a water- or olive oil-based solution; it may also be taken orally or rectally as ozonated water.

**CAUTION**

Make sure to dilute the hydrogen peroxide correctly as it can irritate and burn the sensitive mucosa of the intestines.

enema for treating parasites. The ozonated water destroys the parasites as well as the hard covering that surrounds their cysts or eggs, which are highly resistant to many forms of treatment.

A third approach is to perform an enema with essential oils. Combine two drops of the essential oil of thyme, two drops of oregano oil, and two drops of marjoram oil in a two-quart container of water. This will make two complete enemas utilizing a full quart bag of water. When treating parasites, enemas should be done 2-3 times per week for a period of four weeks; this is followed by a test for ova and parasites (as explained above), followed by a repetition of the enemas and oral anti-parasitics, if necessary.

## Herbs for Parasites

Herbs are a safe and effective alternative to drug therapies for ridding yourself of parasites. They are typically free of side effects and often work better than their synthetic counterparts. Purgative herbs such as pumpkin seeds act as mild intestinal cleansers. Decoctions and powders of pumpkin seeds have shown effects against tapeworm and other intestinal parasites in humans and in animals.[13] A typical dose consists of 10-12 seeds in the morning on an empty stomach for two weeks. If the parasites are systemic and have entered the bloodstream, antibiotic herbs such as *Coptis* (a Chinese herb high in berberine) may also be used.

**Garlic (*Allium sativum*)**—One of the least expensive yet most effective ways to deal with parasites is to use an extract of garlic. Raw garlic and garlic extract have been shown to destroy common intestinal parasites, including roundworms and hookworms. According to Chinese research, in the treatment of 100 cases of amoebic dysentery, the cure rate with garlic was 88%. The study found the purple-skinned bulbous garlic was more effective than the white-skinned variety. In another case, enemas made from tea containing garlic were used for 154 cases

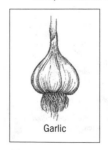

Garlic

of pinworm in children two to nine years old; treatments were repeated on the third and seventh day after the initial treatment. After this period, tests for parasite eggs around the anus were negative (meaning no eggs were found) in 76 of the patients.[14]

Some alternative medicine physicians use freshly juiced garlic (refrigerated after pressing) in the treatment of parasites, dysbiosis, *Candida albicans*, and other infectious microbes. Common dosage is two to

## How to Do an Anti-Parasite Enema

- Measure two quarts of purified, filtered water; don't use tap water or bottled. Bring water to a boil, remove from heat, and steep in a covered pot for 20 minutes.
- Add to the water 4 tsp powdered goldenseal root, 4 tsp powdered thyme (a common kitchen spice), two cloves of crushed garlic juice, 2 tsp of tea tree oil. Let solution cool to body temperature in a covered container.
- Make sure you empty your bowels and bladder prior to the enema. Use K-Y jelly or petroleum jelly (common lubricants found in drug stores) to lubricate the enema speculum (a small tube inserted into the anus) enabling it to easily enter the anus without abrasion. Keep a towel under your buttocks to collect run-off stools and pathogens.
- Hang enema bag above your body so that gravity assists the fluid flow.
- Assume the fetal position and lubricate your rectum, and place enema speculum into rectum. Turn/roll to position on your back with knees up. One hand keeps the speculum in, while the other controls the flow valve.
- Slowly allow the liquid to flow into your colon; stop every three seconds to allow yourself to get used to it. Allow the fluid to enter until you feel a slight cramping or discomfort.
- When your intestines are full, remove speculum, hold your sphincter muscles, get up and get to the toilet. Release bowels, and remain on the toilet seat until all the water has been evacuated.
- Repeat the enema process until you have completely used the water. Clean yourself up. Soak enema speculum in bleach water. Clean the area.
- Do this procedure two to three times a week for four weeks.

three teaspoons in a two-liter bag, which is infused into the patient's colon at the end of a colonic. If doing an enema at home, use 1-2 cloves of garlic, crush them, steep them in a tea for 10-15 minutes with a tight cover, allow this to cool to body temperature, and then put this in the enema bag. Garlic is fairly caustic and if you use too much, you can injure tissues, so it's better to use a small amount. As an oral supplement, two cloves of fresh garlic daily are recommended; in capsule form, 500 mg, twice daily.

**Goldenseal (*Hydrastis canadensis*)**—The alkaloid berberine is found in many plants and in particularly high concentrations in goldenseal. Berberine inhibits the growth of several common parasites that invade the intestine, including *Entamoeba histolytica*, *Giardia lamblia*, *Erwinia carotovora*, and *Leishmania donovania*. In one study, children with giardiasis were given either

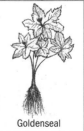

Goldenseal

berberine sulfate (a standardized goldenseal extract) or the drug Flagyl. After ten days, both substances produced similar results: 90% of the berberine-treated group no longer had *Giardia* in their stools compared to 95% of the Flagyl-treated group. Unlike the Flagyl-treated group, however, those receiving berberine suffered no negative side effects.[15] Typical dosage: 500 mg, three times daily.

**Thyme (*Thymus vulgaris*)**—The principle chemical components of thyme are the volatile oils, namely, phenol, thymol, and carvacrol. Thymol is one of the most potent anti-microbial substances known, and even surpasses many of the strongest antibiotics.[16] Thymol's antimicrobial activity is 18 times more powerful than phenol, the major antiseptic used in commercial germicidal cleansers like Lysol®, and can destroy parasites, worms, fungi, bacteria, and many viruses.[17] The recommended dosage is five drops of thyme essential oil diluted in a quart of pure water as an enema solution. You may also take thyme orally at the rate of two or three drops of an oil extract diluted in one cup of water, three times a day for two weeks.

**Grapefruit Seed Extract**—Grapefruit seed extract (GSE) offers some of the benefits of antibiotics (in a natural format) without the side effects. Clinical tests by the U.S. Food and Drug Administration, Pasteur Institute in Paris, and University of Georgia at Athens, have successfully treated bacterial, fungal, and viral infections, such as *Giardia*, amebic dysentery, *E. coli*, *Candida*, and herpes, with GSE.[18] Made from grapefruit seeds and pulp, the medical virtues of GSE were identified in 1964 by Florida physician Jacob Harich, M.D., and later marketed as Citricidal.

Very little is known about the active components of GSE but it contains bioflavonoids (vitamin C enhancers) and hesperidin, a natural immune booster.[19] GSE is effective for allergy patients with intestinal and systemic infections of candidiasis or parasites that cause joint and muscle aches or irritable bowels. While doctors recommend a variety of dosages depending on the stubbornness of the infection, typically a few drops are taken with each meal or diluted in vegetable or fruit juice if the taste is too bitter.[20]

Before beginning any parasite elimination program, consult a qualified health-care professional. This is especially important if you are pregnant.

**Worm Seed (Mexican Tea)**—Epazote (*Chenopodium ambrosoides*), also called worm seed or Mexican tea, is often used in the Caribbean and Central America for worms. Worm seed should never be given to children under the age of six; for those ages six and older, a typical dose of 3-

# Effective Formulas for Parasites

- Biocidin™: This is a complex botanical formula is used to destroy all types of bowel pathogens and is typically taken over the course of six to 12 weeks. Dosage is determined by the health-care practitioner.

- Tricycline: This is a combination of berberine, grapefruit seed extract, and artemesia, also given to destroy all types of bowel pathogens. Typical dosage (practitioner-prescribed): one pill, three times daily, but not taken with food.

- Par Qing: a combination of *artemesia*, anise, cinnamon, and marjoram, for elimination of parasites, both worms and small parasites such as amoebas. Dosage: typically two pills, three times daily, taken with meals.

- Smooth Move Tea: One tea bag can be brewed in one cup of hot water for five minutes; for children, add $1/8$ cup of the brewed tea with apple juice. (This commercially prepared tea is commonly available in natural food stores.)

- Epsom Salts: Known in Germany as *bittersalz*, this inexpensive but bitter-tasting salt of magnesium sulfate heptahydrate is not well-favored by children but can be tolerated by adults, when consumed orally, per directions on package.

- Worm Squirm 1 and 2: Both are encapsulated herbal formulas for ridding the body of parasites; formula number 1 is for roundworms including pinworms, *Ascaris*, hookworms, and whipworms; formula number 2 for tapeworms, flukes, and flatworms and both should not be taken at the same time. Worm Squirm 1 contains *Artemisia annua*, black walnut, cloves, gentian root, ginger, hyssop, mandrake root, and tansy flower; Worm Squirm 2 contains chamomile, male fern rhizome, pink root, pumpkin seeds, and senna.

- PlantiBiotic: This is an antiparasite herbal formula (also effective against *Candida albicans*) that includes barberry (200 mg), berberine (125 mg), citrus seed extract (200 mg), thyme oil (250 mg), oregano oil (250 mg), tea tree oil (100 mg), garlic (50 mg), quassia bark (50 mg), cascara sagrada (50 mg), black walnut hull (50 mg), *Artemesia annua* (50 mg), epazote (50 mg), and cloves (50 mg). The recommended dosage is three pills, three times daily with food, for two months.

> For **grapefruit seed extract**, available as ProSeed™ (in liquid concentrate, Vegicaps®, Feminine Rinse, Ear Drops, Gum Cleanser, and Herbal Cleansing Spray) or a similar line called Seed-a-Sept™ (formulated for physicians), contact: Imhotep, Inc., P.O. Box 183, Ruby, NY 12475; tel: 800-677-8577. For **Biocidin™**: Bio-Botanical Research, Inc., P.O. Box 1061, Soquel, CA 95073. For **Tricycline and Par Qing**: Nutricology/Allergy Research Group, P.O. Box 55907, Hayward, CA 94544; tel: 800-782-4274 or 510-487-8526; fax: 510-487-8682; e-mail: info@nutricology.com; website: www.nutricology.com. For **Worm Squirm 1 and 2**: Arise & Shine, P.O. Box 1439, Mt. Shasta, CA 96067; tel: 800-688-2444 or 530-926-0891; fax: 530-926-8866. For **PlantiBiotic**: Nature's Answer, 320 Oser Avenue, Hauppauge, NY 11788; tel: 800-439-2324 or 516-231-7492; fax: 516-951-2499; website: www.naturesanswer.com.

5 drops per day. Make a tea by steeping 3-4 teaspoons of the dried or fresh herb in one cup of water for 20 minutes; drink one cup per day. Typical dosage: 50 mg, three times daily.

**Chinese Wormwood (*Artemesia absinthium*)**—*Artemesia absinthium* has a long history of use as a vermifuge or "worm expeller," hence its common name, wormwood. It was even prized by Hippocrates to expel worms. Similar in action to the Chinese herb *Artemesia annua*, it is especially effective against *Giardia* and other protozoas, but some caution is advised. It may initially worsen symptoms and cause some intestinal irritation. Although it may be toxic if used alone in large quantities, it is usually mixed in formulas with grapefruit seed extract and other herbs that offset its possible toxic effects. Typical recommended dosage: 150 mg, three times daily.

For more information about **Dr. Hulda Clark's anti-parasite program**, see *Alternative Medicine Definitive Guide to Cancer* (Future Medicine Publishing, 1997; ISBN 1-887299-01-7); to order, call 800-333-HEAL.

Wormwood is also part of the anti-parasite protocol of naturopathic physician Hulda Regehr Clark, N.D., Ph.D. She recommends using a blend of three herbs to flush the parasites out of your system: black walnut hull tincture, wormwood capsules, and fresh ground cloves (to kill the parasites' eggs). This program should only be undertaken with professional guidance from a licensed health-care practitioner.

**Ayurvedic Herbs**—The traditional Indian medical science of Ayurveda has several natural remedies which address specific parasite infections, according to Virender Sodhi, N.D., M.D. (Ayurvedic), of Bastyr University in Bellevue, Washington. For pinworms, Dr. Sodhi recommends bitter melon (*Mormordica charantia*), a cucumber-shaped fruit that is best used cut up and eaten in small pieces with other vegetables because of its bitter taste. Consuming one or two bitter melons a day for 7–10 days, then repeating this after one month, can be effective in the treatment of worms, says Dr. Sodhi. It is easy to tell if there is any recurrent infection, says Dr. Sodhi, as thousands of little white bugs will show up in the stool the day after eating bitter melon if there is pinworm presence remaining.

The herbs embliaribes, vidang, and kamila are most effective for roundworms, according to Dr. Sodhi. "Take one teaspoon of the herb powder extract twice a day with sweetened water or juice to attract the parasites. Do this for seven to ten days and then check your stool. If there is still evidence of infestation, repeat the cycle until you are parasite free."

"Kamila is also effective for tapeworms," says Dr. Sodhi, "as well as betel nut, which can be chewed." The same kind of protocol as with pinworms and roundworms can be used. "Betel nut is also used quite a bit in veterinary medicine, as dog and cats get a lot of tapeworms,

## Important Reminders During Any Parasite Treatment

Whatever treatment you employ to rid your body of parasites, the following recommendations can help ensure that the program is a success:

- If you have children and/or pets, they must be treated at the same time as the adults in the household to prevent re-infection.

- Drink more pure water (not from the tap) than usual to help the body flush out the dead parasites from your system; at least 64 ounces of water per day for a 150-pound adult.

- Sanitize your environment. When you have almost finished treatment, wash all pajamas, bed clothes, and sheets before using them again.

- Eat anti-parasitic foods. According to Ann Louise Gittleman, a nutrition educator in Bozeman, Montana, these include pineapple and papaya, either as fresh juice or in organic supplement form, in combination with pepsin and hydrochloric acid. Avoid all meats and dairy products for at least one week. You can also use pomegranate juice (four 4-ounce glasses daily), papaya seeds, finely ground pumpkin seeds ($1/4$ to $1/2$ cup daily), and two cloves of raw garlic daily.

Do not drink the pomegranate juice for more than four to five days.

- Modify your diet. For people with heavy parasitic infection, nutritionist Gittleman recommends a diet comprised of 25% fat, 25% protein, and 50% complex carbohydrates. You also need a regular intake of unprocessed flaxseed, safflower, sesame, or canola oils (two tablespoons daily) and extra vitamin A. Flaxseed oil is preferable because it has much higher levels of alpha-linolenic acid (an omega-3 essential fatty acid that is commonly deficient in many people) than the other oils.

- Recolonize your intestines. You need to reintroduce beneficial, friendly bacteria (probiotics) into your intestinal system once you have flushed out the parasites, Gittleman advises. The bacterial strains most helpful here are *Lactobacillus plantarum*, *L. salvarius*, *L. acidophilus*, *L. bulgaris*, *B. bifidum*, and *Streptococcus faeceum*, which are available as nutritional supplements. *L. plantarum* is the most effective of these in resolving parasite problems.

too," Dr. Sodhi adds. For *Giardia*, amoebas, *Cryptosporidium*, and other protozoal parasites, the treatment is usually longer than for worms, taking up to several months. The herbs that are most effective for these microscopic intruders are bilva, neem, and berberine, which can be taken in combination.

Dr. Sodhi also recommends bitter melon for protozoal infestations, as well as such nutritional supports as psyllium husk, turmeric, and *L. acidophilus* for the enhancement of the intestinal microflora.

**Virender Sodhi, N.D., M.D., (Ayurvedic)**: 2115 112th Avenue N.E., Bellevue, WA 94004; tel: 425-453-8022; fax: 425-451-2670.

Ayurvedic physicians state that when treating parasites, you must address the immune system; so various herbs and techniques for enhancing the immunity can also be utilized to support the body in its defense against the parasites. Herbs useful for this task, according to Ayurvedic medicine, include ginseng, ligustri berries, and schisandra berries.

## Hygiene
The following hygienic precautions can help you avoid parasitic infection:

### General Hygiene—
- Always wash your hands after using the toilet.
- Wash your hands after working in the garden; the soil can be contaminated with spores and parasites.

### In the Kitchen—
- Do not eat raw beef—it can be loaded with tapeworms and other parasites.
- Do not eat raw fish or sushi—you are likely to get worms if you do.
- Wash your hands after handling raw meat or fish (including shrimp). Do not put your hands near your mouth without washing them first.
- Use a separate cutting board for meat and vegetables. Spores from meat can seep into the board and contaminate vegetables or anything else you put on the board.
- Wash utensils thoroughly after cutting meat.
- Wash vegetables and fruit thoroughly, particularly salad items, as they often harbor parasites. Wash in a few drops of grapefruit seed extract diluted in one gallon of water. Soak for 15-20 minutes. Then soak in fresh water for 20 minutes before refrigerating.

### Pets—
- Do not sleep near your pets since they may harbor worms or other parasites.
- De-worm your pets regularly and keep their sleeping areas clean.
- Do not let pets lick your face.
- Do not let pets eat off your dishes.

### While Traveling—
- Do not drink from streams and rivers.

■ Do not drink the tap water.

■ Start taking grapefruit seed extract (three drops of Citricidal per day or ten drops of Seed-a-Sept four times per day), bismuth (1-2 tsps of Pepto Bismal four times per day), and *L. acidophilus* three days before traveling, and continue them while you travel.

# 9 Supporting the Skin

**A**LLERGY PREVENTION is literally skin deep. The skin is the largest organ of the body and one of the first lines of defense against external pathogens, such as chemicals and poisons, and one of the key pathways in eliminating toxins from the body. As we've learned, effective barrier and detoxification functions are crucial to preventing and reversing allergy and sensitivity.

For all the emphasis Americans place on the appearance of skin—using cosmetics to cover up blemishes, topical ointments to combat pimples, and collagen and botox injections to fight wrinkles—they generally do a poor job of protecting their skin. In fact, many skin-care products actually damage the skin barrier and clog detoxification pores, leading to a host of allergic conditions and other skin problems. Other factors, including essential fatty acid deficiency, humidity, radiation, and stress, impair cutaneous integrity.

In this chapter, we describe how various dietary practices, environmental conditions, and psychological problems affect the skin barrier function. We also offer alternative therapies to restore your skin to health and minimize, even eliminate, skin disorders such as atopic dermatitis, hives, and allergic contact dermatitis.

## Anatomy of the Skin Barrier

The skin is made up of two distinct layers, the epidermis and, beneath it, the dermis. The outermost level of the epidermis, called the stratum corneum (SC), is important for allergy and sensitivity. The SC is a network of cells on the surface of the skin that provides immediate protection from the outside world and helps restrict the loss of water. When SC cells die, they are shed and then replaced by cells that push up from the lowest level of the epidermis, the stratum basale.

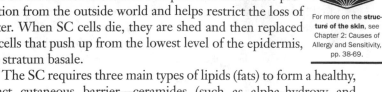

For more on the **structure of the skin**, see Chapter 2: Causes of Allergy and Sensitivity, pp. 38-69.

The SC requires three main types of lipids (fats) to form a healthy, intact cutaneous barrier—ceramides (such as alpha-hydroxy and omega-hydroxy acids), cholesterol, and polyunsaturated fatty acids (essential fatty acids). Microscopic examination of the formation of the SC has found that these three types of fats fill in the space (called domains) between SC cells to make a protective sheet.[1] When the lipids are tightly packed into the spaces between SC cells, potentially harmful substances that touch the skin are unable to squeeze their way through the skin surface and enter the body.

On the other hand, when there are disruptions in the number and compactness of the intercellular lipids, the skin barrier becomes permeable. A sign of this break in the SC lipids is water from the underlying skin layers escaping through the surface of the skin; in clinical terms, this condition is called transepidermal water loss (TEWL). The higher the TEWL measurements, the more permeable the skin barrier.

## Does Skin Permeability Cause Allergic Skin Conditions?

Much research has been done to confirm that intestinal permeability leads to food allergy, manifesting as migraines, gastrointestinal problems, and skin diseases such as hives and eczema. But does skin permeability similarly induce sensitization and cause allergic skin conditions? In the case of allergic contact dermatitis, the answer is obviously yes. When you brush up against poison ivy, oak, or sumac, the urushiol oil released by the plant leaves touches your skin. If your skin barrier function is impaired, the toxin seeps through the gaps between SC cells, enters the blood vessels in the dermis and subcutaneous fatty tissue, and sparks an antibody-mediated reaction. This explains why some people do not suffer with allergic contact dermatitis when exposed to poisonous plants—their skin barriers were intact and able to effectively protect the body from the toxin.

Additionally, research shows that continued barrier disruption exacerbates existing cases of allergic contact dermatitis. In one study, subjects who had previous breakouts of allergic contact dermatitis were treated with acetone, a chemical that is known to cause skin permeability.[3] Within 24 hours of exposure to the acetone, proliferation of Langerhans cells increased by up to 80%; these cells, located in the epidermis, trap and destroy invading antigens. Subjects were then exposed to offending contactants (nickel in jewelry, fragrances in cosmetics, etc.). The allergic response that followed was more severe than usual, due to the increase in the Langerhans cell population. Another study found that a damaged epidermis can be expected to produce a defective stratum corneum, thus resulting in a vicious cycle of continued allergic contact dermatitis reactions, barrier damage, and sensitization to new allergens.[4]

## The Circadian Rhythms of Skin Permeability

Every physiological function in humans is believed to run according to certain innate cycles, whether hourly, daily, monthly, etc. Skin barrier function is no exception. According to a report in the *Journal of Investigative Dermatology*, the degree of skin permeability fluctuates on a circadian (daily) basis. In the study, researchers measured transepidermal water loss, stratum corneum moisture, skin surface pH (acid/base), and skin temperature of 16 healthy volunteers over a 24-hour period. They discovered that permeability in all tested skin sites was higher in the evening and night than in the morning.[2] This may provide clues as to the best time to administer therapeutic aids for restoring skin barrier function.

Hives are usually triggered by injected and oral drugs such as penicillin and aspirin, foods such as strawberries and fish, and inhalants such as pollens, molds, and animal dander. However, this allergic reaction can also be induced by contact with laundry detergents, fabric softeners, and cosmetics, which isn't surprising because these products often contain chemicals that damage the skin barrier, leading to sensitization.

Atopic dermatitis, likewise, can be sparked by numerous allergens—inhaled, ingested, and contactant substances. Food is particularly implicated in the development of eczema. In one recent double-blind clinical test, 87 (81%) of 107 children with atopic dermatitis tested positive to at least one food allergy; eggs were the most common food allergen (70%).[5] This finding suggests that sensitization does not occur through the skin but through intestines. However, another study found that the majority of patients with atopic eczema have normal intestinal permeability function, dismissing the thought the food allergy is the primary cause of eczema.[6] Another study conducted on children with atopic eczema showed that the most common allergens sparking the eczema flare-ups were the inhalants dust mites and cat dander.[7] The researchers of this study, however, found that while the children were more allergic to inhalant substances, sensitization did not necessarily occur through the respiratory tract, as expected. In fact, the researchers concluded that early epicutaneous (through the skin) sensitization to aeroallergens had been enhanced by damage to the skin barrier function.

While other studies have determined that atopic eczema is not always accompanied by skin permeability,[8] it appears that skin barrier default is the primary culprit in initial sensitization. That individuals with eczema develop allergies to substances that enter the body via the gut or respiratory tract suggests that these people become more susceptible to other allergies once the skin barrier has been disrupted. Statistics from the American Academy of Allergy, Asthma & Immunology confirm this—more than 50% of all patients with atopic eczema ultimately develop asthma and approximately 75% develop allergic rhinitis.[9]

# Success Story: Healing an "Incurable" Case of Eczema

Jimmy was 2½ years old when I first met him. I talked mostly to Jimmy's mother because Jimmy wept and moaned constantly. Jimmy was about 90% covered with an intensely itchy as well as painful eczema rash that cracked, bled, and oozed. They had been to pediatricians, allergists, dermatologists, and even some other alternative physicians. Jimmy had undergone many medical tests. All of his practitioners had arrived at a diagnosis of atopic dermatitis and allergy.

## Environmental Control Alleviates Eczema

Eczema patients are more prone to develop inhalant allergies, according to research. Thus, it makes sense that minimizing exposure to inhalant allergens will reduce the symptoms of this skin disease. A report in *Allergy* confirms this thinking. In a study with 45 people with atopic eczema, 28 were enrolled in a comprehensive environmental control program to eliminate house dust mites. Mattresses were encased in Gor-tex bags, high-powered vacuums were used to clean carpets and floors, and benzyl alcohol and tannic acid solutions were sprayed throughout the homes to kill mites and denature allergens. In the control group, light cotton mattress bags, less powerful vacuums, and water sprays were used. No other modifications were made. After six months, most of the 28 patients experienced more significant improvements in their condition than the control patients did; the most severely affected subjects had more remarkable improvements.[10]

For more on **eliminating allergens from your home**, see Chapter 5: Environmental Control, pp. 128-157.

## Psoriasis—An Allergy to Yourself

Psoriasis is a chronic inflammatory skin disease affecting about 2% of the population, especially those between ages 15 and 30. In people without psoriasis, the epidermal cells are replaced approximately every 28 days. However, in people with psoriasis, cells in the epidermis are renewed every three or four days.[11] This accelerated cell turnover causes the epidermis cell thickness to increase by up to nine times. The visible manifestations are thick, scaly, itchy, weepy lesions or pustules, which usually appear on the scalp, elbows, knees, small of the back, and lower legs. However, some psoriatic patients have lesions over much of their body. Some people suffering from psoriasis have symptoms remarkably similar to those of rheumatoid arthritis (joint pain and bone degeneration); however, psoriatic arthritis patients do not have rheumatoid factor, a chemical that indicates rheumatoid arthritis. Topical creams containing tar and phototherapy (sun or light therapy) are often used to minimize symptoms of psoriasis.

Psoriasis, like arthritis, is an autoimmune disease, meaning the patient's immune system is making antibodies to it's own tissue. Psoriasis patients are allergic to themselves, specifically their skin. This inflammatory skin disorder also shares some similarities with atopic dermatitis and other allergic inflammatory skin conditions. As with atopic eczema, psychological stress appears to trigger and exacerbate psoriasis and dealing with psychological issues has been shown to alleviate both disorders.[12] Psoriasis likewise seems to be affected by some foods. In a 1996 study, Italian researchers examined 316 patients with psoriasis. They found that psoriasis was linked to the intake of carrots, tomatoes, fresh fruits, and beta-carotene foods.[13] Furthermore, as with allergic eczema, arachidonic acid (a type of omega-6 fatty acid that can lead to inflammation) has been shown to be involved in the genesis and continuation of psoriasis. Decreasing consumption of foods containing this fat and adding omega-3 essential fatty acids to the diet has produced moderate to excellent results in as many as 58% of psoriatic patients.[14]

Psoriatic patients tend to have poor dietary practices, which could contribute to essential fatty acid deficiency, stress, and other factors that contribute to this disease. In a survey of 219 psoriatic patients and 747 controls, psoriatic patients were found to consume more high-fat and saturated fat foods (high in arachidonic acids) and drink more alcohol than the control group.[15]

Jimmy's doctors had prescribed a multitude of treatments, some of which worked somewhat but only temporarily. Jimmy's mother was frustrated and discouraged, because the doctors' only recommendations were continuation of topical and systemic steroids and three to five years of immunotherapy (allergy shots). But even with these treatments, she was told that her son would suffer from eczema for the rest of his life. Finally, out of desperation, she and Jimmy flew out from the East Coast to my practice in Phoenix, Arizona.

During our initial visit, we confirmed previously noted physical findings of the severe dermatitis and other signs of allergy/sensitivity disease, including dry mucous membranes. Jimmy's mother brought in a first-morning urine specimen, which indicated protein malabsorption, mild dehydration, moderate toxic load, calcium wasting, inadequate vitamin C, and adrenal exhaustion. Basal temperatures were low, indicating low thyroid function. Fecal transit time was 28 hours, indicating constipation and toxic overload. We administered allergy and *Candida* tests, gave Jimmy's mother some information on the Natural Elimination of Allergy Therapy (NEAT) protocol, and recommended Lung Tan Xie Gang, Tri Snake Anti-Itch Pills, and Armadillo Counter Poison Pills, (three patent medicines for eczema); Ultracare for Kids to start detoxification; Similase Jr., a digestive enzyme; a homeopathic stimulation of thyroid, thymus, and adrenal glands; and vitamin C and a multivitamin/mineral supplement to add to the UltraCare for Kids shake. To improve his skin barrier and mitigate inflammation, I recommended that borage oil (high in omega-6 fatty acids) and flaxseed oil (high in omega-3 fats) be added to the shake.

For more on **Natural Elimination of Allergy Therapy**, see Chapter 13: Desensitizing the Immune System, pp. 328-347.

For **Similase Jr.**, contact: Tyler Encapsulations, 2204-8 N.W. Birdsale, Gresham, OR 97030; tel: 800-869-9705 or 503-661-5401; fax: 503-666-4913. For **UltraCare for Kids**, contact: Metagenics, Inc., 971 Calle Negocio, San Clemente, CA 92673; tel: 800-692-9400; fax: 949-366-0818; website: www.metagenics.com.

On the next visit, Jimmy was slightly improved and we started electrodermal screening to find out what he was sensitized to; we also treated him for airborne sensitivities using a specific acupressure protocol to desensitize him. He had an aggravation of his skin condition the night after his treatment, which was resolved by the next morning. He was even further improved by the next visit. However, when we tested and treated him for contactant and other chemicals, he again experienced a flare-up of his symptoms, which is a normal part of the healing process.

At the fourth visit, Jimmy was markedly improved, with the eczema now mostly around his joints. He was no longer crying constantly. We tested and treated him for foods with a similar outcome from the previous visits, except now his rash only flared up behind his ears and around his elbows and wrists. For the last visit, we had his mother bring items from the home environment to test for sensitization. We also repeated all of the previous tests. When I next saw him, Jimmy now had no rash and was acting like a normal, healthy child.

During a six-week span of time, we identified approximately 350 items that Jimmy was sensitized to from a variety of sources—some inhalants, some contactants, and some foods. We helped him repair his barrier functions and restore his support organ functions. We helped to detoxify him, recolonize his gut, and replace his nutrient losses. Then, we desensitized him and gave him strategies to prevent resensitization by keeping his barrier functions intact. He went home a normal little boy with a much-relieved mother who was no longer stressed by her son's condition and had developed strategies to control adverse events and prevent recurrence, without the use of the steroid medications and allergy shots.

# The Causes of Skin Barrier Damage

In general, two mechanisms increase skin permeability: removing/depleting surface lipids and altering the cells in lower levels of the epidermis. The removal or deficiency of lipids means that gaps will open between cells in the stratum corneum. Alterations in epidermal cells can cause defects in the stratum corneum cell structure or other abnormalities in the skin protection barrier. Essential fatty acid deficiency or abnormal metabolism of essential fatty acids, skin-care and cleaning products, ultraviolet radiation, climate changes, hormonal changes, and even psychological stress can lead to skin permeability and increase the risk of sensitization.

### Essential Fatty Acid Deficiency

As we discussed above, three types of fats are responsible for maintaining skin barrier function—cholesterol (SEE QUICK DEFINITION), ceramides (such as alpha-hydroxy acid), and polyunsaturated fatty acids. Usually most Americans have adequate supplies of cholesterol or ceramides for the skin, both from dietary sources and internal metabolism, but they may not get enough polyunsaturated fatty acids, especially essential fatty acids (EFAs—SEE QUICK DEFINITION) that are only available through diet. When these fats are deficient in the diet, fewer are available in the stratum corneum, resulting in an incomplete protective barrier.

The skin barrier requires an abundance of omega-6 essential fatty acids. There are two primary types of omega-6 EFAs, linoleic acid (LA) and arachidonic acid (AA), both of which are only found in foods. Linoleic acid is found in the oils of safflower, sunflower, corn, soy, and sesame. A specialized enzyme converts linoleic acid into gamma-linolenic acid (GLA), a fatty acid that is easily absorbed into the body. Research has found that metabolism of LA into GLA is highly active in the skin epidermis, where GLA is needed to complete the surface lipid structure.[16] GLA is found naturally in evening primrose oil, black currant oil, and borage oil.

Studies have found that dietary deficiency of linoleic acid results in scaly skin disorders and excessive water loss, due to increased skin permeability.[17] However, it is important to note that several studies have found that dietary deficiency of LA is not necessarily to blame for impaired skin barrier function. A study in the *American Journal of Clinical Nutrition* reported that there is no deficit of linoleic acid in most patients with atopic dermatitis.[18] In fact, this study showed that concentrations of linoleic acid tend to be elevated in blood, milk, and adipose tissue, whereas concentrations of linoleic acid metabolites (GLA) are substantially reduced. The researcher concluded that this abnormality is caused by a genetic inability to properly convert linoleic acid to gamma-linolenic acid. Other studies confirm this hypothesis. Researchers have found that individuals with atopic dermatitis tend to have a defect or deficiency in delta-6-desaturase, the metabolic enzyme responsible for converting LA into GLA.[19]

## Changes in Humidity

Changes in humidity—whether seasonal or from going in and out of air conditioning—have been shown to damage the skin barrier. In a recent study, researchers found that seasonal changes in humidity are implicated in exacerbating skin diseases, such as atopic dermatitis and psoriasis. Exposure to changes in environmental humidity (from high to low) seem to cause an increased turnover rate of skin cells, which exhausts the oils in the barrier and exacerbates inflammatory skin lesions and barrier function default.[20]

## Dehydration

Dehydration also impairs skin function. The surface skin is thicker than the interior tissues of the body. Circulation comes to the base of the skin, and the water has to seep upwards through all the strata of the skin to

---

## QUICK DEFINITION

**Cholesterol** is an essential component in cell membranes needed by the body to make bile salts, which help absorb the fat-soluble vitamins (A, D, E, K) and essential fatty acids from the small intestine. Cholesterol, a steroid, is also necessary for steroidal hormones and male and female sex hormones, including pregnenolone, testosterone, estradiol, estrone, progesterone, and cortisol. These are critical for the health of the immune system, the mineral-regulating functions of the kidneys, and the smooth running of the hormonal systems in men and women. Cholesterol is not only obtained through the diet, but produced by the liver, which synthesizes about 3,000 mg of new cholesterol in any 24-hour period, a quantity equivalent to the amount contained in ten eggs. This new cholesterol is used to repair cells; when cholesterol levels get too low, depression, lung disease, and even cancer can result.

**Essential fatty acids (EFAs)** are unsaturated fats required in the diet. EFAs cannot be made in the body and must be obtained through your diet. Linoleic acid is the essential fat; all other oils can be internally metabolized from it. Omega-3 and omega-6 oils are the two most important metabolites of linoleic acid for immune and inflammatory processes. A balance of these oils in the diet is necessary for good health. Fish oils, such as salmon, cod, trout, and mackerel, are rich in omega-3 oils. Linoleic acid, the main omega-6 oil, is found in vegetable oils, including safflower, corn, peanut, sunflower, soybean, and sesame.

## Staph Infections Make Eczema Worse

The severity of atopic dermatitis may be compounded by an overgrowth of bacteria on the surface of the skin. More than 90% of patients with atopic dermatitis show skin colonization of the bacterium *Staphylococcus aureus*, a common bacteria that interferes with the inflammatory process of atopic dermatitis in various ways, which includes the release of great amounts of antigens that provoke inflammation.[21] Eliminating the bacterial infection often improves eczema flare-ups.

In a recent study, researchers screened 21 eczema patients for skin colonization of S. *aureus*, and prescribed three topical treatments—gentian violet (an antiseptic), glucocorticosteroids, or tar solution (both are common eczema medications)—to be applied twice daily for four days.[22] During the treatment period, the patients using gentian violet experienced a dramatic reduction in bacteria and a significant improvement in symptom severity. Those on medication only had decreased bacteria counts after treatment. Natural antiseptics, such as tea tree oil, grapefruit seed extract, or neem oil, may also be effective for ridding the skin of bacterial infections.

reach the outer layer. It's not unlike a flowering plant that must receive adequate water through its roots. The exposed surface of the skin is also constantly losing water due to environmental factors such as sun, wind, and chemicals, to name a few, creating a kind of double jeopardy.

When the body itself is dehydrated, circulation to the base of the outer skin may be shut down as an emergency measure so that water is not lost through evaporation from the skin's surface. If circulation to the base of the skin is shut down, we develop gray skin. Next, the cells of the skin gradually lose structure and go from a plum-like state into a prune-like state. Chronic dehydration shows in the face with wrinkles, lines, and furrows. Any structural change in the cell membrane will affect permeability of the entire skin barrier.

### Ultraviolet Radiation (Sun)

As pollution continually eats away at the Earth's protective barrier, the ozone layer, we are becoming increasingly exposed to the sun's dangerous ultraviolet (UV) rays. We know that both types of UV rays— UVA and UVB—can lead to skin cancer and eye problems if we don't protect ourselves from the harsh radiation. What most people may not realize is that UV radiation also increases skin permeability and can be a significant factor in sensitization.

While many studies have shown that UVB irradiation of mammalian skin is associated with reduced barrier function, one recent study investigated the alterations in stratum corneum lipids caused by daily UVB irradiation in animal skin. The researchers found that TEWL (transepidermal water loss) values were significantly higher in UVB-treated animals than in controls.[24] Further microscopic analysis found abnormalities in the space between stratum corneum cells as well as damaged SC cells.

Additional research has found that these abnormalities were due to a delayed, UVB-induced decrease in cholesterol, fatty acid, and ceramide synthesis in the epidermis.[25] Lipid synthesis was fairly normal between 24 and 48 hours after exposure but significantly declined 72 hours later. Lipid levels recovered after 96 hours, indicating that UVB-induced barrier damage may not be permanent and irreversible.

### Skin-Care Products

Most people know from firsthand experience that abrasives and chemical agents, such as grit and bleach, in household cleaning solutions can irritate the skin. Indeed, they've been shown to damage the skin barrier,[26] and those with eczema and psoriasis are affected more severely.[27] Thus, many people wear protective gloves when using these products. However, numerous skin-care products also contain ingredients that have been clinically proven to damage the skin barrier.

## Water: Too Much of a Good Thing

We need water—in our bodies and in a balanced state in our air—to restore and maintain the skin barrier. However, prolonged immersion in water can be detrimental. In a recent study, immersing skin in water for as little as two hours caused an alteration in the intercellular layers. After six hours, surface lipids began to separate and, after 24 hours, there was extensive loosening of the lipids and SC cells.[23] The researchers concluded that prolonged exposure to water damages the skin barrier similarly to irritant chemicals, leading to skin permeability and susceptibility to sensitization. Most people will never find themselves floating in water for 24 hours; however, taking long baths or swimming for an extended period of time can create conditions for skin permeability.

Sodium lauryl sulfate is a highly irritating chemical that is found in many shampoos, conditioners, body washes, and other skin-care products. Acetone, another well-known irritant, is the main ingredient in nail polish remover. In fact, these two chemicals are routinely used in lab experiments to induce skin permeability. Below, we describe some of the most detrimental chemicals found in skin-care products.

For more on **damaging chemicals found in skin-care products**, see Chapter 5: Environmental Control, pp. 128-157.

# Do Barrier Creams Prevent Latex Glove Reactions?

Allergic reactions to latex gloves have become an epidemic in the health-care profession—it's estimated that latex allergy affects between 5% and 10% of health-care personnel.[28] How many of their patients experience reactions on the other side of the gloves is not known, but it is a major health concern in hospitals and medical offices. Food service and housekeeping employees also often wear latex gloves and are at risk for developing allergies.

To prevent latex reactions, some institutions have begun using nonlatex, nonvinyl gloves; others have provided "barrier" creams that you apply to your skin before slipping on latex gloves. These creams contain zinc oxide, among other ingredients, and are intended to prevent the natural rubber latex (NRL) allergen from touching the skin and setting off a reaction. Do these barrier creams really work?

According to 1998 study conducted in Germany, the answer is no. This study examined 109 people reporting symptoms of latex sensitivity, 66 of whom tested positive for latex-specific IgE antibodies (indicating a true latex allergy), while the rest tested negative for IgE antibody (suggesting sensitivity). Both groups were given two sets of latex gloves—the first pair had a high NRL allergen content; the second pair had a lower NRL content. Both the latex-allergy and latex-sensitive subjects wore both types of gloves, once after applying commercially available barrier cream and once without the barrier cream. The low-allergen gloves did not produce antibody response in either group of untreated glove-wearers, but when the cream was applied, 5% of the latex-allergy group reacted with IgE antibodies. Antibody response to the untreated high-allergen glove was 30% in IgE-allergic subjects and 3% in nonallergic subjects. After applying the barrier cream, 41% of the allergic and 7% of the nonallergic subjects experienced antibody responses to latex.

The researchers concluded that so-called skin-protection creams actually favor the uptake of allergens from gloves, increasing allergic reactions.[29] Using low-allergen latex gloves without barrier creams appears to be the safest choice for latex-sensitive individuals. Additionally, using powder-free latex gloves can reduce the risk for reactions, because the cornstarch powder that lines the gloves acts as a vehicle for transporting latex allergens.[30]

**Sodium Lauryl Sulfate**—Sodium lauryl sulfate (SLS, also known as sodium laureth or lauryl sulfate) is a cleanser found in many skin- and hair-care products and detergents. In one 1998 study, repetitive contact with SLS solutions for three days (simulating typical exposure) was shown to damage the skin barrier.[31] However, researchers were surprised to find that SLS did not cause skin permeability by removing the lipids on the surface of the stratum corneum. Instead, SLS altered the nuclei in epidermal cells and also disturbed SC lipids just beneath the surface. Barrier cream application greatly reduced the damaging effects of SLS—by up to 58% before SLS exposure and 56% after exposure. However, corticosteroid drugs, which are often prescribed for cases of contact dermatitis and eczema, have not been shown to significantly improve barrier function in SLS-damaged skin.[32] Discontinuing use of SLS-containing products is the only way to avoid the permeability caused by this chemical.

**Retinoids (Vitamin A)**—Skin products containing retinoids (natural vitamin A) or retinoic acid (synthetic vitamin A) are very popular in the American marketplace as a means to decrease wrinkling, brown spots, and acne. But anyone who's used products such as Retin-A knows about the side effects—dry skin, peeling, and photosensitivity (adverse reactions to the sun). These drawbacks are due to skin permeability induced by vitamin A.

Several studies have found that retinoic acid loosens the cohesion of cells and lipids in the stratum corneum as well as other levels in the epidermis.[33] While this process, in part, provides for greater elasticity and smoothness to the skin, it also causes barrier dysfunction, increased transepidermal water loss, and scaling. However, further research shows that the natural retinoids retinaldehyde and retinol cause less skin damage than the synthetic retinoic acid.[34]

## The Effects of Alkanes on the Skin

Saturated fats such as alkanes are like plastic bags when applied to the skin. They form a sealed film of grease on the skin barrier, impeding the absorption of oxygen from the air and blocking the elimination of wastes from within the body. Continuous use of skin-care products containing alkanes and other saturated fats contributes to the development of allergy and sensitivity.

The inability to eliminate wastes allows for toxins to accumulate in the subcutaneous connective and fatty tissue. Over time, this leads to lymphatic stress. When the detoxification pathways—lymph, skin, liver, and other organs—are overloaded with toxins, the immune system will tend to overreact because it is overwhelmed with dangerous antigens. Allergic reactions are just one of the many symptoms of a hyperactive immune system caused by toxic overload.

High-quality cosmetics reduce the problem by using other saturated fats, such as beeswax combined with alkane or other oily substances. The skin effects are less obstructive than pure paraffin or paraffin-derivative ointment, but if regularly used, the skin will also become inflexible and start to react.

**Alkanes (Paraffin)**—Alkanes, also known as paraffin, are by-products of petroleum manufacturing commonly used as the base of many topical lotions, cosmetics, and hair-care products. Alkanes are saturated hydrocarbons, which means that by virtue of their complex molecular structure they cannot bind to other molecules. For that reason, they are used as preservatives, since they don't oxidize (mix with oxygen) and become rancid. Alkanes can be purified in the laboratory so that they are nearly free of other substances; they are often the base used in "hypoallergenic" products. A study sponsored by Avon, which sells cosmetics, found that repetitive use of alkane-containing products irritates the skin and contributes to skin permeability.[35]

Moreover, alkanes can confuse the sebaceous glands, whose job it is to regulate the synthesis of fat in the skin. The result is a supposed fat demand of the skin. A typical example for this process is the condition of "housewife hands." Cream (containing paraffin), is rubbed into the hands; they dry out; cream is rubbed in again; they dry out again, and so on. One gets used to putting cream on one's hands, without knowing that fat production of the body is brought to a standstill by alkanes, which are the real cause of fat demand.

## Hormonal Shifts

Hormonal changes in women affect the integrity of the skin barrier. Low estrogen (SEE QUICK DEFINITION) levels, which occur right before menstruation and during menopause, are associated with increased permeability and dry skin. Why is this? Estrogen doesn't appear to have a direct effect on skin barrier function; rather it is the precursor to estrogen, DHEA (SEE QUICK DEFINITION), that helps protect and moisturize the skin.

Research shows that DHEA levels are associated with sebum, an oily substance produced by sebaceous glands located in the epidermis. Sebum is a natural lubricant, working in conjunction with the stratum corneum to combat the effects of a dry climate and other irritants. High levels of DHEA correspond to high amounts of estrogen as well as high production of sebum. Conversely, low levels of this hormone are linked to diminished estrogen and reduced secretion of sebum. DHEA supplementation has been found to relieve dry skin and other skin problems.[36] Estrogen therapy has also been found helpful in restoring skin barrier function.

**Menopause**—Women going through menopause often complain of dry skin and increased skin sensi-

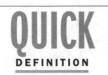

### DEFINITION

**DHEA** (dehydroepiandrosterone) is naturally produced by the human adrenal glands and gonads with optimal levels occurring around age 20 for women and age 25 for men. Then, DHEA levels gradually decline so that a person 80 years old produces only a fraction of the DHEA they did when they were 20. As an antioxidant, hormone regulator, and the building block from which estrogen and testosterone are produced, DHEA is vital to health. Low DHEA levels have been associated with cancer, diabetes, multiple sclerosis, hypertension, obesity, AIDS, heart disease, Alzheimer's, and immune dysfunction illnesses.

**Estrogen** is a female "sex" hormone, produced mainly in the ovaries (some in the fat cells), which regulates the menstrual cycle. Estrogen is important for adolescent sexual development, prepares the uterus for receiving the fertilized egg by stimulating the uterine lining to grow, and affects all the body's cells; its levels decline after menopause. Estrogen slows down bone loss, which leads to osteoporosis, and it can help reverse the incidence of heart attacks. It also improves skin tone, reduces vaginal dryness, and can act as an antiaging factor. There are three natural types of estrogen: estradiol (produced in the ovary); estrone (produced from estradiol); and estriol (formed in smaller amounts in the ovary). Estriol is the least toxic of the three.

tivity to environmental substances and climates, such as changes in humidity. To find out why this occurred, researchers studied 30 women, half on hormone replacement therapy (HRT), the other half not.[37] They found that the women on HRT had better skin barrier function than the control women, even in dry or cold weather. Another study in Belgium found that menopausal women receiving intradermal estrogen therapy had stronger skin barriers.[38]

**Menstruation**—Menopausal women aren't the only ones suffering from skin permeability due to hormone changes. Researchers from the University of California, San Francisco, studied a group of women during a menstrual period to discover the effects of estrogen and progesterone on skin permeability. They found that transepidermal water loss (indicative of increased skin permeability) was higher on the day of minimal estrogen/progesterone secretion (the days immediately preceding the onset of menses) as compared to the day of maximal estrogen secretion (the days immediately preceding ovulation).[39] These findings confirmed that hormone shifts in non-menopausal women also contribute to skin barrier default.

### Psychological Stress

Emotional stress contributes to the development of allergy and sensitivity in many ways, one of which is by increasing skin permeability. In a recent study, Japanese researchers

## Is Anger Skin Deep?

What would anger look like if you expressed it through your skin? According to recent research, it might look like eczema or psoriasis.

An independent study at Columbia Presbyterian Medical Center, in New York City, correlated withheld anger and atopic dermatitis. In this study, 34 adults with atopic dermatitis participated in various psychological tests and were measured against people who did not have this skin problem. The atopic patients felt anger more readily but were less likely to express it; they felt more anxious but less assertive; and they felt less effective in expressing their anger.[40]

The connection between anger and psoriasis was drawn by Madjulika A. Gupta, M.D., at the 19th World Congress of Dermatology in Sydney, Australia, in 1997. Dr. Gupta proposed that early-onset psoriasis may be associated with unexpressed anger. She subjected 137 psoriasis patients to a series of psychological tests that measure how they handled anger. Those people whose psoriasis developed in young adulthood were most likely to have internalized their anger. Such patients were likely to agree with statements such as these: "I keep things in," "I pout and sulk," or "I boil inside but I don't show it." Getting psoriasis before age 40, Dr. Gupta reported, is associated with "greater difficulties with assertion and expression of anger, a personality trait that may adversely affect the patient's capacity to cope with stress."[41]

For more information on **using stress management to mitigate allergic conditions**, see Chapter 14: Mind/Body Approaches to Allergy, pp. 348-373.

attempted to understand the mechanisms responsible for skin barrier damage by subjecting mice to a stressful situation—transferring them to new cages. The researchers measured the skin permeability of these animals and found that when the mice were moved to new cages, levels of the stress hormone corticosterone (a hormone produced by the adrenal glands similar in function to cortisol but not inflammatory) increased. At that time, skin permeability levels also increased. When the researchers administered a sedative to mice before relocating them to other cages, corticosterone levels returned to normal and barrier function was restored.[42] While scientists do not fully understand why stress hormones impair the skin barrier, it's possible that corticosterone somehow loosens or removes skin surface lipids.

## The Skin Barrier of Premature Babies

Preterm infants are at greater risk than full-term babies for contracting disease and infection because their skin barrier has not finished developing. Skin matures toward the end of gestation. However, research has found that most premature infants quickly develop a competent barrier. Estrogen, natural glucocorticosteroids, and thyroid hormone (T3) appear to be the primary forces of skin barrier generation.[43] Thyroid hormone is likely the most important force behind skin construction, according to a recent study which found that hypothyroidism (low or underactive thyroid gland function) significantly delays stratum corneum development in newborn mice.[44]

# Natural Therapies That Support the Skin

Superficial treatment does not stop any allergy. Allergic skin disorders will not be healed by applying a cortisone ointment. More and more patients realize this fact and have been turning to alternative medicine for help in reversing their skin conditions. A 1990 survey found that 227 of 444 (51.1%) of patients with atopic dermatitis and 215 of 506 (42.5%) of people with psoriasis used alternative therapies, such as diet therapy, homeopathy, and herbs, because conventional treatment had failed to relieve their conditions.[45] These numbers are likely higher today, as more people are becoming informed of the safety and efficacy of alternative medicine.

Alternative therapies for the skin focus on repairing barrier function and stimulating detoxification mechanisms. While all allergy and sensitivity sufferers will benefit from these remedies, they are especially important for people suffering from skin allergies. Eczema patients, in particular, need therapeutic help to recover barrier function, because they cannot fully recover from skin damage on their own. In one study, 15 patients with atopic dermatitis and 12 controls were subjected to induced skin barrier damage. Both groups had water loss values up to four times greater than before treatments. The atopic group's epidermis regenerated quicker than the control group's did. However, researchers found that the barrier function in atopic individuals was not completely restored. These findings suggest that repair mechanisms in atopic patients are permanently activated, resulting in faster barrier recovery, but that barrier function cannot be fully repaired due to the deficiency of skin lipids.[46]

Essential fatty acids are crucial to skin barrier repair, but there are many other simple things you can do to support your skin and prevent future allergic flare-ups as well as sensitization to new allergens. Sun protection, hydration, and humidification are a few of the steps; herbs, essential oils, and homeopathic preparations can also improve skin function. Special procedures for aiding the skin's detoxification ability are also useful.

## Essential Fatty Acid Supplements

Both topical and oral administration of essential fatty acids improve skin barrier function. The lipids found in topical creams are absorbed into the stratum corneum and appear to actually fill the intercellular spaces in the skin surface. In topical ointments, a 3:1:1:1 ratio of cholesterol, ceramides, essential free fatty acids, and nonessential fatty acids (such as olive oil) has been shown to accelerate barrier recovery in aged skin, while equal ratios are best for younger skin.[47] Oral supplements of omega-6 EFAs, especially gamma-linolenic acid (GLA), boosts skin cohesion and lipids and prevents transepidermal water loss.[48] Evening primrose oil, naturally high in GLAs, is effective as both a topical and oral supplement. Since patients with atopic eczema often have low levels or metabolic blocks of the enzyme that converts linoleic acid to GLA, GLA supplements are highly recommended. It is important to avoid fats high in arachidonic acids (such as dairy and meat), because these acids produce pro-inflammatory chemicals called prostaglandins, which exacerbate allergic reactions. Furthermore, do not overuse omega-6 EFAs, especially if you are suffering from arthritis, since these fats can contribute to this inflammatory disease. Omega-6 EFAs need to be balanced with omega-3 fats in a ratio of 1:2 for health.

## Topical Drugs Do More Harm Than Good

Topical corticosteriods are among the most frequently used conventional drugs for skin allergies, but research shows that they impair the skin barrier function. A recent study found that cortisone creams deplete the numbers of lipids in the stratum corneum, resulting in progressively greater amounts of transepidermal water loss.[49] Another study of ten volunteers also found that long-term use of these drugs resulted in fewer layers of epidermal cells—9.4 layers compared to the normal 18 layers. Water loss increased compared to the controls. Researchers concluded that long-term use of topical corticosteroids play an important part in the development of barrier dysfunction due to the depletion of skin surface lipids.[50]

For more on the **dangers of conventional allergy medications**, see Chapter 11: Supplements for Symptom Control, pp. 278-303.

**Evening Primrose Oil—**Evening primrose (*Oneothera biennis*) is a yellow wildflower native to North America. It is not a true primrose but rather a member of the willow herb family. Native Americans traditionally used the flower, leaves, and roots to treat bruises, hemorrhoids, even sore throats. In the early 1900s, researchers extracted oil from the seeds and discovered they were rich in gamma-linolenic acid (between 8.8% to 10.5%; 72% is linoleic acid).[51] Today, evening primrose oil is widely used throughout Europe, especially Germany and England, for eczema.

The typical recommended oral dosage of evening primrose oil is 500 mg to 2,000 mg daily for at least 12 weeks; severe cases may require up to 6,000 mg daily. There are a few side effects attributed to this oil, including headache, mild nausea, or soft stools. Patients with epilepsy shouldn't take more than 12 capsules per day. Talk to your doctor if you're on prescription medications before taking evening primrose oil, because certain drugs may increase the effects of evening primrose oil. If you're on anticoagulants drugs, evening primrose oil can enhance blood clotting.

The standard dosage for topical ointments is the same for oral supplements; in fact, you can break open the capsules and apply the oil directly to the skin if you don't have a topical ointment. Use ointments that have a water-in-oil base. If you're using products containing retinoic acid, topical application of evening primrose oil may worsen your skin condition.

**Other Sources of GLA—**Borage seed oil and black currant seed oil are two other sources of gamma-linolenic acid. Borage (*Borago officinalis*) oil contains twice as much GLA (up to 24%) as evening primrose oil; black currant oil is at 18% GLA. However, neither oil has proven to be as effective as evening primrose oil. In a study in which 160 atopic eczema patients were administered with 500 mg of borage oil (23% GLA) daily or a placebo found that the majority of treated patients didn't experience significant improvement in their skin disorder after 24 weeks.[52] While borage oil may be beneficial for some patients, it's not effective for everyone. Borage oil is not recommended for people with epilepsy or for those taking phenothiazine drugs, without medical supervision. Standard dosage is three to four 300 mg capsules taken orally daily.

**A Note on Fish and Omega-3 Oils**—Cold-water fish such as salmon, sardines, mackerel, and trout, which contain oils high in omega-3 fatty acids, have been shown to reduce the severity of skin allergies, while omega-6s provoke symptoms. In a double blind test, 145 patients with moderate to severe atopic dermatitis were randomly assigned to receive 6 g daily of either omega-3 fatty acids (in the form of fish oil) or corn oil (high in linoleic acid, an omega-6 EFA). At the

To learn **how essential fatty acids reduce the allergic symptoms**, see Chapter 11: Supplements for Symptom Control, pp. 278-303.

end of four months, 30% of patients in the fish oil group improved, while 24% of corn oil group improved.[53] Omega-3 fats seem to be more effective than omega-6s, and yet we aren't emphasizing them in this chapter. As you will discover in Chapter 11: Supplements for Symptom Control, omega-3 EFAs are excellent for diminishing the inflammation that occurs in allergic reactions but they are not as important as omega-6 fats in repairing skin barrier permeability.

## Moisturize After Irritant Exposure

While some skin moisturizers contain ingredients that cause skin permeability,[54] certain emollients are recommended to improve barrier function. Moisturizers containing urea (a by-product of protein metabolism found in urine, blood, and lymph fluid), alpha-hydroxy acids, and glycerol are recommended. Be sure to avoid products with retinoic acid (synthetic vitamin A) and other damaging chemicals.

**Urea**—In one study, 15 patients with atopic dermatitis treated one of their forearms twice daily for 20 days with a moisturizing cream containing urea; the other forearm served as a control. On day 21, both forearms were exposed to sodium lauryl sulfate. The next day, researchers measured the transepidermal water loss on each forearm.

The skin pretreated with moisturizer had a significant reduction in water loss and skin permeability than the untreated skin, indicating that urea-containing lotions prevent skin permeability in allergic people.[55] Some moisturizers appear to promote skin barrier integrity in as few as five days.[56]

**Alpha-Hydroxy Acids**—Found in many skin-care products, alpha-hydroxy acids (AHA) are a group of lipids that can strengthen skin barrier function and improve skin appearance, according to clinical studies. However, not all AHAs are effective. Gluconolactone and tartaric acid are two AHAs that have been proven to promote barrier integrity and prevent permeability; another AHA, glycolic acid, does not appear to positively impact barrier function, though it does lead to an increase epidermal thickness in animals.[57]

**Glycerol**—The chemical glycerin, a common ingredient in skin-care products, can be detrimental to the skin barrier, because it tends to draw water from the skin layers to moisturize the skin surface, leading to chronic dehydration. However, research has shown that glycerol, a sugar that is similar to glycerin, actual promotes skin barrier recovery (glycerin is the synthetic version of glycerol). In a recent study, topical application of glycerol accelerated barrier recovery after irritation with sodium lauryl sulfate. According to the study's researchers, glycerol stimulates barrier repair and improves the stratum corneum hydration; its humectant (water attracting) properties did not account for the reduction in water loss.[58] Improvement continued for seven days after treatment. Moisturizers containing natural glycerol (but not the synthetic glycerin) are recommended for barrier recovery.

**Rose Hip Seed Oil**—Skin creams containing rose hip seed oil may also help repair damaged skin. This oil contains traces of retinal, a natural retinol (vitamin A). Unlike the retinol found in products such as Retin-A, rose hip seed oil is bound in a natural, balanced formula and doesn't cause the skin permeability, peeling, and photosensitivity of synthetic forms. This oil also contains a small amount of vitamin C and omega-3 and omega-6 EFAs.

### Herbs for Menopausal Dryness
At menopause, a woman's skin begins to lose its natural moisture as a result of shifts in hormone levels. Adjusting your diet, getting exercise, and taking supplements are important to help offset these changes, but you can also help prevent dry skin by applying moisturizing herbs top-

ically or by taking them as extracts or teas, says medical herbalist and nutrition consultant Amanda McQuade Crawford.

As a tonic to nourish the skin and hair during or after menopause, Crawford suggests combining extracts of wild oat (2 oz), horsetail (2 oz), dandelion root (1 oz raw, 1 oz roasted), dandelion leaf (1 oz), nettle leaf (1 oz), yellow dock root (1 oz), and alfalfa (1 oz). Mix one teaspoon of this blend in a cup of water, diluted juice, or herb tea in the morning and evening, Crawford advises.

For another herbal drink to rejuvenate the skin, combine liquid herbal extracts of wild yam (4 oz), rosemary (4 oz), nettle (1 oz), and licorice root or sarsaparilla (1 oz), says Crawford. This mixture should last about 30 days and should be taken for six months for best results. She recommends a dosage of one teaspoonful in a cup of water, diluted juice, or herb tea, to be taken in the morning and again in the evening.

If you prefer, make a tea from the dried herbs of these same plants, using 5 oz of wild yam root, 4 oz of rosemary flower/leaf, 2 oz of nettle leaf, 2 oz of licorice root or sarsaparilla, and 2 oz of lemon grass leaf. Steep $1/2$ oz of this blend, covered, in $3 1/2$ cups of boiling water for 15 minutes. Strain and drink one cup hot or cold three times a day, Crawford says.

Combining comfrey, sandalwood, calendula, and chamomile makes a healing rinse for the skin. These are wound-healing herbs and extend their benefits to dry or vulnerable areas on the skin, notes Crawford.

## Aromatherapy for Skin Care

According to certified aromatherapist Roberta Wilson, essential plant oils can form the basis of a natural skin-care program using simple preparations easily and inexpensively made at home. The following oils help keep the skin clean yet moisturized and do not cause skin permeability as synthetic products do.

■ Mister: For a floral mist which you can spray on your face throughout the day as a refresher, Wilson suggests mixing the essential oils of lavender (3 drops), rosewood (2 drops), chamomile, neroli, and rose (1 drop each) with distilled water (4 oz). Add the distilled water to a spray bottle, blend in the oils, and shake well before using, says Wilson.

■ Cleanser: To make a cleanser for oily skin, Wilson recommends mixing essential oils of cedarwood and ylang-ylang (1 drop each) with one teaspoon each of water and French green clay powder. Add the

## Sun Protection and Humidity Control

Two simple steps can help prevent skin permeability and sensitization—protecting your skin from the sun and maintaining a constant level of humidity wherever possible. Sunscreen is a crucial component of protection against harmful UV rays. Wearing light, loose clothing covering your legs and arms, as well as a hat and sunglasses, are also highly recommended. As far as humidity control is concerned, obviously it's impossible to regulate the seasons, but you can minimize air moisture fluctuations in your home. Humidifiers and indoor running fountains are useful tools in maintaining balanced humidity.

For more on **sun protection**, see Chapter 4: Prevention of Sensitization, pp. 106-127. For more on **humidifying your home**, see Chapter 5: Environmental Control, pp. 128-157, and Chapter 10: Supporting the Respiratory System, pp. 260-277.

water and oils to the green clay powder in your palm, then blend well until it is pasty. Massage the cleanser into your skin until it feels clean, then rinse with warm water, says Wilson.

■ Rejuvenator: Rejuvenate your facial skin with this blend of essential oils, recommends Wilson. Combine borage oil and vitamin E oil (10 drops each), geranium, neroli, and rosewood (3 drops each), fennel, frankincense, and sandalwood (2 drops each), vetiver (1 drop), and $1^1/_2$ ounces of jojoba oil as a base. Gently massage several drops of this formula into your skin in the morning and evening after cleansing and toning, says Wilson.

You can also use essential oils in baths or apply them in massage to benefit your entire complexion, explains aromatherapy practitioner Chrissie Wildwood. Oils are absorbed into the deepest layers of the skin, where they work to promote healthy skin cells, cell waste elimination, and the retention of moisture, along with aiding capillary function. Research shows that oil baths decrease water loss and skin permeability and moisturize the skin roughness characteristic of atopic dermatitis and psoriasis, so much so that conventional medications are often reduced or discontinued after these baths.[59]

■ Dry Skin: This formula is for skin that tends to feel tight after washing with soap and that flakes and develops facial lines, says Wildwood. She recommends trying any of these three blends. First—blend essential oils of rose otto (1 drop), sandalwood (3 drops), extra virgin olive ($^1/_3$ oz), and macadamia nut ($^1/_2$ oz). Second—mix neroli and sandalwood (2 drops each), rose otto (1 drop), borage oil (2 capsules), and safflower oil ($^2/_3$ oz). Third—combine chamomile (1 drop), lavender (4 drops), avocado oil ($^1/_3$ oz), and peachnut oil ($^4/_5$ oz). Any of these blends will help moisturize dry skin, says Wildwood.

■ Aging Skin: Generally, this is a skin type that needs nourishing and toning, explains Wildwood. Here again, she offers three aromatherapy blends. First—mix the essential oils of sandalwood (4 drops), frankincense (2 drops), passionflower (2 capsules), wheat germ (¹/₅ oz), and sunflower seed (1 oz). Second—combine rose otto and myrrh (1 drop each), avocado (¹/₃ oz), and sunflower seed (¹/₂ oz). Third—blend neroli (2 drops), myrrh and geranium (1 drop each), macadamia nut (¹/₃ oz), and apricot kernel (¹/₂ oz).

# Steps for Skin Detoxification

Skin, as an extremely important detoxification organ, is an essential element of the whole detoxification and elimination system of the body. As in all other organs of the detoxification and elimination system, the skin should liberate the body from toxic substances. The pores and glands are the skin's main pathways of elimination, through which toxic chemicals can be excreted via either sweat or sebum (oil secreted by the skin).[60] When these secretions are blocked, it can lead to detoxification problems.

The body's elimination organs can also help each other and take the place of an overstressed organ. Skin plays an important part in the elimination process, as it has to take over part of detoxification if the liver and kidneys can't fulfill their functions. This is the origin of many skin diseases, which in reality are extreme responses to the elimination process. As we learned in previous chapters, toxic overload is a major contributor to allergy and sensitivity.

To promote your skin's ability to detoxify, you need to detoxify your skin. Stephen B. Edelson, M.D., director of The Environmental and Preventive Health Center of Atlanta, in Georgia, emphasizes the importance of skin detoxification—especially sauna therapy—with his allergy patients.

## Dry Skin Brushing
To enhance the skin's ability to detoxify, use a loofah sponge or dry skin brush. Brush the skin with long strokes towards the heart, before bathing or showering. Brushed skin is better able to eliminate toxins from the body, as oils and dead skin are removed and pores are unclogged. Toxins are transferred into the main lymphatic drainage ducts, which go directly to the liver for elimination. White blood cells also migrate into the skin after brushing and enhance the function of the immune system.

To proceed, simply begin gently brushing from the ends of the arms with long strokes that sweep towards the trunk of the body. Do all sides of the arms. Then brush the head and neck with downward strokes towards the clavicle (collar bone). Brush the feet and legs upward towards the groin area; again, be sure to brush all areas of the legs. As you brush the trunk, use upward-sweeping motions towards the heart. The ideal time to perform the dry skin brushing is prior to showering; then jump into the shower to remove the dead skin cells. Be sure to clean the brush thoroughly with soap and water and then hydrogen peroxide after each use.

## Sauna (Heat Stress Detoxification)

Using a sauna can effectively clear the body of fat-soluble toxins. Studies of fat biopsies before and after a heat stress detoxification protocol revealed an average of 21.3% reduction in the body levels of 16 toxic chemicals, including PCBs and PBBs, with a 64%-75% reduction in harmful toxins.[61] After discontinuing the heat and detoxification therapy, the study found that toxins in patients continued to decrease for up to four months. William Rea, M.D., director of the Environmental Health Center in Dallas, Texas, has published documentation showing that his detoxification program, which includes fasting, juicing, sauna therapy, exercise, and lymphatic drainage, produced a reduction of various pesticide residues ranging up to 66%.[62] Dr. Edelson recommends that allergy patients do at least 15 minutes of aerobic exercise preceding sauna therapy to "improve circulation so that the chemicals will more easily leave the fats and move to the liver."

For information on **medically supervised sauna detoxification**, contact: Stephen B. Edelson, M.D., The Environmental and Preventive Health Center of Atlanta, 3833 Roswell Road, Suite 110, Atlanta, GA 30342; tel: 404-841-0088; fax: 404-841-6416; website: www.ephca.com. Walter J. Crinnion, N.D., Healing Naturally, 11811 N.E. 128th Street, Suite 202, Kirkland, WA 98034.

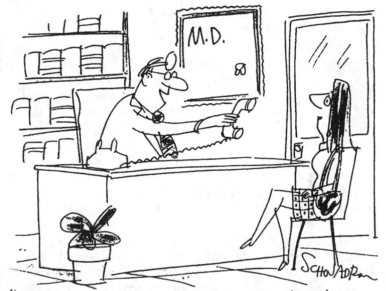

"I NOW OFFER NUTRITIONAL COUNSELING. HERE'S A RECORDING OF MY MOM'S RECIPE FOR CHICKEN SOUP."

# CHAPTER

# 10

# Supporting the Respiratory System

**E**ACH DAY, WE INHALE 23,000 times; that adds up to almost 3,000 gallons of air moving throughout our respiratory system every day.[1] As we know, there's more to our air than oxygen and carbon dioxide. Outdoors, the air is heavily contaminated with toxins and pollutants—vehicle exhaust, smog, heavy metals, and industrial and agricultural petrochemicals, as well as pollens and mold spores. Indoor air can be up to 100% more polluted than outdoor air,[2] as such irritants as cigarette smoke, volatile organic compounds, animal dander, dust mite and cockroach casings, and mold spores, among other substances, are recirculated in tightly sealed buildings.

Fortunately, our bodies have developed a unique respiratory defense system, which, when healthy, keeps harmful substances out while allowing oxygen in. This is called the mucous membrane barrier. However, as we've seen with the digestive and skin barriers, various dietary and external factors can damage the mucous membrane system and lead to sensitization. A lack of humidity and oxidative stress, due to poor diet and environmental toxins, can cause mucous membrane permeability and pave the way for reactive airway disease/asthma, allergic rhinitis, and chemical sensitivities. Humidification, antioxidant supplementation, and herbs can restore the integrity of the respiratory tract and eliminate allergy and sensitivity.

# Mucous Membranes: Defense of the Respiratory System

The respiratory system is an intricate network of multiple passageways and organs, including the nose and nasal cavity, sinuses, throat (pharynx, larynx, trachea), tubes called bronchi, and alveoli in the lungs. This system supplies the body with oxygen, which is necessary for the function of every cell and organ, and also expels carbon dioxide (a by-product of oxygen metabolism) from the body. Even before humans began polluting the world's air with petrochemicals and other hazards, the respiratory system encountered potentially harmful substances (antigens) in the air, including pollens, mold spores, insect parts, animal dander, viruses, and bacteria. To ensure that these and other foreign particles don't enter the bloodstream and risk harming the body, the respiratory tract is lined by a protective tissue called the respiratory epithelium, which comprises the surface of the sinuses, nose, and lungs. The respiratory epithelium, in turn, is protected by a barrier called the mucous membrane, or mucosa.

The mucous membrane is a layer of cells topped by millions of tiny hairlike projections called cilia and coated by mucus, a watery substance secreted by the epithelium. This combination of structures and substances is one part of the respiratory tract's filtration and cleaning system. When we inhale, nose hairs and lymph tissue filters the air and traps large foreign particles. As the air enters the throat, nasal cavity, and sinuses, finer foreign air particles and bacteria adhere to the mucosa. The cilia, beating in a wavelike fashion, then move the trapped particles and some of the mucus toward the pharynx (located in the upper throat behind the tongue and nasal cavity). This process is called mucociliary clearance. In a healthy person, mucus and trapped particles are cleared every ten minutes. From there, the particles are expelled by coughing, or swallowed so they can be destroyed by stomach acid.

## The Protective Role of Airway Surface Liquid

Mucus is not merely a holding facility for antigens. It is part of the airway surface liquid of the mucous membranes, which has important immunologic functions. Airway surface liquid contains immunoglobulins (antibodies), enzymes, and other lipids (fats) and proteins that are specifically designed to bind with and neutralize foreign substances.

Inhaled antigens, such as cigarette smoke and vehicle exhaust, can form free radicals. A free radical is an unstable molecule of oxygen with an unpaired electron that steals an electron from another molecule and produces harmful effects, including cell death and tissue damage. Free radicals are formed when molecules within cells react with oxygen (oxidize) as part of normal metabolic processes. The airway surface liquid contains certain enzymes and amino acids called antioxidants ("against oxidation") that protect cells against harmful free radicals. These antioxidants readily react with oxygen breakdown products and neutralize them before damage occurs. The major antioxidants in mucus function through the enzymes glutathione perioxidase and superoxide dismutase. Vitamins C (ascorbic acid) and E (tocopherol), beta carotene, and the minerals selenium and zinc are also secreted by the epithelial cells.

Immunoglobulins in the airway surface liquid, as well as those secreted by epithelial cells (secretory IgA), also protect the respiratory system from various bacteria and viruses. Mucus is usually clear; however, when we have a bacterial or viral infection, mucus may be yellow or green. This discoloration is caused by a proliferation of antibodies and white blood cells, which are mobilized to attack and destroy pathogens that adhere to or penetrate the mucous membranes. This is also the reason why we accumulate large quantities of mucus when experiencing an allergic reaction.

# What Causes Mucous Membrane Dysfunction?

Environmental factors are mostly to blame for breakdowns in the mucous membrane barrier function. The respiratory system is well equipped to handle direct assault, but it has its limits. The respiratory barrier, like our skin and intestinal wall, must be properly nourished and maintained in an environment conducive to health and regeneration. Without a good diet, adequate detoxification abilities, and a supportive environment, the mucous membrane system can be damaged, become permeable, and literally open the door to sensitization. A dry climate, toxic overload, and antioxidant deficiencies all cause barrier dysfunction.

### Lack of Humidity

The mucous membrane and its components need ambient moisture to do their job. Moisture keeps the mucus sticky and the cilia moving at a rapid, uniform pace. Experiments have shown that breathing dry air (low relative humidity) results in excessive water loss by the mucosa and diminished mucus adhesiveness as well as reduced or irregular ciliary beating.[3] This results in slower and less-efficient mucociliary clearance.

If free radicals, viruses, bacteria, and other pathogens are allowed to accumulate on the mucous membranes due to inadequate mucociliary clearance, they can break down the mucous membrane. Free radicals, if left unfettered, can destroy cells and tissue. Bacteria and viruses can multiply and unleash toxins that diffuse the epithelium and damage or destroy it, further inhibiting clearance.[4] The result is a breakdown in mucous membrane integrity and increased risk of sensitization to the inhalants encountered most frequently.

Unless you use a humidifier or live in a perpetually humid climate, sleep sets up the potential for respiratory problems. As you sleep, you breathe constantly, without taking in any fluids or food—substances that provide moisture for your airways during the waking hours. The bedroom is often dry in terms of relative humidity; this is especially true in newer houses and apartments that have been built for energy efficiency, with tightly sealed windows and central heating and cooling systems, which minimize moisture circulation. This lack of humidity depletes mucus and impairs ciliary function, and can put you at an increased risk for sensitizing to substances in your bedroom air—animal dander, dust mite casings, down feathers, and others.

## Environmental Pollutants

According to research, it's no coincidence that respiratory allergies have skyrocketed this past century. Since the turn of the twentieth century, automobiles, manufacturing plants, and agricultural enterprises have released billions of pounds of toxins into the air. The majority of Americans are exposed to air pollution. Approximately 107 million live in counties with unhealthy air, according to the U.S. Environmental Protection Agency.[5] Countless others are bombarded by dangerously high volatile organic compounds (VOC) levels re-circulated in approximately 30% of new or renovated buildings—"sick buildings." Common allergens such as dust mites and cockroaches, as well as cigarette smoke, are also trapped inside the air ducts of these buildings.

Inhaling these environmental pollutants wreaks havoc on the mucous membranes and leads to sensitization. For example, research shows that lead, found in car and industrial emissions, depresses enzymes needed for production of the respiratory antioxidants glutathione peroxidase (an enzymatic variation of the amino acid glutathione) and superoxide dismutase, increasing asthma risk.[6] Diesel exhaust readily forms into free radicals within the respiratory system, causing tissue damage including loss of surface membrane integrity and DNA damage in airway cells.[7] Sulfur dioxide, a major pollutant from vehicle exhaust, alters and reduces mucus secretion and ciliary activity. In a state of chronic exposure, the mucosa becomes inflamed, cilia beat more slowly, and areas of abnormally thin or even broken epithelial lining develop. This condition is similar to leaky gut, in that foreign particles are allowed entry into the bloodstream, increasing the risk of sensitization and leading to the development of asthma and allergic rhinitis.[8] Inhaling tobacco smoke reduces mucus secretion and diminishes ciliary activity, leading to increased epithelial permeability and higher risk of sensitizing to commonly inhaled substances such as dust mites.[9]

Certain medications also disrupt respiratory barrier function. Anticholinergics, aspirin, anesthetics, and benzodiazepines (tranquilizers) have been shown to depress mucociliary clearance as well as cough clearance (ability to fully cough up antigens).[10] This is problematic as it allows toxins and free radicals to accumulate in airway passages and break down the mucous membranes.

## Oxidative Stress and Allergy/Sensitivity

When you are deficient in antioxidants or when your ability to detoxify is impaired, free radicals run unchallenged throughout the respiratory system and the rest of the body, damaging cells. They tend to affect the immune, endocrine, and nervous systems, damaging mitochondria, interrupting communication among cells, and depleting key nutrients and antioxidants. This is called oxidative stress. A key marker of oxidative stress is low levels of glutathione in the body.

Glutathione is found in high levels in the respiratory tract lining fluid. Glutathione is a tri-peptide, a small protein consisting of three amino acids, that functions as a principle antioxidant, scavenging free radicals and toxins that would otherwise damage and destroy cells. Further, glutathione regulates the activities of other antioxidants, such as vitamins A, C, and E.

Various dietary factors determine the levels of glutathione in the respiratory tract. Vitamin C helps increase glutathione levels.[11] The amino acid cysteine, found in poultry, yogurt, oats, egg yolk, red peppers, broccoli, Brussels sprouts, and wheat germ, is converted to glutathione in the body. Dietary deficiency of selenium has been shown to impair glutathione activity.[12]

Antioxidant deficiency, whether due to toxin exposure or poor diet, is directly linked to increased oxidative stress in the respiratory tract and higher incidences of asthma and allergic rhinitis. Studies have found that patients suffering from bronchial reactivity and asthma have low glutathione levels in the mucous membranes and a high degree of oxidative stress in the respiratory tract.[13] Further studies have shown that mild asthmatics have abnormally low concentrations of vitamins C and E in their lung lining fluid as well as substantial oxidative stress.[14] It has also been discovered that subjects with the lowest intake of vitamin C and manganese (an antioxidant mineral) have a fivefold higher risk of bronchial allergy and asthma than those with the highest dietary intake of these nutrients; low intake of zinc and magnesium is also associated with increased risk of bronchial allergy.[15] An excess of dietary iron has been shown to promote free-radical production and increase the risk of asthma.[16]

Antioxidant deficiency has also been linked to chemical sensitivity. In one study, patients with multiple chemical sensitivity (MCS) showed low levels of the antioxidants vitamin C, selenium, copper, zinc, and others. Subsequent antioxidant supplementation reversed MCS symptoms in 25% of the patients.[17]

## A Vicious Cycle

Oxidative stress doesn't just lead to sensitization—it also contributes to the continuation and exacerbation of allergy symptoms. Free radicals in the airways lead to mucous membrane permeability and sensitization. Sensitization activates certain immune cells that stimulate production of free radicals as well as inflammatory chemicals and antibodies. This leads to airway reactivity, such as reactive airway disease and allergic rhinitis. Over time, the increased free-radical load—from both external and internal sources—leads to a vicious cycle of toxic overload in the respiratory tract, more inflammation and high pulmonary pressures causing lung tissue damage, and more severe allergic reactions. The result is the irreversible condition of asthma.

During an allergic reaction, the immune system mobilizes the release of various antibodies and inflammatory chemicals as well as white blood cells called neutrophils. Neutrophils in the airway trigger the secretion of free radicals, in particular a type of free radical called superoxide.[18] Research has shown that the more superoxide radicals present in the respiratory tract, the greater the airway obstruction in asthma.[19]

Another problem posed by free radicals in the respiratory tract is that they spark the release of phagocytes, white cells that "eat" and destroy antigens.[20] The problem with phagocytes is that they don't eat only antigenic cells but also tissue cells, which causes the tissue damage commonly associated with allergic inflammatory diseases such as asthma (lung tissue) or arthritis (joint tissue). Over time, tissue damage causes permanent asthma and also increases the risk of sensitizing to other inhalants.

## Success Story: Supplements, Herbs, and Air Purification Reverses Asthma

Isabel, 15, was a highly athletic young woman, involved as an important player in a competitive team sport at her high school. She had suffered from asthma since she was nine, and now it was getting progressively worse. Isabel depended on regular high doses of bronchial inhalants and prednisone.

She told Eugene Zampieron, N.D., co-director of the Naturopathic Medical Center of Middlebury, Connecticut, that she was most likely to experience an asthma attack during times of physical exertion (playing soccer), when she felt anxious, and when the weather was cold and damp. At such times, Isabel said, her heart seemed to race and she felt "as if my chest was going to explode." Dr. Zampieron notes that "some combination of weather, humidity, temperature, and barometric pressure seems to have a negative effect on many asthmatics."

Although Isabel wheezed when she exhaled, Dr. Zampieron determined that there was no infection in her lungs. The lungs of asthmatics are prone to infection from the trapped mucus that accumulates there, says Dr. Zampieron. He next checked Isabel, through a hair analysis, for signs of excess copper. This heavy metal interferes with the functioning of the thyroid and adrenal glands, depletes the body of vitamin C, contributes to the inflammation of the lungs, and compromises the liver's ability to detoxify substances, especially histamine, which is released in abundance during an asthma attack, explains Dr. Zampieron.

The hair analysis showed that Isabel had high copper levels and that she was deficient in magnesium, selenium, manganese, and molybdenum. Where did she get the excess copper and why was she deficient in these other trace minerals?

"In New England, the water tends to be very hard, full of minerals, including copper, and it's transported to homes through old copper pipes which probably leach," says Dr. Zampieron. "In addition, you inhale copper through the steam produced when you shower. Copper competes with other 'good' minerals such as zinc, selenium, and manganese." Other family members seemed to be affected by the copper as well; Isabel's brothers had symptoms of attention deficit disorder, which is linked to high copper levels.

As a teenager, Isabel tended to eat too many refined, sugar-based foods, which explained her micronutrient shortfalls. Molybdenum deficiency has been correlated with asthma, says Dr. Zampieron. Isabel's selenium deficiency was troublesome because this trace mineral is needed to stop the release of inflammatory substances that otherwise produce the bronchial constriction and oxygen deprivation so feared by asthmatics. So, too much copper and too little selenium both helped to generate Isabel's asthma, and, uncorrected, they made it worse.

During an asthma attack, several things happen, explains Dr. Zampieron. The smooth muscles in the bronchi (major air passages in the lungs) go into spasm; the large airways get inflamed, accompanied by water retention, the secretion of mucus (which can plug up smaller airways), and an influx of various inflammatory cells (such as lymphocytes, platelets, and other immune system cells) that contribute to bronchial spasm.

People suffering from asthma are often deficient in magnesium. This mineral helps to relax and calm the smooth muscles of the bronchi that have contracted or are spastic, as in an asthma episode. Studies have shown that low dietary intake of magnesium is linked with impaired lung function, wheezing, and a tendency for the bronchi to be hyper-reactive to asthma triggers. In fact, giving magnesium intravenously (at the rate of 2 g hourly, up to 24 g maximum) is now a clinically accepted method for halting an acute asthma attack.

Dr. Zampieron next sought to find out if Isabel had food allergies. Chronic allergies to foods can contribute to asthma, he says. In Isabel's case, these foods were, principally, cow's milk (she drank about one-half gallon of milk every day), wheat, yeast, and certain natural chemicals found in animal products. Specifically, two fatty acids called arachidonic and stearic acid; a high consumption of animal products can account for high levels of these substances in the body, says Dr. Zampieron.

"As an athlete, Isabel drank a lot of milk, believing it to be a quick, high energy, rich protein food that was good for her physical performance. The fact of the matter was that this product acted to her detriment." Dr. Zampieron found

For more on **how magnesium treats asthma**, see Chapter 11: Supplements for Symptom Control, pp. 278-303.

that Isabel also was highly allergic to bananas; bananas are high in serotonin, a neurotransmitter that increases levels of an intracellular messenger called cyclic GMP (guanosine monophosphate). While this is technical, it's a point important to understanding how Dr. Zampieron uses nutrients and herbs to alleviate asthma. In the cells of the body, there are two substances whose job is to block or allow the contraction of smooth muscles. One is called cyclic GMP (which helps contraction) and the other, slightly different, cyclic AMP (adenosine monophosphate, which helps expansion). When muscles aren't contracting, they're relaxing, which is what an asthmatic wants, and one way for this to occur is to have more cyclic AMP, says Dr. Zampieron. In Isabel's case, this translated into not eating bananas.

Other dietary recommendations included completely eliminating all dairy products, beef, and chicken from Isabel's diet. She substituted soybean products (such as soy cheese for her pizzas), goat's milk cheese, and fish. Cold-water fish consumption is helpful for asthmatics because fish such as salmon contain omega-3 fatty acids, which can help decrease the inflammation and diminish the levels of arachidonic acid (an omega-6 oil) that contribute to the inflammation, says Dr. Zampieron.

At one point, Isabel told Dr. Zampieron that she had trouble sleeping at night because "I'm allergic to my room." A laboratory test for substance allergies showed that she was in fact allergic to dust mites. To deal with this, Dr. Zampieron suggested she get an air purification unit for her bedroom.

"The approach here is to starve the dust mites by decreasing the amount of dust in the air," explains Dr. Zampieron. All the allergenic particulates you typically find in indoor air, such as dust mites, pet dander, molds, hair, "stick" to the negative ions generated by the air purifier and fall to the floor. Then, if you carefully vacuum the floor (with a non-allergenic vacuum bag) and use wet rags to clean all the other surfaces, you stand an excellent chance of eliminating dust mites from the room, Dr. Zampieron says. It's also advisable to remove all carpets from an asthmatic's living space, as these are major collection points for allergens.

He next recommended anti-asthma supplements for Isabel. The amino acid N-acetyl-cysteine, for example, would decrease the thickness and stickiness (called viscosity) of her bronchial fluids, enabling more free, relaxed movement of the lungs during breathing. To further support the relaxing of Isabel's lung muscles, Dr. Zampieron put together a special herbal formula. This included a form of wild basil (known in Jamaican folk medicine for its anti-asthma benefits), ammi-visnaga (known in Egypt as khella, and related to carrots), and *Ginkgo biloba*. Both basil and ammi-visnaga contain substances that relax smooth muscles and block the release of histamine; ginkgo helps to dry out the lungs, relax smooth muscles, and curtail the release of serotonin, which initiates the inflammation process.

Another herb Dr. Zampieron used with Isabel was *Coleus forskohlii* extract. This herb is a smooth muscle relaxant, lowers normal or elevated blood pressure, and increases levels of cyclic AMP, needed for muscle relaxation. As a complement to the *Coleus forskohlii*, Dr. Zampieron recommended that Isabel drink 3-4 cups daily of decaffeinated, organically produced green tea. This natural tea contains substances (related to caffeine) that relax and expand the bronchi and enhance the levels of cyclic AMP in the smooth muscles. "This herb works well, synergistically, with the forskohlii," says Dr. Zampieron.

An additional herb that he judged helpful for Isabel was licorice root, in extract form. This herb helps support the body's production of cortisol, a natural anti-inflammatory agent; using it would help Isabel gradually get off the cortisone and beta-blockers she was taking for her asthma.

Dr. Zampieron recommended an alternative inhaler containing homeopathic remedies selected for asthma, including *Arsenicum album*, which would address the fear and anxiety associated with an asthma attack. The preparation contained homeopathically prepared adrenal gland extract to help Isabel's adrenal glands accommodate the switch from synthetic cortisone to cortisol secreted under the stimulation of the licorice; it also contained homeopathic histamine, which functions as an anti-histamine.

For more on **herbs for asthma**, see Chapter 11: Supplements for Symptom Control, pp. 278-303. For more on **homeopathic remedies**, see Chapter 12: Homeopathic and Physical Therapies, pp. 304-327.

Isabel's response to Dr. Zampieron's program was "very rapid and dramatic," he recounts. Within three weeks, Isabel's mother commented on the positive changes she observed in her daughter. Isabel's soccer coach also remarked on Isabel's enhanced athletic abilities and stamina. Before, Isabel would start wheezing about halfway through the game and have to be taken out by her coach, now she was able to go the entire game without any signs of asthma.

Eugene Zampieron, N.D., A.H.G.: Naturopathic Medical Center of Middlebury, 900 Straits Turnpike, Middlebury, CT 06762; tel: 203-598-0400; fax: 203-263-2970.

Six months after starting Dr. Zampieron's program, Isabel was able to discontinue all her conventional drugs. She was able to reduce her intake of the herbs by about half, too. "This is an effective protocol for asthma," says Dr. Zampieron. "The combined effects of the herbs, dietary changes, and air purification were the stabilizing factors. Isabel can perform athletically and not go into an asthma attack."

# Alternative Therapies to Restore Mucous Membrane Integrity

In most cases, restoring the respiratory barrier function can be readily achieved by humidifying the sleeping space and supplementing the diet with antioxidants. These steps have been shown to be effective in diminishing allergy and sensitivity symptoms. Humidifying the sleeping space and reducing your exposure to environmental and indoor pollutants are also highly recommended. Detoxifying the respiratory tract will aid in properly eliminating free radicals from the airways.

### Humidify the Sleeping Space

Although certain aeroallergens, such as dust mites and molds, thrive in humid conditions, it is highly recommended that individuals with respiratory allergies and sensitivities humidify their bedrooms. As we've seen, a dry environment alters and diminishes mucociliary clearance and can lead to mucous membrane permeability and sensitization.

For optimum mucosa integrity, the indoor air should be kept at 35% to 45% relative humidity, according to Robert S. Ivker, D.O., author of *Sinus Survival*. Even if you live in a damp climate, humidifiers are a good idea during the winter months, as many heating systems can dry out the indoor air. To test your humidity levels, purchase

 a special measuring device called a hygrometer at your local hardware store.

For more on **reducing exposure to toxic inhalants**, see Chapter 5: Environmental Control, pp. 128-157.

There are various types of tabletop room humidifiers. These units can humidify a medium- to large-size room, and cost from $30 up to $200. According to Dr. Ivker, evaporative humidifiers are popular and affordable, but unfortunately can become host to bacteria. Evaporative units are also available for humidifying the entire house. Cool-mist units require distilled water or special cartridges to filter out minerals from the water supply, and can spray white dust in the room. Steam-mist models (vaporizers) are effective, but may burn you if you get too close to the mist or if the unit tips over. Warm-mist models, on the other hand, pose no burning danger, require no distillation or filtration

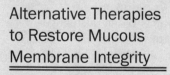

## Alternative Therapies to Restore Mucous Membrane Integrity

- Humidify the Sleeping Space
- Purify Your Air
- Supplement with Antioxidants
- Take Demulcent Herbs
- Detoxify the Respiratory System

system, and kill bacteria, but they may use more electricity than other models.

Central (in-duct) units are also available for house-wide humidification. They are attached to the central heating system's furnace, and cost several hundred dollars. There are two problems with these models—they do not humidify individual rooms as well as tabletop units, and some of the devices use a tray of standing water as a reservoir, which can promote bacteria and mold growth. However, some models do not have reservoirs attached.

For more information about **humidifiers**, contact: Bionaire USA, 233 Fortune Blvd., Milford, MA 01757; tel: 800-253-2764; website: www. bionaire.com.

Less-expensive options include placing a small fountain in your room—as long as the water is constantly running, no mold or pathogenic bacteria can grow in it. Hanging a wet towel on a hanger in the bedroom can also add moisture to the ambient air, or just place a pie-pan of water where air from your bedroom duct will hit it.

## Purify Your Air

As the average American spends an estimated 90% of the time indoors, the quality of indoor air becomes crucial. Unfortunately, indoor air pollution ranks near the top of the list of polluted environments. Toxic substances such as pollens, dust mites, mold spores, allergens, sulfur dioxide, tobacco smoke residues, carbon tetrachloride, benzene, chloroform, chemical gases, and formaldehyde are now commonly found in tightly sealed indoor environments. These can produce mild to serious irritations in the eyes, throat, and lungs, and generate headaches, sinus problems, wheezing asthma, and allergy attacks.

In nature, a thunderstorm can clean up the stagnant air in a local environment by way of ionization and ozone release. Look for air purification units that imitate the refreshed air quality of the thunderstorm by using ozone to reduce the amount of most of the common indoor airborne pollutants. These devices use an unobtrusive fan to distribute negative and positive ions to cover an indoor area between 20-2,500 square feet, depending on the size of the unit.

The ions (produced by a pulsating negative/positive ion field generator) help remove particulate matter from the air. The ozone (the amount released is adjustable, burns up most of the organic polluting materials and odors in the air. Newer models also have ozone monitors and an automatic shut-off, in case levels reach anywhere near toxic levels. The combination of ionization and ozonation oxidizes airborne pollutants and knocks down

For **ion/ozone air purification units**, contact: U.S. Complementary Health, Inc., 3441 E. Tierra Buena Lane, Phoenix, AZ, 85032; tel: 602-493-1637.

floating particulate matter. Ozone is possibly the best method for removing odors.

Other air purification systems use HEPA (high-efficiency particulate arrestor) to filter out miniscule particles. These are likewise effective in reducing exposure to toxic inhalants.

## Antioxidant Supplements

Supplementing with antioxidants, especially N-acetyl-cysteine (NAC), beta carotene, vitamins C and E, and selenium, have been shown to improve mucous membrane integrity and mitigate respiratory allergy and sensitivity symptoms. As discussed in Chapter 7: Healing Leaky Gut Syndrome, some studies have shown that the absorption of oral glutathione supplements is limited.[21] However, other studies have found that oral glutathione is indeed absorbed by the body.[22] Glutathione is best absorbed orally when combine with anthocyanidins (bioflavonoids). The only sources of this patented combination are the SCAVE products available in Europe, and Recancostat, available from Tyler Encapsulations. You can also increase the availability of glutathione by increasing the precursors that the body needs to manufacture glutathione, including foods in the cabbage family as well as onions and garlic.

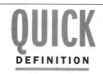

For **glutathione supplements combined with anthocyanidins**, contact: Tyler Encapsulations, 2204-8 N.W. Birdsale, Gresham, OR 97030; tel: 800-869-9705 or 503-661-5401; fax: 503-666-4913.

# QUICK
### DEFINITION

**Amino acids** are the building blocks of proteins. There are more than 22 amino acids linked in various combinations to form 1,600 basic proteins necessary for body structure and the formation of antibodies, hormones, enzymes, organs, and cell membranes. Some amino acids are manufactured in the body while others (the essential amino acids) must be obtained from dietary sources.

**N-acetyl-cyteine**—N-acetyl-cysteine (NAC) is a sulfur-containing amino acid (SEE QUICK DEFINITION) that is readily converted in the body to cysteine, an amino acid that acts as an antioxidant, shields the liver from toxic heavy metals, and helps prevent infections by augmenting the actions of vitamin C. Cysteine is a precursor of glutathione. NAC itself is also a potent antioxidant in the airways—it scavenges hydrogen peroxide, a damaging free radical, and prevents lung tissue damage.[23] In clinical studies, supplementing with NAC has been shown to prevent tobacco smoke–induced oxidative damage on respiratory cells,[24] reverse the free-radical damage of diesel exhaust,[25] and decrease the severity of lung smooth muscle reactivity to toluene, an environmental pollutant.[26] It also inhibits the phagocyte burst that occurs during allergic reactions.[27]

NAC has been used for decades for treating respiratory illnesses because of its excellent mucolytic action. Mucus is necessary to protect the respiratory tract from irritants, but overproduction can also foster bacterial infection and become an obstruction to breathing freely. NAC helps reduce the viscosity of mucus so this it may be coughed up more easily.[28] RDA: none; therapeutic dose: 500 mg, three times daily.

**Beta Carotene**—Beta carotene is converted by the body to vitamin A as needed. It is a primary antioxidant that helps protect the lungs and mucous membranes. Studies have shown that asthmatics have a low concentration of beta carotene (pro-vitamin A) in their airways, indicating high oxidative stress.[29] Food sources: carrots, sweet potatoes, squash, cooked spinach, most leafy green vegetables, yellow fruits and vegetables, fish liver oil. RDA: none; therapeutic dose: 10,000-50,000 IU. Prolonged ingestion of high doses may cause a benign yellowing of the skin, especially of palms and soles. Avoid while taking the prescription drug Accutane, especially during pregnancy.

**Vitamin C**—Vitamin C (ascorbic acid) is a powerful antioxidant and anti-inflammatory. It is a major component of the

## Guidelines for Amino Acid Supplementation

When buying amino acids look for USP pharmaceutical grade, L-crystalline, free-form amino acids. The designation *USP* means that the product meets the standard of purity set by the United States Pharmacopeia. The term *free-form* refers to the highest level of purity of the amino acid. The *L* refers to one of the two forms of most amino acids, designated D- and L- (for example D-lysine or L-lysine). The L-form amino acids are proper for human biochemistry, as proteins in the human body are made in this form.

We don't recommend taking individual amino acid supplements for indefinite periods, because this can create an imbalance of other amino acids and may contribute to the development of other health conditions. Consult your physician before taking amino acid supplements.

airway surface lining and protects the mucous membranes from oxidative stress. It is particularly helpful in fighting the free radicals generated by vehicle emissions.[30] It also promotes glutathione production.

Asthmatics tend to have low concentrations of this and other antioxidants in their lung lining fluid.[31] Vitamin C supplements have been used with great success in improve mucous membrane function and minimizing asthma symptoms. Vitamin C is also found in abundance in the adrenal glands, and appears to be necessary in the production of the adrenal hormone cortisol, which shuts off inflammatory reactions in the respiratory tract and elsewhere.[32]

Food sources: most fruits and vegetables, especially oranges, grapefruit, kiwi, lemons, avocado, and parsley. Supplements: the most

For more on **how vitamin C and other antioxidants help allergy sufferers**, see Chapter 11: Supplements for Symptom Control, pp. 278-303.

cost-effective form of vitamin C is ascorbic acid, which is extracted from rosehips or acerola. There is also a new form of vitamin C called ester-C, which is purported to stay in the body longer, thereby increasing absorption. It is best to take supplements that contain bioflavonoids, antioxidant pigments such as citrus bioflavonoids, quercetin, catechins, hesperidin, rutin, and proanthocyanidins, which boost the amount of vitamin C inside cells. RDA: 60 mg; therapeutic dose: 500-5,000 mg daily.

**Vitamin E**–Vitamin E protects cell membranes from oxidative damage and acts as an anti-inflammatory, blocking the activity of an enzyme that provokes inflammation. Levels of vitamin E are typically low in the lung lining fluid of those with asthma, which allows free radicals to damage the mucous membranes.[33]

Food sources: cold-pressed oils such as sunflower and safflower, almonds, hazelnuts, and wheat germ. Supplements: vitamin E is actually a group of compounds called tocopherols. When purchasing supplements of vitamin E, avoid products that contain vitamin E in the DL-alpha tocopherol acetate form—this means that it is a petroleum-based synthetic form of the vitamin. The natural form of vitamin E will be designated with the letter "D." Avoid taking iron supplements at the same time of day as vitamin E supplements as they mutually prevent absorption. Drink filtered water (no chlorinated water) and avoid "bad" polyunsaturated fats, since these may destroy vitamin E. RDA: 30 IU; therapeutic dose: up to 3,000 IU daily.

**Selenium**–The importance of selenium, a mineral that is often deficient in people with respiratory allergies, is its activity as an antioxidant and anti-inflammatory agent. Selenium works in conjunction with vitamin E in cell membranes to fight free radicals.[34] Selenium can also protect against the absorption of heavy metals, such as aluminum, mercury, and lead.[35]

Food sources: the small amount of selenium needed by the body is often hard to obtain through the diet because foods are now grown in mineral-poor soils.[36] If grown in fertile soil, grains are a good source of selenium, as are organic liver, meat, and fish. Supplements: avoid multimineral supplements that contain sodium selenite, an organic salt that is not well absorbed. Organic selenium from yeast or the chelated mineral (seleno-methionine) are better sources. RDA: 26 mcg; therapeutic dose: 200-1,000 mcg daily. Precautions: Selenium toxicity is possible but rare, as only very small amounts are needed by the body. An overdose can cause hair loss, nail malformations, weakness, and slowed mental function.[37]

## Demulcent Herbs

*Demulcent* is a term used by herbalists to describe an herb that has a protective effect on the mucous membranes. Most of the herbs that contain demulcents have large amounts of mucilaginous materials—gummy, slimy chemicals that have a direct action on the lining of the respiratory tract, especially the throat, soothing and minimizing irritations.

**Marshmallow (*Althea officinalis*)**—Marshmallow root contains 25% to 35% mucilage. It is used by herbalists to soothe sore throats, relieve lung congestion, and reduce inflammation of the respiratory mucosa. It is usually taken as a tea: take several teaspoons of the root, cover with boiling water, and steep for 20-30 minutes to extract all of the medicinal components.

**Slippery Elm Bark (*Ulmus fulva*)**—Slippery elm, obtained by removing the bark from the branches of the slippery elm tree, has been used a demulcent for the respiratory as well as gastrointestinal systems. Slippery elm is available as a tincture or capsules, or a decoction can also be made: simmer the bark very gently, one part of the bark to eight quarts of water; bring to a boil and let it brew for 20-30 minutes; drink 2-3 cups daily.

**Mullein (*Verbascum thapsus*)**—The flowers and leaves of the mullein plant are used to treat inflammation of mucous membranes. The herb contains mucilage, as well as flavonoids and other chemicals that soothe the respiratory tract. Additionally, mullein has mild expectorant activity, meaning it aids in the coughing up of mucus and antigens. The dried leaves were traditionally smoked like tobacco to treat asthma and coughs; however, asthmatics are advised not to smoke anything. As a tea, steep two teaspoons of dried flowers and leaves in one cup of hot water for 10-15 minutes. Drink up to eight cups daily.

**Deglycyrrhizinated Licorice (DGL)**—Deglycyrrhizinated licorice (DGL) is a type of licorice root preparation that removes a chemical component responsible for increasing water retention with regular licorice root. DGL is well documented in clinical trials to heal gastric ulcers as well as Tagamet and other frequently prescribed anti-ulcer drugs.[38] It does this by soothing the mucosa and improving the integrity of the mucous membrane.[39] Respiratory mucus only differs from digestive tract mucus by the cilia found in the respiratory system. Thus, DGL supplementation is useful in restoring respiratory mucosa integrity. Therapeutic dosage: two to four 380 mg chewable tablets, 20 minutes before meals; take for 8-16 weeks.

## Detoxify the Respiratory System

During the energy crisis in the 1970s, building construction practices changed: homes, offices, schools, and all buildings were insulated and sealed tightly. This method saves a great deal of energy, but tends to trap indoor air pollution, including pollens, oils, dry cleaning fluid (a known liver toxin), and other allergens. Chemicals, such as benzene (a carcinogen), are released from paint, new carpets, drapes, and upholstery. Formaldehyde vapors rise up from plywood, new cabinets, furniture, carpets, drapes, wallpaper, and paneling. All enter the body through the lungs. Asthma sufferers may need to detoxify for symptomatic relief.

**Herbs for Lung Detoxification**—Herbs are frequently used to target specific aspects of lung contamination and detoxification:

■ Fenugreek and horehound help decrease production and thickness of mucus secretions; a typical dose is 500 mg daily.

■ Wild cherry bark is an expectorant that helps remove mucus and congestion; typical recommended dose is 250 mg daily.

■ To strengthen lung tissue, use the herbs mullein (500 mg), elecampane (500 mg), and grindelia (250 mg).

Use caution with eucalyptus oil, because many people have allergies or sensitivities to eucalyptus tree pollen.

■ Eucalyptus and thyme oil (2-3 drops each) are antiseptics that kill microbial organisms; a combination of these herbs can be taken as a tincture ($^1/_2$ tsp, three times per day).

**Inhalation Therapy**—Steam inhalation can be very helpful for detoxifying the lungs. To a pot of boiling water, add two to three drops of eucalyptus and thyme oils. Remove the pot from the stove and place your head above the steam. Create a "tent" by covering your head with a towel and inhale the steam vapors. The steam arising from inhalation therapy is very hot. Be sure to keep your head far enough above the steam so as not to get burned.

**Exercise**—Exercise helps the lungs by increasing the perfusion of blood, which causes an enhanced intake of oxygen and *qi* (vital life-force energy) and increased expiration of waste products. Aerobic exercises, such as running, cycling, and walking, can help clear the lungs. However, aerobic activity needs to be done in fresh, clean air—running in a polluted environment only increases the overall body burden of toxins (and may trigger asthma attacks in some people) and should be avoided. Yoga breathing techniques are excellent for cleansing the lungs and increasing oxygen levels in the body.

For more information about **yoga**, see Chapter 14: Mind/Body Approaches to Allergies, pp. 348-373.

# Supplements for Symptom Control

**A**LTERNATIVE MEDICINE CAN'T CURE allergy or sensitivity overnight. It took months, even years, of poor diet, toxic overload, and other factors to break down barrier functions and overwhelm the immune system. Similarly, it may take weeks, months, perhaps years, to fully restore health.

As you undergo the therapies discussed in this book, you will invariably suffer relapses of your allergy or sensitivity. However, there are numerous ways to minimize, even prevent allergy/sensitivity symptoms. We have divided these symptom control measures into two chapters. This chapter focuses on dietary supplements for symptom relief, including vitamins, minerals, bioflavonoids, essential fatty acids, and Western and Chinese herbs. Chapter 12 covers homeopathic and physical therapies, such as acupuncture, acupressure, and special therapies for asthma.

## In This Chapter

- Success Story: Supplements to the Rescue
- Nutritional Supplements
- Essential Fatty Acids
- Botanical Medicines
- Chinese Herbal Medicines
- The Dangers of Conventional Allergy Treatment

If you are currently taking prescription medications for your symptoms, check with your physician before self-treating to identify any possible contraindications. It's important to note, however, that the therapies suggested in these two chapters are as effective—if not more effective—as conventional drugs in relieving allergy symptoms. In fact, many allergy drugs have adverse, even dangerous side effects that can impair your body's ability to get well again. We discuss the major caveats of these drugs in this chapter.

| Allergy/Sensitivity | Recommended Therapies |
| --- | --- |
| Allergic Rhinitis/Sinusitis | Nutritional Supplements, Botanical Medicines, Chinese Herbs, Homeopathy (Chapter 12), Nasal Irrigation (Chapter 12), Meridian Therapy (Chapter 12) |
| Asthma/Reactive Airway Disease | Nutritional Supplements, Essential Fatty Acids, Botanical Medicines, Chinese Herbs, Homeopathy (Chapter 12), Meridian Therapy (Chapter 12), I.R.R. Therapy (Chapter 12), Buteyko Therapy (Chapter 12) |
| Atopic Dermatitis | Essential Fatty Acids, Botanical Medicines, Chinese Herbs |
| Hives | Chinese Herbs, Homeopathy (Chapter 12), Meridian Therapy (Chapter 12) |
| Allergic Contact Dermatitis | Chinese Herbs, Homeopathy (Chapter 12) |
| Migraine/Headache | Baking Soda/Heparin, Botanical Medicines, Chinese Herbs, Oriental Bodywork (Chapter 12) |
| Ear Infection (Otitis media) | Homeopathy (Chapter 12), Meridian Therapy (Chapter 12) |
| Gastrointestinal Symptoms | Botanical Medicines, Chinese Herbs |
| Joint Inflammation (Allergy-induced arthritis) | Essential Fatty Acids, Meridian Therapy (Chapter 12), Osseous Manipulation (Chapter 12) |

# Success Story: Supplements to the Rescue

Most allergy patients are misdiagnosed, states allergist Doug Kaufman, M.D., who shares a clinical practice with Dave Holland, M.D., in Dallas, Texas. If physicians would ask the right questions, he says, they would find "there is often a dietary or fungal basis to their patients' problems."

## Emergency Care for Anaphylactic Shock

Anaphylaxis, or anaphylactic shock, is a life-threatening IgE-mediated allergic reaction that requires immediate medical care. Approximately 700 people die each year from anaphylactic shock, sparked by insect stings, medications (especially injectables), foods, and latex.[1] If you think you're having an anaphylactic response to a substance, it's crucial that you go to an emergency medical facility immediately.

Gastrointestinal problems, such as nausea, vomiting, cramping, abdominal pain, and diarrhea, are common symptoms of anaphylaxis and should not be dismissed as the stomach flu if you're prone to severe allergic reactions. Other symptoms of anaphylaxis are headaches, swelling of the tissue, itching, hives, flushing, nasal congestion, wheezing, upper airway swelling, pain beneath the sternum (breastbone), fainting, or seizure. Up to one-third of patients may experience symptoms hours or days after the initial anaphylactic episode.

To order **Medic-Alert items**, contact: Medic-Alert, 2323 Colorado Avenue, Turlock, CA 95382.

Adrenaline (epinephrine) injections are the primary emergency treatment for anaphylaxis. Doctors may also use corticosteroids, antihistamines, and other medications to control these reactions. Patients who know they are susceptible to anaphylaxis should carry emergency adrenaline kits at all times. Kits such as the Ana-Kit, EpiPen, or EpiPen EZ, are available with a doctor's prescription. If you have nothing else, Primatene Mist, available over the counter, can be used as it contains epinephrine. It's also wise to carry an identification card that lists drug allergies and wear a Medic-Alert bracelet or necklace that contains information about your medical condition, in case of severe shock or unconsciousness. Natural remedies are highly effective for many allergic conditions but anaphylaxis is not one of them.

He cites the case of Lorraine, 52, who had initial symptoms of sinusitis, chronic joint and muscle aches (fibromyalgia), and migraine headaches. Previous allergy tests had already identified 15 substances to which she was seriously allergic; avoiding these had not helped. Kaufman decided it was more expedient to take immediate steps to block the allergic reaction, rather than try to identify yet more allergens.

To do this, he relied on a substance called quercetin, a bioflavonoid, which is one of several vitamin C "helper" substances that enhance the beneficial activities of vitamin C and increase its absorption by the liver, kidneys, and adrenal glands. A typical dosage for quercetin is 200-400 mg, three times daily, taken 20 minutes before meals. Quercetin tends to block allergy receptor sites that bind the allergic proteins, says Kaufman. He suggested a carbohydrate-restricted eating plan for Lorraine as well, temporarily eliminating all sugars, grains, and fruits from her diet to minimize intake of any food-borne fungal materials.

He also had Lorraine take psyllium hulls every day to cleanse and empty her colon; blackstrap molasses to help reduce her sugar cravings; chromium picolinate to help stabilize her blood sugar; grapeseed extract (200 mg, two times daily for two weeks, then 100 mg, three times daily for several months) as a general antioxidant; glucosamine sulfate to treat her joint aches and arthritic symptoms; and a conventional drug called Nystatin to reduce the fungal infection in her intestines.

**Doug Kaufman, M.D.:** The Douglas Plaza, 8226 Douglas Avenue, Suite 522, Dallas, TX 75225; tel/fax: 214-369-7722.

There are two therapeutic goals in this case, explains Kaufman. First, you want to starve the fungus of all nutrient sources. "We see complete allergy remissions by following a particular type of diet that starves the fungus." Second, you want to bolster the patient's immune system, because, in large measure, "allergy indicates an immune system that is deficient," says Dr. Kaufman. All immunoglobulins are made from B lymphocyte cells in the immune system. A faulty diet, such as one high in alcohol or certain fats, can suppress immune function by hampering the formation of new T cells, central to an ability to respond to infections, says Dr. Kaufman. "As you begin to restore the patient's immune response, allergies and other autoimmune complexities tend to start clearing up."

As the fungi in Lorraine's system began to die off, she temporarily felt worse, which is a common and expected reaction, says Dr. Kaufman. After three days of this "healing crisis," she started feeling much better: her energy began to improve and her sinus swellings abated. After about six weeks on the program, Lorraine's migraine headaches were gone and her joint aches were "vastly improved," says Kaufman. "Lorraine complied with the program. As patients like her notice their symptoms of many years beginning to leave, you couldn't pry them off this program."

# Nutritional Supplements

Perhaps the simplest way to relieve allergy and sensitivity symptoms is by taking nutritional supplements. Dietary supplements are readily available in health food and vitamin stores and also in supermarkets, as more and more people are realizing that the typical American diet is sorely deficient in many necessary vitamins, minerals, and other nutrients. Supplements come in powder, tablet, capsule, and liquid forms; be sure to read labels to avoid buying products with fillers, such as cornstarch and gelatin, to which you may be allergic or sensitive.

## Vitamin C (Ascorbic Acid)

Both an antioxidant (SEE QUICK DEFINITION) and anti-inflammatory, vitamin C has been shown to improve and block asthma attacks and allergic rhinitis symptoms. Researchers have found that asthmatics tend to have up to 50% lower concentrations of vitamin C than non-asthmatics.[2]

A 1992 study published in the *Journal of the American College of Nutrition* showed that taking 2,000 mg of vitamin C per day may reduce blood histamine levels by up to 38%, thus blocking inflammation.[3] Infusions of vitamin C have also been shown to promote the production of cortisol, an adrenal hormone that suspends allergic reactions.[4] High doses of vitamin C (2,000 mg or more) have been shown to quickly arrest bronchial symptoms in asthma and allergic rhinitis, and even prevent symptoms from occurring in the first place.

A 1997 study examined the effects of vitamin C on 20 asthma (exercise-induced) patients between the ages of 7 and 28 years. These subjects had at least a 15% reduction in their forced expiratory volume after a standard exercise test on a treadmill. As part of the study, patients stopped taking their regular asthma medications or using bronchodilators 12 hours before the test. Half of the patients were randomly assigned to receive 2 g of oral vitamin C one hour before a seven-minute exercise session on the treadmill; the rest were given a placebo. Vitamin C prevented airway restriction in five of the treated patients. These five patients continued taking oral vitamin C (500 mg per day) for two weeks; four of them experienced remission of their asthma during this time.[5] In another study, 2,000 mg of oral vitamin C given to 16 patients with allergic rhinitis for two consecutive days proved to be significantly more effective than a placebo in reducing bronchial reactivity.[6]

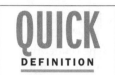

**DEFINITION**

An **antioxidant** (meaning "against oxidation") is a natural biochemical substance that protects living cells against damage from harmful free radicals. Antioxidants work against the process of oxidation—the robbing of electrons from substances. If unblocked or left uncontrolled, oxidation can lead to oxidative stress, causing cellular aging, degeneration, arthritis, heart disease, cancer, and other illnesses. Antioxidants in the body react readily with oxygen breakdown products and free radicals, and neutralize them before they can damage the body. Antioxidant nutrients include vitamins A, C, and E, beta carotene, selenium, coenzyme Q10, pycnogenol (grape seed extract), L-glutathione, superoxide dismutase, N-acetyl-cysteine, bioflavonoids, and anthocyanidins (berries, cherries, etc.). When antioxidants are taken in combination, the effect is stronger than when they are used individually.

A **free radical** is an unstable, toxic molecule of oxygen that destroys healthy molecules. The process develops when molecules within cells react with oxygen, or oxidize. Free radicals then begin to break down cells, especially the cell membranes, and can harmfully alter proteins, enzymes, and even DNA. Sources include pesticides, industrial pollutants, and tobacco smoke.

Vitamin C is also an important factor in helping remove environmental toxins from the body. Vitamin C is also necessary in the formation of collagen, and can help rebuild joint tissue damaged as a result of allergy-induced arthritis. Take vitamin C with bioflavonoids for maximum absorption.

Food sources: most fruits and vegetables, especially oranges, grapefruits, kiwis, lemons, avocados, and parsley. Supplements: the most cost-effective form of vitamin C is ascorbic acid, which is extracted from rosehips or acerola. There is also a new form of vitamin C called ester-C, which is purported to stay in the body longer, thereby increasing absorption.[7] RDA: 60 mg; therapeutic dose: 500-5,000 mg (to bowel tolerance); in patients with exercise-induced asthma, take vitamin C approximately 30 minutes to one hour before exercise for maximum protection.

Possible side effects: essentially nontoxic in oral doses. However, excessive ingestion may cause abdominal bloating, gas, flatulence, and diarrhea. Many alternative medicine practitioners recommend taking vitamin C to "bowel tolerance" (amount tolerated before diarrhea occurs). Acid-sensitive individuals should take the buffered ascorbate form of vitamin C supplement.

## Vitamin E (Tocopherol)

Vitamin E protects cell membranes from oxidative damage and acts as an anti-inflammatory, blocking the activity of an enzyme that provokes inflammation. It also inhibits mast cell degranulation, the biochemical process that releases histamine and other inflammatory chemicals during an allergic response. It helps maintain the elastic quality in cells, which, in turn, increases elasticity in muscles, important for allergy-induced arthritis.

As with vitamin C, levels of vitamin E are typically low in asthma patients.[8] Studies have shown that supplementation of vitamin E enhances the function of T lymphocytes and elevates amounts of B cells in asthma patients.[9] These effects appear to stabilize the hyperactive immune system and prevent asthma attacks. In addition, high doses of vitamin E supplements have been shown to inhibit allergic rhinitis nasal symptoms.[10]

Food sources: cold-pressed oils such as sunflower and safflower, almonds, hazelnuts, and wheat germ. Supplements: vitamin E is actually a group of compounds called tocopherols. When purchasing supplements of vitamin E, avoid products that contain vitamin E in the DL-alpha tocopherol acetate form—this means that it is a petroleum-based synthetic form of the vitamin. The natural form of vitamin E will be designated with the letter "D". Research has shown that the natural form of vitamin E has better antioxidant protective properties and recent research indicates that mixed tocopherols may, in fact, be the best. Avoid taking iron supplements at the same time of day as vitamin E supplements as they mutually prevent absorption. Drink filtered water (no chlorinated water) and avoid polyunsaturated fats, since these may destroy vitamin E. RDA: 30 IU; therapeutic dose: 200-800 IU; up to 3,000 IU per day has shown no negative effects, although prolonged ingestion of high doses may produce adverse skin reactions and upset stomach.

## Vitamin B5 (Pantothenic Acid)
Vitamin B5 is involved in the production of adrenal hormones, such as cortisol, and also helps metabolize fat and carbohydrates. In large doses (up to 1,500 mg per day), vitamin B5 has an antihistamine effect[11] as it promotes cortisol release, thus reducing the symptoms of allergic reactions. Vitamin B5 is also an excellent aid in reducing the effects of stress on the body.

Food sources: liver, meat, chicken, whole grains, and legumes; eating a variety of foods can ensure adequate levels of vitamin B5. RDA: none; therapeutic dose: 10 mg to 2,000 mg. Extremely high doses (10,000 mg+) will produce diarrhea.

## Bioflavonoids
A bioflavonoid is a pigment within plants and fruits that acts as an antioxidant to protect against damage from free radicals and excess oxygen. In the body, bioflavonoids enhance the benefits of vitamin C and are often formulated with this vitamin in supplement form. Originally called vitamin P (until 1950), these vitamin C "helper" substances include citrin, hesperidin, rutin, quercetin, epicatechin, flavones, and flavonols. When taken with vitamin C, bioflavonoids increase the absorption of vitamin C into the liver, kidneys, and adrenal glands. Acting as antioxidants, they also protect vitamin C from destruction by free radicals. Bioflavonoids also have a unique ability to bind and strengthen collagen structures, which are vital for the integrity of connective tissue in cases of allergy-induced arthritis.

There are more than 4,000 classified bioflavonoid compounds occurring in different types of food. The bioflavonoid called anthocyanidin give the deep red or blue color to blueberries, blackberries, cherries, grapes, and hawthorn berries, increases the release of the anti-inflammatory prostaglandins in the gastrointestinal system;[12]

this could prove useful in fighting leaky gut syndrome and gastrointestinal reactions.

Food sources: fruits such as grapefruit, lemon, oranges, apples, apricots, pears, peaches, tomatoes, cherries, blueberries, cranberries, black currants, red grapes, plums, raspberries, strawberries, hawthorn berries, and other berries; vegetables such as red cabbage, onions, parsley, rhubarb; herbs such as milk thistle and sage; grape skins, pine bark, red wine, and green tea. Supplementing with all types of bioflavonoids is recommended for allergy and sensitivity sufferers; however, quercetin has shown particular promise in reducing symptoms.

**Quercetin**—A bright yellow pigment, quercetin has outstanding anti-inflammatory properties useful in treating allergic inflammation.[13] A natural bioflavonoid and antioxidant, quercetin stabilizes mast cells and basophils, thus suppressing the release of histamine, leukotrienes, and other substances that cause inflammation in an allergic response.[14] Quercetin is useful in helping correct intestinal permeability (leaky gut syndrome) and associated food allergies.[15] It has also been found effective in treating nasal/eye symptoms of allergic rhinitis, as it corrects metabolic impairments in essential fatty acid, and other fats needed by lymphocytes.[16] Quercetin also supports the function of vitamin C.

Food sources: onions and green tea. Supplements: quercetin works best when combined with the enzyme bromelain.[17] Therapeutic dose: 200-1,000 mg daily.

## Magnesium

A cofactor in more than 300 enzymatic reactions involving energy and nerve function, magnesium stimulates adrenal and immune function, relaxes smooth muscles, and serves as a natural bronchodilator and antihistamine. Numerous studies prove that intravenous administration of magnesium can stop acute asthma attacks when conventional drugs have failed.

In one study, ten children suffering from acute asthma attacks (peak expiratory flow averaged at less than 60%) were treated with an intravenous infusion of up to 2 g of magnesium, while a control group of ten received a saline placebo. None of the patients had responded to earlier conventional treatment with beta-2 agonists or corticosteroids. Thirty minutes after treatment, the magnesium group experienced significant improvement in peak expiratory flow and a great reduction in asthma symptoms, compared to the control group. This improvement persisted for at least 90 minutes following treatment.[18] Inhaled magnesium (3 mL) has also proved as effective as nebulized salbutamol (a conventional drug) in blocking bronchial constriction in severe asthma attacks.[19]

Oral supplementation of magnesium is also useful in minimizing asthma symptoms. In a double-blinded, controlled study conducted at City Hospital in Nottingham, England, researchers placed 17 asthmatic subjects on a low-magnesium diet for a week, after which they administered oral magnesium supplements (400 mg daily) to some subjects while treating the rest with placebo tablets. A week later, the researchers provoked all subjects with an asthma-inducing irritant. The magnesium-treated group experienced a significant reduction in asthma symptoms compared to the placebo group.[20]

Conventional asthma drugs, especially glucocorticoids (prednisone, hydrocortisone, etc.) have been shown to disrupt magnesium absorption, leading to magnesium deficiency in asthmatics.[21] Magnesium deficiency can cause anxiety, muscle tremors, confusion, irritability, and pain. Processed food or foods cooked at high temperatures can be depleted of their magnesium content.

Food sources: tofu, nuts and seeds, and green leafy vegetables, especially kale, seaweed, and chlorophyll. Supplements: magnesium is absorbed well when taken as an oral supplement and will increase the measurable levels inside red and white blood cells. Magnesium glycinate, fumarate, or citrate are usually better absorbed with less of a laxative effect. Epsom salts (magnesium sulfate), an old-fashioned remedy, is an excellent addition to a bath, but has a strong laxative effect if taken as an oral supplement. RDA: 400 mg; therapeutic dose: 500-1,000 mg. Precautions: very high doses of magnesium (30,000 mg) may be dangerous if kidney disease is present. Doses of 400 mg or higher may produce a laxative effect, causing diarrhea.

## Essential Fatty Acids

The kinds of fats that make up your diet directly affect the severity of allergic inflammation and other symptoms. There are "good" and "bad" dietary fats, and if your diet contains too many of the bad fats, it may be making your allergy symptoms worse or helping to create it in the first place. The inflammatory process can become uncontrollable or over-reactive when certain dietary factors skew the delicate balance of inflammation-mediating substances. Prostaglandins (SEE QUICK DEFINITION), which can either cause or decrease inflammation, are composed of different fatty acids. The type of prostaglandins (anti- or pro-inflammatory) manufactured by the body depends upon what kinds of fats make up your diet, as well as on the presence of certain enzymes and nutrients (vitamins C, B3, and B6, magnesium, and zinc).

Essential fatty acids (EFAs—SEE QUICK DEFINITION), which are derived only from the diet and cannot manufactured in the body, are the building blocks of both pro- and anti-inflammatory prostaglandins. In healthy individuals, the body balances these prostaglandins to ensure adequate immune response and to limit inflammatory responses.

The two principle types of essential fatty acids are omega-3 and omega-6. Deficiencies in EFAs, particularly the omega-3s, are quite common in America because of modern food processing techniques. Humans evolved on a diet that contained small but roughly equal amounts of omega-3s and omega-6s. When the food supply began to change about one hundred years ago to more processed foods, the amount of omega-3s in many commercial products declined. At the same time, the domestic livestock industry began to use feed grain, which happens to be rich in omega-6 fatty acids and low in omega-3s. Because of these changes, the American diet now has 20 to 25 times more omega-6s than omega-3s, rather than the ideal 1:2 ratio.

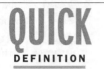

**DEFINITION**

A **prostaglandin** is a hormone-like, complex fatty acid that affects smooth muscle function, inflammatory processes, and blood vessel functions, particularly in the lungs and intestines. Eating too many trans-fatty acids (found in processed foods such as margarine) reduces production of helpful prostaglandins.

**Essential fatty acids (EFAs)** are unsaturated fats required in the diet. Omega-3 and omega-6 oils are the two principal types. The primary omega-3 oil is alpha-linolenic acid (ALA), found in flaxseed and canola oils, as well as pumpkins, walnuts, and soybeans. Fish oils, such as salmon, cod, and mackerel, contain the other important omega-3 oils, DHA (docosahexaenoic acid) and EPA (eicosapentaenoic acid). Linoleic acid is the main omega-6 oil and is found in most vegetable oils, including safflower, corn, peanut, and sesame. The most therapeutic form of omega-6 oil is gamma-linolenic acid (GLA), found in evening primrose, black currant, and borage oils. Once in the body, omega-3 and omega-6 are converted to prostaglandins, hormone-like substances that regulate many metabolic functions, particularly inflammatory processes.

Prostaglandins that cause inflammation are formed when the diet is high in animal fats, which contain high amounts of arachidonic acid. Arachidonic acid is a long-chain polyunsaturated omega-6 fatty acid, found primarily in animal foods such as meat, poultry, and dairy products. When the diet is abundant in arachidonic acids, these are stored in cell membranes. An enzyme transforms these stored acids into pro-inflammatory prostaglandins and other chemical messengers called leukotrienes, which instigate inflammation. If there is an overabundance of arachidonic acid or "bad" fats, then more pro-inflammatory agents will be produced by the body. This process is called the arachidonic acid cascade.

The arachidonic acid cascade has been implicated in provoking asthma attacks, as pro-inflammatory prostaglandins and leukotrienes

For more on **essential fatty acid supplements for skin barrier function**, see Chapter 9: Supporting the Skin, pp. 236-259.

have been found to constrict bronchial passages, increase airway membrane permeability, cause airway swelling, and promote secretion of mucus.[22] This inflammatory process also leads to or exacerbates headaches, skin rashes, and arthritic pain.

Many allergy/sensitivity patients, and most people in general, do not consume enough of the beneficial omega-6 EFAs found in vegetable oils, but eat too much of arachidonic acids, found in animal fats. Beneficial omega-6-fatty acids (linoleic acid and gamma-linolenic acid) are metabolized into anti-inflammatory prostaglandins necessary to prevent autoimmune disease, as well as keep the skin barrier intact. Most people also have an enzyme block (delta-6-desaturase) that does not let them properly metabolize omega-6-fatty acids. Borage oil, black currant oil, and evening primrose oil (in that order) contain the highest levels of beneficial omega-6 EFAs. Dietary consumption of all omega-6 fats needs to be in balance. Allergy patients should limit intake of foods containing arachidonic acid (animal fats) and eat more vegetable oil.

Anti-inflammatory prostaglandins are produced from omega-3 fatty acids. The primary omega-3 fatty acid is alpha-linolenic acid (ALA), which is abundant in flaxseed oil. Three tablespoons of unheated flaxseed oil can be put on salad, steamed vegetables, or other foods. Purchase oils that are "expeller pressed," not just "cold pressed." Check the expiration date and adhere to it; flaxseed oil can rapidly turn rancid and should be stored in the refrigerator. Organic, whole flaxseeds can also be used to add a nutty flavor to cereals, vegetables, or casseroles; place a few tablespoons in a coffee grinder to release the seeds' oils. Purslane (*Portulaca oleracea*), often considered a weed, is actually a nutritious vegetable high in omega-3 fatty acids. Less than one cup supplies a full day's supply of ALA. Purslane also contains vitamin E, a potent antioxidant that is necessary for the formation of the anti-inflammatory prostaglandins, as well as vitamins A and C.

Other types of omega-3 fatty acids include eicosapentaenoic acid (EPA) and docosahexaenoic acid (DHA), which are chemically closer to becoming prostaglandins than ALA. Food sources high in EPA/DHA include salmon, bluefish, bass, trout, organ meats, and brown and red algae. High cooking temperatures can destroy the EFA content in certain foods and oils, so baking or grilling fish is a preferable cooking method to frying. For allergy patients, we recommend supplementing with all three forms of omega-3s (ALA, EPA, and DHA).

Clinical research has proven that dietary supplementation of omega-3 EFAs is especially effective in reducing asthma symptoms. In one study conducted by Italian researchers, seven atopic patients suffering from seasonal asthma were administered oral supplements of omega-3 fats (3 g per day) for 30 days. The researchers found that forced expiratory volume significantly improved and bronchial reactivity decreased as a result of omega-3 EFAs. The test subjects then stopped taking omega-3 supplements for 30 days, at which time their lung function had returned to low, pre-treatment values and airway constriction increased.[23]

## Dietary Recommendations for Improving the Body's Fat Intake

■ Eat foods rich in the three types of omega-3 fatty acids: alpha-linolenic acid (ALA)—the oils flaxseed (58%), chia seed (30%), poppy seed (15%), pumpkin seed (15%), canola, walnut, and soy, purslane and cattail, and dark green leafy vegetables;[24] eicosapentaenoic acid (EPA)—cold-water fish, salmon, mackerel, halibut, and Chinese snake oil; docosahexaenoic acid (DHA)—cold-water fish and commercial supplements containing vegetable sources of DHA.

■ Obtain an adequate supply of niacin, vitamins B6 and E, zinc, and magnesium to enhance fatty-acid metabolism. Beans, especially lima, soy, great northern, kidney, and navy, poultry, and fish contain these important nutrients as well as omega-3 fatty acids. Be sure to check for food allergies first.

■ Reduce carbohydrate intake and avoid all refined sugars, processed foods, margarine, hydrogenated oils, and gluten-containing foods such as wheat, oats, and barley.

■ Incorporate certain spices and herbs into the diet, such as fresh mint leaves, thyme oil, and ginger; these foods contain substances that will help stabilize fats in the cell membranes.

■ Avoid all fats and oils containing very-long-chain fatty acids, such as mustard, peanut butter, peanut oil, and canola oil.

**Fish Consumption Can Benefit Allergy, But Be Cautious**—Increased use of fish, both as a whole food and as fish oil supplements, is a sound beginning in relieving allergic symptoms. Research shows that fish oils compete with arachidonic acid, which otherwise produces inflammation. Studies have found that fish and fish oil supplementation can alleviate minor respiratory problems in some cases of severe asthma.[25]

But while fish, especially salmon and other cold-water fatty fish, have high levels of beneficial EFAs, there are a few problems associated with eating fish. Increasingly, the salmon reaching the North

American market are farm-raised rather than caught from rivers and streams. Commercially produced or "farmed" fish have a less desirable fatty-acid profile than wild fish; specifically, researchers have found that farmed fish are lower in omega-3s.[26] Seafood and fish products are becoming increasingly less healthy. According to research conducted by Vincent Buyck, Ph.D., of the College of Complementary Medicine and Sciences, in Washington, D.C., as water temperatures rise, some microorganisms mutate into forms that can cause disease. When these microorganisms are ingested by seafood or fish (and subsequently by humans), they present a threat to human health.[27] Additionally, seafood and fish may be contaminated due to living in polluted waters.

Eating fish that is boiled or baked is preferable to eating it fried. Foods that are fried have a high level of polychlorinated phenols, a toxic by-product caused by heating oils to frying temperatures. These phenols increase inflammation and can worsen allergy symptoms.[28]

## Common Foods That May Contain Hydrogenated Fats and Trans-Fatty Acids

- Margarine, Crisco
- Diet foods
- Mayonnaise
- Crackers and chips
- Cookies, cakes and cake mixes, pastries, and doughnuts
- Candy
- Packaged breads
- Canned, creamed soups and gravy
- Breakfast cereals and frozen waffles
- Microwave popcorn
- Frozen entrees, French fries, fish sticks, and chicken nuggets

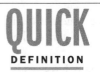

### DEFINITION

**Hydrogenated and trans-fatty acids** refer to a synthetic process in which natural oils are broken down into a semi-solid fat by adding a hydrogen atom to an unsaturated fat molecule. This process is widely used to prolong the shelf-life of commercial baked goods, packaged foods, most salad oils and dressings, margarines, and cooking oils such as corn and safflower. The molecules that make up these fats, called trans-fatty acids, are known to interfere with the healthy functioning of our bodies due to their unusual molecular shape.

## Avoid the "Bad" Fats

Hydrogenated fats and trans-fatty acids (SEE QUICK DEFINITION) can directly contribute to inflammation. We recommend avoiding foods that contain these fats, which are, unfortunately, a common ingredient in most refined foods. Read the labels of packaged foods before you buy to determine if they contain hydrogenated fats. In the list of ingredients, you will see them described as either "hydrogenated" or "partially hydrogenated" oils. The "Nutrition Facts" label will also provide you with amounts of saturated and unsaturated fats.

The membrane of every cell is a thin envelope of fats that encases and protects the internal biochemical components. Within this fatty envelope are thousands of proteins that facilitate communication and transport—acting like a gate—across the cell membrane. The ability of the cell wall to change shape, so that life-sustaining nutrients can be absorbed and wastes expelled, is dependent upon fatty acids.[29] Normal fatty acids (cis-fatty acids) have a "rounded" shape and help to form a strong yet flexible membrane surface. But trans-fatty acids have a "straight" shape, which forms a weak, brittle cell wall that cannot efficiently transport nutrients and wastes. A weak cell wall can break or become distorted, leaving it vulnerable to attack by free radicals.[30] As we've seen, free radicals and oxidative stress are implicated in skin and mucous membrane barrier default.

It is estimated that as a nation we consume more than 600 million pounds of trans-fatty acids a year, mostly in the form of frying fats and margarine. Trans-fatty acids contribute to EFA deficiency, as they interfere with the enzyme systems that convert EFAs into the unsaturated fatty acid derivatives that are needed for brain, sense and sex organs, and—particularly important for the allergy sufferer—adrenal function.[31] Trans-fatty acids also have been shown to inhibit the production of anti-inflammatory prostaglandins.

## Curb an Allergic Migraine Fast

At the onset of a migraine headache that has been triggered by a sensitivity to foods or chemicals, dissolve two tablets of Alka-Seltzer Gold in a glass of water and drink it. The drink creates an alkaline (opposite of acidic) environment in the body which has the effect of neutralizing the allergic reaction and preventing the migraine from fully taking hold. One-half teaspoon of baking soda in a small glass of water provides similar results.

Clinical trials have shown that inhaling heparin, a natural substance the body produces to prevent blood clotting, can reduce the allergic response associated with migraines.[32] Heparin normalizes the immune system's levels of basophils, lymphocytes, and T cells (which are lower in migraine patients), and can be inhaled to stop a headache in progress.

# Botanical Medicines

Various herbal remedies have shown excellent results in reducing allergy/sensitivity symptoms. Particularly effective are anti-inflammatory herbs such as stinging nettle, *Ginkgo biloba*, and licorice.

**Stinging Nettle (*Urtica dioica*)**—Stinging nettle, a perennial herb indigenous to Europe and North America, is often regarded as an annoying—and irritating—weed, for its leaves do indeed sting. As an herbal remedy, nettle leaf and/or root is effective in treating anemia, benign prostatic hyperplasia, skin ailments, and diuresis. Herbal preparations containing the freeze-dried leaves have also been found to relieve allergic rhinitis symptoms. In a double-blind study, 69 patients with allergic rhinitis were randomly given either a freeze-dried preparation of stinging nettle (two 300 mg capsules daily) or a placebo. In the treatment group, 58% rated it moderately effective in alleviating the symptoms of rhinitis, compared to only 37% in the placebo group.[33] There are no known side effects. Recommended dosage: two 300 mg capsules daily.

**Ephedra (*Ephedra sinica* or Ma huang)**—Ephedra has been a major herb in traditional Chinese medicine for more than 5,000 years; it is particularly useful for relieving asthma symptoms, including wheezing, coughing, and bronchial inflammation, as well as nasal congestion. Its active constituents are ephedrine, which is similar in structure to the epinephrine (adrenaline) produced in the body and used as treatment

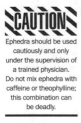

in anaphylactic shock, and pseudoephedrine, which is somewhat weaker than ephedrine.[34] These components facilitate bronchodilation, decongestion, and other anti-inflammatory responses.[35]

Ephedra should be used cautiously and only under the supervision of a trained physician. Do not mix ephedra with caffeine or theophylline; this combination can be deadly.

Ephedra has been the focal point of much controversy lately, due to its potential side effects. In fact, the Food and Drug Administration has considered regulating the use of this herb. Excessive intake of ephedra can be dangerous, resulting in insomnia, high blood pressure, glaucoma, motor disturbances, impaired cerebral circulation, and urinary disturbances. This herb should not be used by anyone with hypertension, high blood pressure, heart disease, thyroid disease, diabetes, prostate problems, or by anyone taking monoamine-oxidase (MAO) inhibitor antidepressant drugs. Recommended dosage: 15-30 drops of tincture four times daily (check with a doctor first).

**Ginkgo biloba**—The ginkgo tree is one of the oldest living trees on earth. Its leaves contain biochemical compounds responsible for ginkgo's healing properties.[36] Clinical and laboratory tests have shown that standardized *Ginkgo biloba* extract (standardized to 24% ginkgo flavoglycosides) has significant benefit in the treatment of increased intestinal permeability. Ginkgo protects the intestine by reducing the oxidative damage in the intestinal lining due to free-radical activity. Additionally, ginkgo extract has been shown to suppress the function of platelet-activating factor (PAF), a chemical that mediates allergic inflammation and is particularly responsible for skin reactions. The ginkgo flavo-glycosides compete with PAF for binding sites on blood cells, thereby inhibiting the inflammatory events induced by PAF.[37] Recommended dosage: 300 mg, two times daily.

**Licorice Root (*Glycyrrhiza glabra*)**—Licorice is a traditional herbal remedy with an ancient history. Glycyrrhizin (glycyrrhetinic acid) is believed to be the primary active constituent. Modern research has shown that it has beneficial effects on the endocrine system, adrenal glands, and liver; it acts as a systemic anti-inflammatory.[38] It also stimulates interferon (a cytokine with antiviral activity) and enhances the body's production of cortisone.[39] Studies have shown that licorice is helpful in relieving the symptoms of atopic eczema because of the herb's promotion of cortisone.[40]

Licorice is also particularly effective in helping to repair leaky gut syndrome. Its efficacy is thought to be due to flavonoid derivatives of licorice called steroidal saponin glycosides, which exert a protective effect. Licorice root has also been shown to reduce the gastric bleeding caused by the use of NSAIDs. If the use of NSAIDs is necessary, gastric mucus damage has been reduced by giving simultaneous dosages of 500 mg of deglycerrated licorice.

Licorice is not recommended for people with heart disease, liver disease, hypertension, or pregnant women. If diuretics or heart medications containing digitalis have been prescribed, licorice should be avoided. People taking glucocorticoid drugs should not use licorice without the supervision of a physician, due to the herb's effects on natural cortisone production. Recommended dosage: up to six 400-500 mg capsules per day or 20-30 drops of tincture three times per day.

> **CAUTION**
>
> Because licorice root mimics some of the adrenal hormones so closely, it can cause retention of sodium and water and thus raise blood pressure. This is not normally a concern, but if you tend to have a blood pressure problem, it is best to use a type of deglycerrated licorice (DGL), which will help in the regeneration of stomach and intestinal cells, without the increase in water retention.

For an **herbal remedy containing licorice root**, contact: Alternative Therapy, Inc. ("Allergy"), 1664 Fairlawn Avenue, San Jose, CA 95125; tel: 800-311-7922. For **herbal remedies containing ephedra**, contact: Nature's Way Products, Inc., 10 Mountain Springs Parkway, Springville, UT 84663; tel: 800-962-8873 or 801-489-1500; fax: 801-489-1700; website: www.natureswway.com. Nature's Herbs, 600 East Quality Drive, American Fork, UT 84003; tel: 800-437-2257 or 801-763-0700.

**Chinese Skullcap or Scute (*Scutellaria baicalensis*)**—Japanese research has yielded new information that Chinese skullcap root has significant anti-allergenic and antioxidant properties.[41] The active ingredient, baicalin, is responsible for its anti-inflammatory action. It destroys an enzyme system, which inhibits the release of antibodies and prevents the allergic response. Chinese skullcap has been shown to block highly inflammatory end products of the arachidonic acid cascade and is useful in relieving atopic dermatitis, asthma, and bronchial constriction due to allergy. Recommended dosage: 10-30 drops of tincture per day.

**Feverfew (*Tanacetum parthenium*)**—Feverfew, a member of the aster family, has been used for more than 2,000 years to treat fevers, headache, menstrual irregularity, and externally for pain. Herbal preparations containing fresh or dried leaves have been clinically proven to relieve migraine headaches. In fact, feverfew can be more effective at controlling pain and inflammation than aspirin or NSAIDs (nonsteroidal, anti-inflammatory drugs).[42] It blocks the production of inflammatory chemicals and slows the migration of certain white blood cells to the inflamed area, thus modulating inflammation and pain. A double-blind study from England determined that feverfew was effective in reducing the pain of migraine headaches and was also useful for rheumatoid arthritis, which is commonly induced by food allergies.[43] The effectiveness of feverfew is dependent upon adequate levels of parthenolide, the active ingredient. The preparations used in the clinical trials in migraine headaches had a parthenolide content of 0.40%-0.66%.

If you're allergic to members of the aster family, do not use feverfew. Possible side effects include mouth ulcers, tongue inflammation, lip swelling, and occasional loss of taste, which subside upon feverfew withdrawal. Do not use if you're pregnant. Recommended dosage: three 300-400 mg capsules per day; 15-30 drops of tincture per day.

### Botanical Medicines for Gastrointestinal Symptoms
A major symptom of both true allergies and sensitivities/intolerances is gastrointestinal upset, including bloating, gas, abdominal pain, diarrhea, and nausea. Demulcent herbs can alleviate these symptoms. *Demulcent* is a term used by herbalists to describe an herb that has a protective effect on the mucous membranes. Most of the herbs that contain demulcents have large amounts of mucilaginous materials— gummy, slimy chemicals that have a direct action on the lining of the intestines, soothing irritations. In general, all mucilage-containing demulcents minimize irritation down the whole length of the bowel, reducing the sensitivity of the digestive system to gastric acids, relaxing painful spasms, and decreasing leaky gut and digestive inflammation and ulceration.[44]

**Marshmallow (*Althea officinalis*)**—Marshmallow root contains 25% to 35% mucilage. The root of the plant is used by herbalists for any inflammation of the gastrointestinal system. It is usually taken as a tea:

take several teaspoons of the root or leaves, cover it with boiling water, and steep for 20-30 minutes to extract all the medicinal components. Six cups of this tea a day can be useful in severe cases of leaky gut.

**Slippery Elm Bark (*Ulmus fulva*)**—Slippery elm bark, obtained by removing the bark on the branches of the slippery elm tree, has been used as a demulcent for the respiratory and gastrointestinal systems. Its traditional use is in ulcers, colitis, irritable bowel, infections, and diarrhea.[45] Slippery elm is available as tinctures or capsules, or a decoction can be made where the bark is very gently simmered, one part of the bark to eight quarts of water; bring to a boil and let it simmer for 20-30 minutes; drink 2-3 cups a day.

**Cabbage Juice**—Raw, green, organic cabbage juice contains high amounts of glutamine, an essential amino acid that aids in the metabolism of gastrointestinal cells. Cabbage juice can be made in combination with other vegetables that are effective in reconstructing a healthy gut mucosa, such as chickweed and plantain banana. Put them together to make an excellent healing juice. Four to eight ounces a day is advisable.

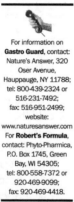

For information on **Gastro Guard**, contact: Nature's Answer, 320 Oser Avenue, Hauppauge, NY 11788; tel: 800-439-2324 or 516-231-7492; fax: 516-951-2499; website: www.naturesanswer.com For **Robert's Formula**, contact: Phyto-Pharmica, P.O. Box 1745, Green Bay, WI 54305; tel: 800-558-7372 or 920-469-9099; fax: 920-469-4418.

**Okra (Hibiscus)**—Okra, a mucilaginous vegetable that is under utilized as a food source, contains ingredients that soothe and restore the irritated gastrointestinal tract. It is included in several commercial herbal formulas, such as Gastro Guard (from Nature's Answer) and Robert's Formula (from Phyto-Pharmica).

**Fenugreek**—Crushed fenugreek seeds contain 28% mucilin and make an excellent demulcent. The use of this medicinal plant dates back to the Egyptians and the Greek physician Hippocrates. Fenugreek seeds can be steeped as a tea or used in capsules. To make tea, use one teaspoon of fenugreek to one cup water. In capsule form: one capsule (250 mg) 2-3 times daily with hot water.

**Aloe Vera Cocktail**—This is an excellent formula for any upper gastrointestinal inflammation. You'll need 1$^{1}/_{2}$ oz aloe vera juice, one capsule or one dropperful (tincture) of Robert's Formula, and one capsule deglycerrated licorice. Open capsules and put powder in aloe juice. Shake and drink before meals and bedtime.

# Chinese Herbal Formulas

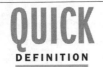

**QUICK**
**DEFINITION**

**Qi** (pronounced CHEE) is a Chinese word variously translated to mean "vital energy," "essence of life," and "living force." In Chinese medicine, the proper flow of *qi* along energy channels (meridians) within the body is crucial to a person's health and vitality. There are many types of *qi*, classified according to source, location, and function (such as activation, warming, defense, transformation, and containment). Within the body, *qi* and blood are closely linked, as each is considered to flow along with the other. *Qi* may be stagnant (non-moving), deficient (partially absent), or excessive (inappropriately abundant) from a given organ system. *Qi* has two essential qualities: yang (active, fiery, moving, bright, energizing) and yin (passive, watery, stationary, dark, calming).

Traditional Chinese medicine (TCM), practiced for more than 5,000 years, is complex and often difficult for Westerners to understand. One important concept in Chinese medicine is the free-flowing motion of *qi* (SEE QUICK DEFINITION) and blood (including lymph and other fluids) through channels, or meridians, in the body. A Chinese medicine physician considers the flow of *qi* in a patient through close examination of the patient's pulse, tongue, body odor, voice tone and strength, and general demeanor, among other elements. Underlying imbalances and disharmony in the body are described in terminology analogous to the natural world (heat, cold, dryness, or dampness). The concept of balance, or the interrelationship of organs, is central to TCM. Disease arises when obstructions occur to impede the flow of *qi* and thus disturb the regulation of related organs and body systems. Symptoms of allergy and sensitivity are related to obstructions in varying organ meridians; not all symptoms are caused by the same *qi* blockages.

Chinese herbs are classified by energetic functions (distinguished as cold, hot, dry, and damp) and the organs that their energies affect (lung, kidney, or liver). Similarly, the diseases that affect the human body are classified accordingly—by excess or deficient energy and organ imbalances. A trained TCM practitioner can determine whether your symptoms are classified as an excess of heat, cold, dryness, or dampness, and may prescribe herbs to balance the excess quality.

**Apricot Seed (*Pruni armeniacae* or Xing Ren)**—An antitussive (cough suppressant) and expectorant, the mature seed of the apricot tree is used in many Chinese formulas to relieve coughing and wheezing; it also has laxative effects. A bitter, warming herb, it can be toxic in high doses (50-60 kernels are toxic for adults; ten kernels are toxic for children).

**Astragalus (*Astragali* or Huang Qi)**—Astragalus root has been studied extensively for its cardiovascular effects and antibacterial properties. It is a sweet, slightly warming herb that stimulates healing and draining of edema and pus. It also dilates blood vessels and improves circulation of the skin, among other effects. It's a good, overall immune booster.

**Centipede (*Centipeda minima* or Shi-Hu-Sui)**—An acrid, warming herb, centipede has been clinically proven to have anti-inflammatory properties. In a 1991 study, it was found that centipede's active ingredients (including three types of flavonoids, various EFAs, and proteins) inhibited histamine release in cutaneous allergic reactions.[46] It is traditionally used to relieve stuffy nose, cough, and sinusitis.

**Corydalis (*Corydalis ambigua* or Yan Hu Suo)**—The root of the corydalis plant is widely used in TCM to relieve pain. More than 20 alkaloids have been extracted from this bitter, warming herb. The alkaloid corydaline B is believed to be responsible for raising the pain threshold and relaxing muscles, while other substances called tetradydropalmatine and bulbocapnine have been shown to calm the central nervous system, acting as a very mild anesthetic.[47]

**Chrysanthemum Flower (*Chrysanthemi morifolii* or Ju Hua)**—A slightly bitter, slightly cold herb, the flower of the chrysanthemum is used singly or in combination with other herbs. It has a hypotensive effect, meaning it is able to lower blood pressure by dilating blood vessels, and relieve the rapid onset of inflammatory conditions, including headaches and red, painful, tearing, or dry eyes. Avoid if you have diarrhea.

**Ginseng (*Panax ginseng* or Ren Shen)**—Western researchers have studied ginseng root for its many effects, including mental improvement, fatigue relief, and stress reduction through stimulation of the adrenal and pituitary glands. In the case of allergy, ginseng in an antihistamine and is able to inhibit tissue swelling and inflammation, as well as tonify the lungs. Overuse of ginseng can lead to headaches, insomnia, and increased blood pressure. Chinese medicine considers this a slightly bitter, warming herb.

**Magnolia Flower (*Magnolia liliflorae* or Xin Yin Hua)**—The flower of the magnolia tree is an acrid, slightly warming herb used to treat symptoms of sinus infection, inflammation, nasal congestion, and headache. It is a hypotensive and also has sedative effects.

**Perilla Seed (*Perillae semen* or Tsu Su Tsu)**—The extracted oil of the seed of the perilla plant is frequently used in formulas to relieve asthma symptoms, including cough and phlegm. It is an acrid, warming herb. Perilla seed oil is high in omega-3 fatty acids, particularly alpha-linolenic acid. In a clinical study, seven asthmatic subjects were fed perilla seed oil supplements for four weeks while a control group consumed corn oil (omega-6 EFA) supplements. At the end of four weeks, the perilla seed group had a significant increase in peak expiratory flow, indicating that airway constriction was greatly reduced. Levels of leukocytes (which cause inflammation during an allergic reaction) were also diminished in the blood of the perilla seed group, while they increased in the corn oil group. The researchers concluded that perilla seed oil is useful for asthma due to its leukocyte suppression and pulmonary improvement functions.[48]

**Xanthium (Xanthii or Can Er Zi)–** This slightly bitter, warming fruit of the xanthium (cocklebur) plant is used in formulas to treat headaches, sinus discharge, pain, arthritis with numbness, skin disorders, and itching. It is effective for chronic allergic rhinitis and is also an antibacterial. Among its active constituents are linoleic acid (an omega-6 EFA) and vitamin C. Many people are sensitized to cocklebur pollen.

## Patent Medicines

The Chinese herbs described above are typically sold in combination remedies with other herbs. Referred to as patent medicines, these remedies are standardized formulas based on recipes that have been used for more than 2,000 years. Now available as pills, ointments, or tinctures, patent medicines are easier to take then the traditional tea beverages made from the same ingredients. It is important to find a reliable manufacturer of patent medicines, one who doesn't include ingredients from endangered species, artificial colorings, sugar coatings or contaminants. Reputable manufacturers provide a list of ingredients and the symptoms that these ingredients can benefit on the label of their product. Follow the directions carefully and consult with a health-care practitioner before beginning a course of Chinese herbs. Specific patent medicines that are useful in allergy relief include the following:

**Bi Yan Pian–**Also known as "Nose Inflammation Pills," this combination of 12 herbs is used to relieve sneezing, itchy eyes, facial congestion, and sinus pain. It is recommended for cases of acute and chronic allergic rhinitis, sinusitis, and other nasal allergies. Among the herbs in this formula are magnolia flower, xanthium fruit, licorice root, and chrysanthemum flower. Recommended dosage: four tablets, four times a day.

**Chuan Qiong Cha Tiao Wan–** Also known as "Ligusticum with Green Tea Mix Pill," this combination of eight herbs is used to relieve nasal congestion, headache, and allergic rhinitis. It's best when taken with green tea, a known antioxidant. Licorice root is among its ingredients. Recommended dosage: eight pills, 3-5 times a day.

**Tablet Bi-Tong–**Also known as "Nose Open Tablet," this combination of eight herbs is used to stop pain, sneezy, watery eyes, and nasal congestion accompanying allergic rhinitis. Centipede and chrysanthemum flower are included. Recommended dosage: four pills, three times a day.

**Clean Air Tea–**Also known as "Clear Qi, Expel Phlegm Pills," this formula contains eight herbs, including apricot seed and Chinese skullcap root, and is useful in treating bronchial congestion, sinus congestion, and asthma with expectorated phlegm or nasal discharge. Recommended dosage: six pills, three times a day.

**Chuan Ke Ling–**Also known as "Asthma Cough Efficacious Remedy," this four-herb formula helps relieve labored breathing with cough; it is indicated for chronic asthma. Licorice root is among the main ingredients (30%). Recommended dosage: 3-4 tablets, 2-3 times a day.

**Lung Dispersing Water–**This Chinese patent formula of nine herbs, including magnolia flower and perilla seed, is used for clearing cough and breathing difficulties due to asthma. Read label for dosage.

**Chi Kuan Yen Wan–**Also known as "Bronchitis, Cough, Phlegm, Labored Breathing Pills," this 13-herb combination is used to treat a dry cough with sticky phlegm in asthma. It contains apricot seed. Recommended dosage: 20 pills, twice daily.

**Wan Nian Chun Zi Pu Ziang–**Also known as "Thousand Year Spring Nourishing Syrup," this is a combination of eight herbs that improves strength in those with asthma and arthritis. Ginseng root is among its ingredients. Recommended dosage: 10 cc with water, once daily.

**Qing Bi Tang–**Commonly known as Nasal Tabs or Pueraria Combination, this 13-herb formula is indicated for acute and chronic sinus congestion, allergic rhinitis, and headache. It contains ephedra, magnolia flower, and licorice root. Read above for cautions about ephedra. Recommended dosage: 2-4 tablets, three times a day.

**Saiboku-To**—This combination of ten herbs has been found to reduce the bronchial spasms and other symptoms of steroid-dependent asthma.[49] It contains licorice root, perilla seed, magnolia flower, and Chinese skullcap. Read label for dosage.

**Kai Yeung Pill**—Also known as "Pit Viper Dispel Itching Pill," this 12-herb formula relieves skin itching and is especially useful for cases of eczema and allergic contact dermatitis. It contains astragalus root, ginseng root, and xanthium fruit. Recommended dosage: 30 pills, three times a day. Avoid during pregnancy.

**Zemaphyte**—A ten-herb combination, this patent medicine has been proven to relieve the symptoms of atopic dermatitis in several randomized, double-blind, placebo-controlled trials. In one of the studies, Zemaphyte significantly improved eczema symptoms within eight weeks. The researchers found that the herbal preparation was able to block interleukin (an inflammatory chemical) receptors as well as decrease adhesion of inflammatory chemicals on vascular cells.[50] Read label for dosage.

For more information about **Chinese herbal medicine**, contact: American Association of Oriental Medicine, 433 Front Street, Catasauqua, PA 18032; tel: 888-500-7999 or 610-266-1433; fax: 610-264-2768; website: www.aaom.org. To order **patent medicines for allergy**, contact: China Herbs, 6333 Wayne Avenue, Philadelphia, PA 19144; tel: 800-221-4372; fax: 215-849-3338. Crane Herb Company, 745 Falmouth Road, Mashpee, MA 02649; tel: 800-227-4118 or 508-539-1700; fax: 508-539-2369; website: www.craneherb.com.

**Armadillo Anti-Itch Pills**—This formula contains 20 herbs, including astragalus root, chrysanthemum flower, xanthium fruit, and Chinese skullcap root. It is useful for alleviating skin itching, inflammation, or pain characterizing weepy eczema, allergic contact dermatitis, and hives. Recommended dosage: four pills, three times a day.

**Tri-Snake Counter Poison Pills**—This ten-herb formula relieves itching due to allergic contact dermatitis, hives, and eczema. Astragalus root and ginseng root are included. Recommended dosage: 4-5 pills, twice daily. Avoid during pregnancy.

**Corydalis Yanhusus Analgesic Tablets**—Aslo known as "Corydalis Stop Pain Tablets," this two-herb combination is recommended for a wide variety of pain, including sinus and other headaches, sinusitis pain, and joint inflammation. It contains 66% corydalis root. Recommended dosage: four pills, three times a day.

### Patent Formulas for Gastrointestinal Symptoms

In Chinese medicine, there are several excellent patent formulas that have a soothing effect on the digestive system:

**Pill Curing Formula**—Pill Curing Formula helps cramping, abdominal pain, diarrhea, irritation, and mucousy stools. It is a TCM alternative to Pepto Bismal. It is made up of many ingredients, including chrysanthemum flowers. Read label for dosage.

**Shenling Baizhupian**—Shenling Baizhupian is a classic patent medicine formula for digestion, erratic loose stools, and symptoms of irritable bowel. It includes licorice root. Read label for dosage.

**Yunnan Paiyao**—Yunnan Paiyao is a valuable first-aid remedy for internal and external bleeding; studies indicate that it can cause blood to clot 33% faster. The main ingredient is pseudo ginseng root. When taken internally, Yunnan Paiyao has been shown to stop internal bleeding in the gastrointestinal system and is used for the treatment of gastrointestinal inflammation. Recommended dosage: 200 mg, twice daily on an empty stomach.

# Dangers of Conventional Allergy Treatment

Pharmaceutical medications are often the first step of allergy treatment in a conventional medical setting. However, research shows that antihistamines, cortisone, and other frequently prescribed allergy drugs have many adverse consequences.

Antihistamine drugs, both topical and oral, are the most commonly prescribed and administered allergy medication. They block some if not all of the histamine released during an allergic reaction; histamine does not cause allergic reactions but it does incite such classic allergy symptoms as runny nose, watery eyes, sneezing, and itchy skin. While antihistamine drugs generally relieve these symptoms, they have numerous drawbacks. Among the side effects of regular doses of antihistamines are drowsiness, dizziness, lack of coordination, fatigue, blurred or double vision, mood changes, delusions, hallucinations, insomnia, constipation or diarrhea, urinary frequency or difficulty, coughing, palpitations, tightness in the chest, headache, and tingling or weakness in the hands. Birth defects have also been linked to the use of antihistamines by pregnant women.

A recent study conducted by University of Iowa researchers, published in *Annals of Internal Medicine* (backed by Aventis, maker of the second-generation fexofenadine antihistimane drug Allegra®), found that standard doses of allergy drugs containing the antihistamine diphenhydramine (as found in Benadryl®) may impair people's ability to safely drive more than alcohol (because of drowsiness).[51] Another antihistamine commonly prescribed for allergies, astemizole (Hismanal®), can have possible adverse side effects on the cardiac system. Sedating histamines (such as Benadryl®, Tavist®, Chlor-Trimeton®, Zyrtec®, Atarax®) may have various adverse effects, such as headaches, nervousness, anxiety, blurred vision, dizziness, nausea or vomiting, urinary retention, and cardiovascular problems including palpitations, arrhythmias, and hypertension. Moreover, antihistamines have a dramatic impact on childhood learning ability. In one study, children who took diphenhydramine-containing drugs such as Benadryl® for hay fever scored approximately ten points (45 points out of 60) lower than children who did not (54 points out of 60) on a test.[52]

## Asthma Drugs

Although some of the frequently prescribed asthma drugs can be life-saving in an emergency, overuse or long-term use of most asthma medications can produce severe side effects. Oral corticosteroids, such as prednisone, may over a period of time increase a patient's risk for osteoporosis, diabetes, immune depression, adrenal suppression, cataracts, facial swelling, candidiasis, and a loss of minerals such as potassium, calcium, and magnesium, among other problems. Inhaled cortisone may also have serious side effects. In one study, taking inhaled corticosteroids in quantities of over 1.6 mg per day for three months significantly increased the risk of glaucoma or ocular hypertension in elderly patients.[53]

There is also strong evidence that long-term use of inhaled corticosteroids can slow growth in asthmatic children, as cortisone drugs reduce collagen synthesis in children.[54] This can occur with doses of beclomethasone at 400 micrograms (0.4 mg) or more daily, or budesonide at 800 micrograms (0.8 mg) or more daily. Fluticasone appears to be without adverse effects on growth when used in conventional doses but may have adverse effects when used in higher doses. It is not known at this time whether this growth suppression ultimately affects final adult height.

Inhaled cortisone can also suppress normal adrenal function and cause excessive weight gain; in clinical studies, 0.5 mg of fluticasone per day caused depleted cortisol levels and increased weight gain.[55]

Corticosteriods are also implicated in increased risk for osteoporosis or bone loss, since these drugs hamper absorption of magnesium and calcium, minerals necessary for strong bones.

Theophylline, which is related to chemicals found in coffee and chocolate and stimulates the heart and central nervous system, according to asthma specialist Richard N. Firshein, D.O., "can help a patient through a difficult period but can easily reach toxic levels," and is dangerous to anyone with a liver disorder. Additionally, he reports it has been linked to the onset of learning disorders and nervousness.[56]

Of even more concern today, however, may be studies showing an increased death rate from the use and misuse of the beta-agonist sprays. According to a 1992 report published in *The New England Journal of Medicine*, a pattern of increasing use over time is an important predictor of serious or fatal asthma attacks, as is doubling your monthly use, increasing your usage by one canister a month, or inhaling a total of more than one-and-a-half canisters per month.[57] As to the latest symptom relievers for asthma (the anti-leukotriene, anti-IgE, anti-cytokine, and anti–platelet-activating products), "further research is needed," emphasizes researcher John W. Georgitis, M.D.[58]

# CHAPTER

# 12

# Homeopathic and Physical Therapies

**I**N CHAPTER 11, WE REVIEWED the nutritional and herbal remedies that alleviate symptoms of allergy and sensitivity. In this chapter, we'll focus on the homeopathic and physical therapies that likewise provide quick and often lasting relief from asthma, allergic rhinitis, hives, allergic contact dermatitis, ear infections, headaches, and other symptoms. Some of these therapies are easy enough to do at home. However, as with any medical intervention, it is best to seek the advice of a licensed alternative medicine practitioner before turning to self-treatment.

## Success Story: Homeopathy and Osseous Manipulation Relieve Allergies

### In This Chapter

- Success Story: Homeopathy and Osseous Manipulation Relieve Allergies
- Homeopathic Remedies
- Nasal Irrigation
- Meridian Therapy
- Osseous Manipulation
- Special Therapies for Asthma

When Patricia, a 24-year-old student, came to see chiropractor and homeopath Norman Allen, Ph.D., D.C., of Toronto, Canada, she had been suffering with a long list of symptoms for most of her life, but they had become more severe during the previous 18 months. Among her problems were vertigo, tremors, an inability to relax, abdominal pains after eating, dizziness, flushing, cramps at night that caused her to wake up, cold extremities, an inability to tolerate fats, and, most distressing to her, such severe diarrhea that she was afraid to eat or travel in a car. In fact, the motion of a car made her diarrhea worse. Since she was terrified to put food in her mouth due to her digestive dysfunction, she was seriously underweight and appeared virtually anorexic.

Patricia's history revealed a chronology of allergic reactions exacerbated by antibiotics and chemicals in the environment. At birth, she was immediately intolerant to cow's milk. At the age of 11, she had a severe chemical reaction to the oil-based paint at school, which provoked vomiting, shaking, numbness in her legs, and loss of weight. Soon after, she was advised by her physician to eliminate dairy from her diet, which was a step in the right direction, but not enough to reverse the downward spiral. She became fatigued easily. At 12, she developed ovarian cysts, followed by tinnitis (ear ringing) at 16.

Birth control pills were prescribed to manage her cysts and menstrual cycle, and she took them for the following seven years. During this time, she had bouts of debilitating fever, vomiting, and cramps. At 19, she incurred a series of bladder and kidney infections for which she was given many rounds of antibiotics, including Bactrim and Macrodantin. After that, her chronic diarrhea started, and she became practically housebound. By 23, her nausea had taken on a new ferocity, and she was debilitated by constant flu-like symptoms. A colonoscopy and gastroscopy proved negative. Not surprisingly, since her eating was sparse and digestion fraught with problems, blood tests revealed she was deficient in several nutrients, including vitamin B12 and folic acid.

After an extensive history, Dr. Allen decided upon a three-pronged approach to Patricia's problems. First, he recognized that the combination of her digestive symptoms, chemical sensitivities, and long-term use of antibiotics and birth control pills suggested that she had dysbiosis (an imbalance of intestinal flora) and the probability of serious food allergies. Rather than test for individual sensitivities, he immediately put her on a non-allergenic seven-day rotation diet, in which individual foods were eaten only once a week. In this way, if Patricia did react to any of the foods on her diet, it would be easier to determine which food it was. Also, a rotation diet lessens the chance that a person will develop new allergies to an over-consumed food.

"Diet is a very important part of the general management of allergies," explains Dr. Allen. "It's often difficult to control what we inhale. But one thing we can control is what we eat, which has an effect on our immune system and our body's toxicity."

In Patricia's case, Dr. Allen had her eliminate all toxic foods from her diet and replenish her nutrients with fresh, organic fruits and veg-

For more on **rotation diets**, see Chapter 6: Therapeutic Diets, pp. 158-183. For more on **dysbiosis**, see Chapter 7: Healing Leaky Gut Syndrome, pp. 184-211.

etables, rotated on a weekly basis to avoid developing allergies to them. Since she had trouble digesting fats, Dr. Allen decided to have her bulk with carbohydrates. The ones he found to be least allergenic for her were rice, millet, yams, potatoes, tapioca, arrowroot, and amaranth (non-glutenous grains).

The next step in Dr. Allen's treatment program was to find a homeopathic remedy that specifically fit Patricia's symptoms. One of the reasons homeopathy works so well for allergy patients is that it is an energy treatment and hence has no allergens to which patients may react. Homeopathic prescribing is based on the total symptomatic picture and individuality of the patient. "The key to finding a remedy for Patricia was her flushing, which was so vivid, and a diarrhea made worse from motion," says Dr. Allen. This indicated to him the need for *Ferrum* (an iron).

"Patricia was a very sensitive person so we started the *Ferrum* at a low 6C potency and she gradually worked up to a 30C potency over the next several months. We worked together over a period of 18 months but, after the first visit, she showed some immediate improvement and, after four days, reported an 80% relief from her diarrhea, flushing, and cramping."

As a sign that the *Ferrum* was working, Patricia had a "healing crisis" a week after she first took it, which included burping, nausea, vomiting, cramps, and diarrhea. This almost totally resolved itself about four days later and she continued to improve. She was no longer in constant pain and could continue her studies without fear of sudden diarrhea.

Next, Dr. Allen prescribed the homeopathic remedy *Pulsatilla* 200C, a commonly used remedy for women, which was selected in part because of Patricia's tendency toward weepiness, and *Sulfur* 1M to clear her system of blockages. Later on in the treatment, Patricia added *Veratrum album* (slowly increased from 6C to 200C), which had a strengthening effect on her when alternated with the *Ferrum*. One of the characteristics of a patient who might be able to benefit from *Veratrum* is that of cold extremities, a symptom Patricia had experienced frequently.

The third course of action taken by Dr. Allen was somatic. He used craniosacral therapy to facilitate a release of any structural problems or hidden emotional problems that might impede the healing process. As Dr. Allen gently aligned Patricia's craniosacral system, exerting light pressure to clear it of restrictions, and using the gentle rocking motion inherent to the therapy, Patricia became more and more relaxed. In addition, Patricia found that the therapy had other psychological benefits as well. After the ten-week treatment was over, she had dealt with a deep-seated fear of abandonment (a primal human fear which can be triggered by overwhelming situations).

**Norman Allan, Ph.D., D.C.:** Medical Arts Building, 170 St. George Street #607, Toronto, Ontario, M5R 2M8 Canada: tel: 416-928-9272; fax: 416-955-1741.

Patricia's return to health allowed her take on a stressful professional apprenticeship program and regain her vibrant, energetic personality. She and Dr. Allen are cautiously adding foods back into her diet, still rotating and testing each one for an allergic response. While this stringent diet might seem difficult to some people, Patricia knows what it was like to be practically house-bound and she is grateful for her returned health. "Every once in a while she'll 'cheat,'" says Dr. Allen, "but cheating to her is usually something like having too many buckwheat noodles, a part of her rotation. Occasionally, she'll party and expose herself to something that will cause a reaction. What we learned very quickly is that the reactions aren't any milder, but they're brief and she bounces back to health within a day or so."

# Homeopathic Remedies

Homeopathic medicine, established in Germany in the 18th century, is based on three principles: like cures like (Law of Similars); the more a remedy is diluted, the greater its potency (Law of Infinitesimal Dose); and an illness is specific to the individual (a holistic medical model). Prescribing considers all of an individual's symptoms and signs. According to homeopathy's founder, Dr. Samuel Hahnemann, disease can be permanently and rapidly reversed by using a medicine that is capable of producing (in the human system) the most similar and complete symptoms of the disease in a healthy person. Each homeopathic medicine is "proven" or tested in healthy people and their symptoms recorded. When treating ill patients, a homeopathic practitioner matches the patient's symptoms with a remedy that produced similar symptoms in a healthy person when "proven."

Treating "like with like" works effectively to reverse disease because the homeopathic remedy works on an energetic level (having been diluted to the point that no chemical components remain). Dr. Hahnemann found that the more a substance was diluted and shaken, the higher its potency. Homeopathic remedies are prepared in a series of dilution steps using water and succussing (vigorous shaking). Potency levels are designated with "X" and "C". The "X" means that the homeopathic remedy has been serially diluted on a 1:10 scale (one part substance to nine parts water) and the "C" means the remedy has been diluted on a 1:100 scale (one part substance to 99 parts water). A number value is placed before the scale designator to identify how many dilutions the remedy has undergone. A remedy designated "6X" has undergone six dilutions at one part substance to nine parts water; a remedy that is designated "12X" has undergone 12 dilutions and is stronger than the 6X remedy. Common potencies available over-the-counter are 6X, 12X, 30X, 6C, 12C, and 30C. Lower potencies tend to have a greater effect on the physical plane, while higher potencies affect the mental/emotional plane.

Classical homeopathic remedies are prescribed for a patient based on each person's unique and distinguishing symptoms. This individualized prescription considers not only the physical symptoms but also the mental and emotional states as well. This is vastly different from conventional medicine, which will generally give one medicine to every patient for a specific disease condition. In homeopathy, any number of homeopathic remedies could be prescribed for that condition, but a specific remedy can be identified after reviewing the patient's individual symptoms.

## Building the Totality of Symptoms

The main symptom profile includes physical complaints, the effect of motion and temperature on pain, food cravings, and personality or emotional disposition. In homeopathy, the subjective quality of how a pain "feels" is extremely useful in identifying a remedy. When pursuing homeopathic treatment, pay attention to your pain and try to match it to the following categories:

- Sharp: stabbing, cutting, stitching, piercing, pricking, splinter-like, stinging
- Shooting: radiates from one location to another
- Stiff: constricted or contracted
- Pressing: squeezing, compression, crushing, pinching
- Changeable: wandering in any direction or is hard to locate
- Burning: cold or hot needles
- Lame: dislocated, broken, sprained, or paralytic area
- Other types of pain: throbbing or pulsating, digging, twisting, drawing, pulling

Frequency and duration of symptoms are also important. Do they occur regularly at a particular time or in correlation with the weather? Do they come on strongly and persist for only a short time? Physical signs are also part of the patient profile. The affected areas may be swollen and discolored (red, white, pale, waxy, or bruised), or hot or cold to the touch. Homeopaths also consider what aggravates the condition. It is unusual for many Americans to consider that their emotional disposition factors into their physical ailments, but in homeopathy, these qualities are as important as the location and duration of pain. Homeopaths look for the following emotional patterns: restlessness, irritability, quick to overreact, or cries easily. A strong desire for rest or remaining still, a constant need for motion or activity, desire to be outdoors, or fear of crowds help construct the personality profile.

## Homeopathy for Allergies—Not a "Placebo Effect"

As with many alternative therapies, conventional medicine has been hasty to dismiss the beneficial results of homeopathy as "placebo effect"—that is, that relief was psychosomatically induced, much as people experience symptomatic relief from placebos used in clinical studies. However, recent research has shown that homeopathy is effective—and not because of the patients' belief in the modality.

In one study, 20 steroid-dependent asthma patients were administered a subcutaneous treatment of a commercial homeopathic combination remedy every five to seven days while 20 others received a placebo. The homeopathy-treated group was able to reduce their steroid use by 100%, while the placebo group was not. The researchers concluded that the homeopathic remedy may have an anti-inflammatory effect on the respiratory system.[1] A similar study examining the effects of a combination homeopathic preparation called Traumeel S (from Heel/BHI) on 103 steroid-dependent asthma. All homeopathic-treated patients were able to considerably reduce their medication while experiencing significant improvements in muscle power and sense of well-being. The placebo-treated group enjoyed no such benefits.[2]

Several studies have proven the efficacy of *Galphimia glauca* in treating eye and nasal symptoms (pollinosis) of hay fever.[3] In one, 201 patients with pollinosis were either given *Galphimia glauca* or a placebo. After two weeks, 65% of the homeopathic group experienced significant improvement or cure of eye symptoms and 66% of nasal symptoms cleared. In the placebo group, 44% had relief from eye symptoms and 44% from nasal symptoms. After five weeks, there was a 77% improvement in the homeopathic group for all symptoms compared to only 51% in the placebo group.[4]

Homeopathy has also been shown to be effective in reducing the pain and relapse of ear infections. In a 1997 study, 103 children with acute otitis media were prescribed single homeopathic remedies (including the ones below), while 28 were treated with conventional antibiotics. The homeopathic-treated group experienced pain relief in an average of two days (compared to three days in the antibiotic group). At the end of treatment, 70.7% of the children in the homeopathic group were free from recurrence a year after treatment, with only 56.5% free in the antibiotic group. The maximum number of recurrent infections in the remainder of the homeopathic group was three; the maximum in the antibiotic group was six.[5]

## Common Homeopathic Remedies for Allergies and Allergic Conditions

There are many remedies that can be effective in treating allergic reactions, depending upon the type of allergy, time and location of reaction, affinity for warmth or cold, and emotional state. If a remedy is well suited for your condition, you will experience immediate improvement or, in some cases, a healing crisis (a brief worsening of symptoms followed by improvement). If symptoms persist, however, it indicates an incorrect potency, dosage, or remedy, or perhaps deeper underlying problems. As with all medicinal substances, one should be cautious in self-prescribing homeopathic remedies and seek professional medical advice before beginning a homeopathic course of treatment. The standard recommended dose for each of the remedies below is three tablets of 6C or 30C every four hours until you see improvement. Repeat dosage if symptoms reappear. Be sure to follow the directions on the product labels.

For information about **homeopathy**, contact: Homeopathic Educational Services, 2124B Kittredge Street, Berkeley, CA 94704; tel: 510-649-0294; fax: 510-649-1955; website: www.homeopathic.com. For **referrals to homeopaths in your area**, contact: North American Society of Homeopathy, 1122 East Pike Street #1122, Seattle, WA 98122; tel: 206-720-7000; fax: 206-329-5684; website: www.homeopathy.org.

### For Asthma—

■ *Ammonium carbonicum*: Indicated for severe asthma, accompanied by exhausted breathing, shortness of breath with wheezing, bronchial constriction and congestion, difficulty in expectorating, burning in chest, cough with palpitations, slow labored breathing, bubbling sounds, lung swelling, and slimy sputum with specks of blood. Symptoms worsen around 3 a.m., on cold, cloudy days, in the damp open air, during menstruation. Symptoms improve while eating, lying on abdomen, or in dry weather.

■ *Aralia racemosa*: Indicated for dry cough with first sleep, asthma on lying down at night, tickling in throat or sensation that something is stuck; strong, spasmodic cough, constriction of chest, whistling while breathing; frequent sneezing, hay fever accompanied by excessive water nasal discharge and salty, bitter taste in mouth. Also feel raw burning behind sternum; may become drenched with sweat during sleep. Symptoms worsen between 9 p.m. and 11 p.m., after a nap, or being in a draft. Symptoms improve while lying with head high or sitting up.

■ *Arsenicum album*: Indicated for wheezing cough that may be alternately dry and loose; cough worsens during drinking and while lying on back, accompanied by burning in the chest, darting pain in the upper portion of the right lung, bloody sputum, and scanty, frothy expectoration. Feel very restless and anxious, chilly, need for warm water but only drinks in sips; also can't lie down due to fear of suffocation or death. Symptoms worsen between 11:30 p.m. to 3 a.m., when consuming cold drinks, or in cold air.

■ *Arsenicum iodatum*: Indicated for hay fever–induced asthma; dry, hacking cough with little or difficult expectoration (yellow/green foul-smelling mucus); "air hunger" (difficulty getting deep breath), short of breath, burning heat in the chest. Feel thirsty and chilly. Symptoms worsen in dry, cold weather or when it's windy and foggy, after indoor exertion, eating apples or breathing tobacco smoke. Symptoms improve in the open air.

■ *Cuprum metallicum*: Indicated for spasmodic asthma alternating with vomiting; cough with gurgling sound, feel like suffocating, painful chest constrictions and spasms, loud rattle in chest; breathing worsens while bending backward. Symptoms worsen around 3 a.m., when angry, in hot weather, or when raising arms. Symptoms improve upon consuming cold drinks.

■ *Ipecac*: Indicated for constant constriction in chest; persistent or suffocating cough with every breath that causes nausea, vomiting; may cough until blue in the face; rattle in chest without expectoration; voice may be hoarse. Feel thirstless and chilly. Symptoms worsen in warm or damp weather, with a moist warm wind, after overeating, or lying down. Symptoms improve in open air.

■ *Kali nit*: Indicatied for dry, short, hacking cough in the morning accompanied by chest pain and bloody, sour-smelling sputum, constriction in chest and right lung, severe shortness of breath (can't hold breath long enough to drink), heart palpitations. Feel burning internally but cold externally. Symptoms worse when walking in cold, damp weather, lying with head low, or eating veal. Symptoms improve with gentle motion and drinking sips of water.

■ *Lachesis*: Indicated for dry, fitful coughs, sensation of suffocating while lying down, painful larynx; breathing almost stops when falling asleep; feel like you must take a deep breath. Feel thirsty and cold. Symptoms worsen upon waking, consuming warm drinks, swallowing, going from cold to warm weather. Symptoms improve in open air, upon consuming cold drinks, and when bathing.

■ *Lobelia*: Indicated for asthma attack accompanied by weakness in the stomach and preceded by prickling all over, rattle in chest, difficulty in expectorating, chest constriction causing shortness of breath. Feel sensation of pressure in chest. Symptoms worsen after sleep or smoking. Symptoms improve after rapid walking, in the evening, in warm places, or after eating a little.

■ *Natrum sulphuricum*: Indicated for asthma attacks in damp or cold air; cough with thick green mucus, hold chest while coughing, feel pain in left part of lower chest, need to take a deep long breath. Recommended for children.

■ *Pulsatilla*: Indicated for asthma marked by dry cough at night that loosens up in the morning, thick yellow/green mucus, shortness of breath, pressure on and soreness in chest, and "air hunger." Feel smothered when lying down, thirstless, discouraged, desirous of sympathy, and whiny. Symptoms worsen in warm room or warm air, in the evening, before menstruation and during pregnancy, and after eating rich foods and fats. Symptoms improve in open air, with erect posture, or upon crying.

■ *Sambucus*: Indicated for children that awaken with throat spasm or feeling of suffocation; also mucus obstruction, spasmodic cough, whistling while breathing, difficulty in expectorating, chest pressure accompanied by stomach pressure or nausea. Wake up sweating profusely but feel dry, burning heat while asleep. Not thirsty. Symptoms worsen in dry, cold air, during sleep, after consuming cold drinks or eating fruit, or while head is low. Symptoms improve while sitting up, wrapped up, and in motion.

■ *Spongia tosta*: Indicated for dry, barking, deep cough accompanied by severe dryness in airways, including larynx (which is also painful to touch), wheezing, panting, grabbing throat when swallowing. Symptoms worsen during inhalation and before midnight, in a dry, cold wind, upon being awakened, after raising arms, or by using voice. Symptoms improve when lying with head low, after eating, and after coughing.

■ *Sulphur*: Indicated for difficult and irregular breathing, violent cough with mucus rattling, shortness of breath at night, burning and pressure in chest, pains shoot to back, rapid morning pulse, red/brown spots over chest. Feel thirsty and chilly. Symptoms worsen at night and while standing and bathing. Symptoms improve while sitting up.

## For Allergic Rhinitis/Hay Fever—

■ *Allium cepa*: Indicated for excessive, bitter nasal discharge; red, burning eyes, excessively watery eyes with stinging tears; severe sneezing especially while entering a warm room, cough, hoarseness; headache, burning and sore eyelids/lips/nostrils. Symptoms worsen in a warm room both in the evening and morning (pollination times). Symptoms improve in cool, open air.

■ *Arsenicum album:* Indicated for persistent sneezing, thick watery nasal discharge, dull throbbing headache, tickle on inside of nose, congested nose, burning or bleeding of nose; burning, inflammation of eyes with bitter tears, red, scabby lips; sensitivity to smells and food odors and to light. Feel chilly; have burning thirst for cold drinks, sip drinks. Symptoms worsen after midnight, after exertion, smoking, in wet or cold weather, during weather changes. Symptoms improve with hot food and drink, when wrapped up, with head elevated, sitting up, and sweating.

■ *Arsenicum iodatum:* Indicated for sneezing, nasal irritation with persistent sensation of needing to sneeze, swollen and sore nose aggravated by sneezing, thin, watery irritating discharge, burning in nose and throat. Feel thirsty and chilly. Symptoms worsen in dry, cold weather or in windy, foggy weather. Symptoms improve in open air.

■ *Arum triphyllum*: Indicated for sneezing that worsens at night, persistent sneezing without relief, prickling in nose, dull throbbing headache, sore nostrils, obstructed nasal passage so must breathe through mouth, blood in discharge, constant picking of nose until it bleeds, chapped face and lips; hoarse voice, stinging eyes, asthmatic breathing. Feel thirsty but drinking is painful. Feel drowsy, nervous, and irritable. Symptoms worsen in cold, wet winds, in the evening, while lying down, or while talking.

■ *Arundo*: Indicated for hay fever that begins with itching in nostrils and roof of the mouth that causes sneezing; burning and itching in ear canals, eczema behind ears.

■ *Dulcamara*: Indicated for constant sneezing; swollen watery eyes, especially in open air, stuffy nose, thick yellow mucus; diarrhea accompanies hay fever in the summer, nose aches, frequent urination. Feel thirsty and chilly. Symptoms worsen in sudden temperature changes, in autumn, in cold wet places, and before storms. Symptoms improve in warm heat.

■ *Euphrasia*: Indicated for hay fever concentrated in eyes, with watery, yellow discharge, swollen lids, mucus on cornea, sore eyes with pressure; frequent sneezing with bland (not bitter) nasal discharge; dry hard cough. Symptoms worsen in sunlight and wind, in a warm room, during the evening, and while lying down. Symptoms improve in open air, by blinking, and by wiping the eyes.

■ *Gelsemium*: Indicated for summer hay fever accompanied by sneezing in the morning, violent sneezing, thin watery discharge; dull headache and fever, heavy, drooping eyelids, double vision; stuffy nose with very watery, streaming discharge, red, sore edges of nostrils, swallowing is painful in the ears, hot face but cold feet and hands, chills up and down the spine. Feel thirstless. Symptoms worsen in warm, humid, foggy weather (spring and summer), before thunderstorms, and after hearing bad news. Symptoms improve after profuse urination, sweating, bending forward, or being in the open air.

■ *Galphimia glauca*: Indicated for excessive mucus secretions from nose and eyes, swelling of the eyelids, sneezing; shooting pains in the stomach. Feel hypersensitive to weather changes. Also recommended for skin allergies (eczema, hives).

■ *Natrum muriaticum*: Indicated for hay fever with watery or discharge like raw egg whites, loss of smell and taste, difficulty breathing, stuffy nose that alternates between streaming with discharge and congestion, sneezing in the early morning, sore nose, burning and watery eyes with swollen eyelids, bursting headaches. Feel thirsty and chilly. Symptoms worsen between 9 a.m. and 11 a.m., in the sun and heat, after experiencing an upsetting situation. Symptoms improve in open air, after sweating, upon resting, deep breathing, and cool bathing.

■ *Nux vomica*: Indicated for runny nose triggered in daytime and outdoors, prolonged violent sneezing, stuffy nose at night, nose feels congested but discharge streams out of one nostril, crawling sensation in the nostrils; eye/nose/face irritation, itching in throat, itching in middle ear, sniffles, scratchy sensation in the throat in early stages. Can't tolerate sunlight (photophobia), especially in morning. Symptoms worsen in the early morning, in cold open air or drafts, after consuming coffee and other stimulants, eating rich foods, being sedentary, with overwork, and fatigue. Symptoms improve indoors, in the evening, in warmth, and after consuming hot drinks.

■ *Psorinum*: Indicated for stinging in right nostril followed by excessive sneezing, burning followed by increased discharged that relieves burning, stopped-up nose, persistent postnasal drip, red eyelids, bitter tears. Feel sensitive to drafts; chilly, anxious; feel hungry or well before attack; sweat profusely. Symptoms worsen in cold air or after bathing, during weather changes, in the winter. Symptoms improve in the heat, while lying with head low, after washing, and after sweating.

■ *Sabadilla*: Indicated for violent sneezing attack, excessive itching in the nose, much water discharge from nose and eyes that worsen when smelling flowers; tearing in open air and with bright lights, severe frontal headache, muffled cough, tickling in nose that spreads, itching of the palate, dry mouth but no thirst. Crave hot things; feel chilly. Symptoms worsen in open air, cold air, or with cold drinks. Symptoms improve with warmth and warm drinks.

### For Allergic Contact Dermatitis—

■ *Anacardium*: Indicated for very itchy rash that feels better in hot water/bath, blistering eruptions, yellow discharges oozing from blisters, crusting. Itching worsens after scratching.

■ *Croton tiglium*: Indicated for excessive itching, dry/hard/tight skin, rash mostly occurring on the face and genitals, painful scratching, poison ivy rash accompanied by explosive diarrhea. Symptoms worsen upon washing.

■ *Rhus toxicodendron*: Indicated for poison ivy rashes with water-filled blisters and extreme itching. Feel very restless; experience joint stiffness. Symptoms worsen with cold baths or showers, scratching, at night, or at rest. Symptoms improve with hot baths or showers.

### For Hives—

■ *Apis*: Indicated for hives due to insect stings; large, swollen, red hives that sting, burn, and hurt, excessive itching at night; swollen, puffy face and eyelids. Symptoms worsen with heat and hot water. Symptoms improve with cold water.

■ *Rhus toxicodendron*: Indicated for hives accompanied by joint stiffness, fever, and chills; intense itching; hot, burning pain. Symptoms worsen in cold damp weather or if you become chilled when hot and sweaty, with overwork. Symptoms improve in heat and warmth, in dry weather.

■ *Urtica urens*: Indicated for hives from eating shellfish or touching stinging nettles, prickly heat sensation, itching, burning, stinging rashes that are raised and red. Symptoms worsen in cool, wet air and after cold bathing. Symptoms improve in warmth.

### For Ear Infections—

■ *Aconite*: Indicated for very painful ear infections with high fever; bright red ears, very sensitive to noise. Symptoms worsen with cold, dry weather, upon pressure or touch, during teething, when exposed to noise or light. Symptoms improve with rest. Use within 24 hours of onset.

■ *Belladonna*: Indicated for sudden-onset, right-sided ear infections accompanied by high fever and red face, throbbing headache; light and noise sensitivity, hot, dry skin and mouth, glassy eyes. Symptoms worsen in drafts, to touch, and in motion. Symptoms improve with bed rest in dark, quiet room.

■ *Chamomilla*: Indicated for ear infection occurring during teething, pain in hot ears, hypersensitivity to pain and music, one cheek may be red-hot and the other pale; hearing may be lost during infection, green diarrhea during teething. Child is whiny, irritable, wants to be carried. Symptoms worsen during teething, in cold wind, at night, and around 9 p.m.

■ *Hepar sulphuris*: Indicated for painful infection with thick pus behind eardrum, sour-smelling discharge, darting pain in ears, perforation of eardrum. Child wakes up at night in pain, feels irritable. Symptoms worsen in drafts and wind. Symptoms improve in heat.

■ *Mercurius*: Indicated for sharp, stinging pains accompanied by increased drooling, bad breath, and foul-smelling sweat; very sensitive to heat and cold, yellow/green or bloody discharge, ear pain worse when swallowing or blowing your nose; pain in teeth and gums, white coating on tongue. Symptoms worsen at night, in damp cold, in drafts, or while sweating. Symptoms improve in mild temperature and at rest.

■ *Pulsatilla*: Indicated for congested ears that ache more at night, thick yellow/green discharge from nose, ears, and lungs, red and swollen ears. Feel no thirst; child is whiny and clingy. Symptoms worsen in warmth and stuffy rooms, if feet get wet, after eating rich foods. Symptoms improve if walking in open air.

■ *Silica*: Indicated for chronic ear infections; eardrum may rupture and be full of pus; swollen lymph nodes; irritating, thin, foul-smelling discharge, blocked ears better when yawning or swallowing; sensitive to noise, painful inflammation of mastoid bone behind ear, low energy. Symptoms worsen in cold, damp climates and to touch. Symptoms improve in warmth and heat.

For **individual and combination homeopathic remedies,** contact: Apex Energetics, 1701 East Edinger Avenue, Suite A-4, Santa Ana, CA 92705; tel: 800-736-4381. BioEnergetics, Inc., P.O. Box 127, Sandy, OR 97055; tel: 800-334-4043 or 503-668-7478. Biomed Comm, Inc., 2 Nickerson Street, Suite 102, Seattle, WA 98109; tel: 888-637-3516 or 206-284-3433. Boiron, 6 Campus Blvd., Building A, Newtown Square, PA 19073; tel: 800-264-7661 or 610-325-7464. Dolisos, 3014 Rigel Avenue, Las Vegas, NV 89102; tel: 702-871-7153; website: www.dolisos.com. Heel/BHI, Inc., 1160 Cochiti Road S.E., Albuquerque, NM 87123-3376; tel: 800-621-7644 or 505-293-3843; website: www.heelbhi.com. Liddell Laboratories, 1036 Country Club Drive, Moraga, CA 94556; tel: 800-460-7733 or 925-377-3000. P & S Labs, 210 West 131st Street, Los Angeles, CA 90061; tel: 800-624-9659.

**Commercial Combinations—**There are several manufacturers that offer combinations of homeopathic remedies to relieve the various symptoms that accompany allergies. You can find these combination medicines at health food stores and some pharmacies, or buy them directly from the manufacturer. A homeopathic nasal spray, containing *Luffa operculata*, *Galphimia glauca*, histamine, and sulfur (made by Heel/BHI), has been shown to be as effective and tolerated as well as cromolyn sodium, which is conventionally used to relieve nasal symptoms of hay fever.[6] Carefully read the symptom list and efficacy claims of these combinations to make sure they'll work with your unique condition.

# Nasal Irrigation

Nasal irrigation can relieve the nasal congestion and swelling common in allergic rhinitis and sinusitis. It washes debris from the nose and shrinks swollen mucous membranes. Irrigation with a simple saline solution has been found to immediately reduce histamine levels; these levels were maintained for at least 30 minutes after treatment in clinical trials on allergic rhinitis patients.[7] Follow the directions below to perform your own nasal irrigation; this protocol was developed by Barbara E. Wilder, R.N., M.S.N., C.P.N.P.[8] You can repeat this process two or three times a day. Don't worry if you feel a mild burning sensation when you first start nasal irrigations—it will diminish after a few days. If you're using nasally administered medications, irrigate before using inhalers.

■ Wash a one-quart glass jar thoroughly and fill it with one quart of purified water. Add 2-3 heaping tablespoons of pickling/canning salt (not table salt) and one teaspoon of baking soda (pure bicarbonate). Stir before each use; cap and store at room temperature. For children, use 1½ teaspoons of salt and gradually increase to 2-3 teaspoons so as not to irritate their nasal passages. The solution keeps for one week.

■ Pour some of the solution into a clean bowl. You may warm it slightly in the microwave but do not heat until too hot.

■ Using a bulb ear syringe, large medical syringe (30 cc), or a Water Pik device, squirt solution into each nostril, making sure that you aim toward the back of the head not the top of the head. It's best to stand over a sink or even in the shower. Some of the salt-water solution may get into your mouth; spit it out. Swallowing a little of the solution is not harmful.

## Magnatherm for Respiratory Allergies

**M**agnatherm is a form of unassisted short-wave diathermy (electrically induced heating of tissues) that may be used over the sinuses or lungs to relieve congestion. Treatments, which last for 10-15 minutes, help open swollen passages and create drainage in these areas. Many physical therapists, allopaths, chiropractors, and naturopathic physicians have the equipment to perform magnatherm.

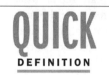

## QUICK
### DEFINITION

**Acupuncture meridians** are specific pathways in the human body for the flow of life force or subtle energy, known as *qi* (pronounced CHEE). In most cases, these energy pathways run up and down both sides of the body, and correspond to individual organs or organ systems, designated as Lung, Small Intestine, Heart, and others. There are 12 principal meridians and eight secondary channels. Numerous points of heightened energy, or *qi*, exist on the body's surface along the meridians and are called acupoints. There are more than 1,000 acupoints, each of which is potentially a place for acupuncture treatment.

■ For children, you can used a nasal steroid container or other spray bottle and squirt the solution repeatedly into each nostril. Let the child sit or stand up during the irrigation—don't force them to lie down.

### Nasal Hyperthermia (Vapor Inhalation)

Inhalation of heated water vapor is a folk remedy for allergic rhinitis that has been proven to be clinically effective in reducing congestion and histamine levels for up to four hours following treatment. Vaporizers can heat water to various degrees; between 41° C and 43° C is the optimal temperature for vapor therapy. In one study, 30 rhinitis patients underwent three hyperthermic treatments in three weeks, in which they spent 20 minutes inhaling vapor from water heated to 43° C; 20 minutes inhaling vapor from water heated to 41° C, and nasal irrigation. All patients experienced symptom relief from the vapor systems but not from the nasal irrigation; 41° C was the more comfortable temperature.[9]

# Meridian Therapy

Meridian therapies, such as acupuncture or acupressure, work to balance the flow of *qi* (vital life energy) through energy meridians (SEE QUICK DEFINITION). These meridians run throughout the body and are associated with different organs—if there is a block in the energy meridian, it will be expressed as health problems in the organs associated with the blocked meridian. Blocked *qi* can be released by applying pressure to the specific points along the energy meridians. Acupuncture uses needles, while acupressure (such as shiatsu and *Jin Shin Do*) uses rubbing, kneading, or other types of pressure from the fingers and hands. Both types of stimulation can be effective in alleviating the symptoms of allergy and sensitivity. Research has shown that long-term use of acupuncture can prevent symptoms from recurring in many individuals.

## Acupuncture

Acupuncture is an integrated healing system developed by the Chinese over 5,000 years ago. The treatment is administered by an acupuncturist using hair-thin, stainless-steel needles, generally presterilized and disposable; these are lightly inserted into the skin at any of more than 1,000 locations on the body's surface, known as acupoints. Acupoints are places where *qi* can be accessed by acupuncturists to reduce, enhance, or redirect its flow. These acupoints exist on meridians, the body's specific pathways for the flow of energy. In most cases, these energy pathways relate to individual organs or organ systems, designated as Lung, Small Intestine, Heart, and others. Acupuncture is employed for a wide variety of conditions, including pain relief, arthritis, migraines, allergy, and asthma.

Conventional medicine has been slow to accept that this millennia-old therapy is effective, primarily because, until recently, there has been a lack of well-designed clinical studies testing acupuncture.

## How Acupuncture Works for Pain Control

Scientists have attempted for the past several years to understand how acupuncture relieves pain and inflammation. They now believe that acupuncture needles trigger the nervous system and procure the release of pain-killing and anti-inflammatory chemicals in the body.[10] Currently, this is how acupuncture is believed to affect human physiology:

- The acupuncture needle stimulates a sensory nerve in a muscle.
- This stimulation prompts electrical impulses to travel along the spinal cord nerve.
- This nerve signals other nerve cells to release endorphins, naturally produced chemicals that dull pain (endorphins are among the pain-killing opioids released during an allergic addiction reaction).
- Meanwhile, the brain releases neurotransmitters (brain chemicals) to block the pain pathways.
- Then the pituitary gland delivers the endorphins and various anti-inflammatory chemicals into the brain tissue and bloodstream, leading to a cessation of pain.

For more on the **allergic addiction syndrome**, see Chapter 6: Therapeutic Diets, pp. 158-183.

However, in the past decade, dozens of placebo-controlled studies have proven the efficacy of acupuncture in immediately relieving symptoms of asthma, allergic rhinitis, hives, arthritis, even chemical sensitivity, among other disorders. In fact, regular courses of acupuncture have shown to be long-term preventatives against allergy flare-ups. In one study, acupuncture was significantly more effective than conventional immunotherapy in preventing relapses of symptoms in 143 patients with IgE-mediated allergies (asthma, allergic rhinitis, and hives).[11]

**Asthma**–Several studies show that acupuncture is a powerful tool in relieving asthma symptoms, both for the short and long term. In one study, 17 patients with a long-standing history of asthma were treated with acupuncture. After ten weeks of acupuncture therapy, more than 70% of the patients reported a significant improvement in their asthma symptoms, which continued for six months after starting treatment.[12] In another study, 94 patients with asthma who were treated with acupuncture experienced a significant reduction in symptoms compare to 49 patients who served as controls. The researchers examined both sets of subjects and found that acupuncture reduced bronchial hyper-reactivity, normalized blood chemicals (acetylcholine), promoted the function of cell beta-adrenergic receptors (like beta-agonists), and elevated concentrations of T lymphocytes and other important immune cells.[13] Another study concluded that delayed and immediate allergic asthma attacks could be inhibited by acupuncture, due to acupuncture's effect in significantly lowering secretory IgA and IgE production.[14]

**Allergic Rhinitis**–Acupuncture has been shown to be particularly effective in reducing rhinitis symptoms and even desensitizing patients to allergen exposure. In a 1998 study, 24 allergic rhinitis patients, were treated with either real acupuncture (using rhinitis-specific acupoints) or placebo acupuncture (nonspecific points) for nine treatments. For two months following treatment, the subjects recorded their symptoms. The real acupuncture group experienced a significant reduction in allergy symptoms compared to the placebo group.[15]

In another study, 102 patients with allergic rhinitis were treated with acupuncture needles containing allergen extracts for two sessions. One the third session, the patients were exposed to the allergen. Allergic reactions were significantly reduced compared to pre-treatment levels. The researchers followed these patients for two years, at which time it was determined that 72.2% of the patients no longer reacted to the test allergens, while 23.6% had improved significantly. This outcome was better than that of the control group.[16]

**Hives**–While controlled scientific research is lacking, acupuncture has been clinically observed to relieve the symptoms and prevent relapses of urticaria (hives). According to a 1998 report in the *Archives of*

*Dermatology*, the most effective acupoints are Large Intestine 11 (LI 11), Spleen 10 (SP 10), and Spleen 6 (SP 6).[17]

**Chemical Sensitivity**—Symptoms of chemical sensitivity and environmental illness may also be effectively reduced with acupuncture. In one 1995 study, 20 patients with symptoms (mostly skin reactions) of environmental illness (multiple chemical sensitivity) were treated with acupuncture. The researchers found that cortisol levels increased in all patients as a result of the acupuncture treatments, resulting in a significant decrease in symptoms.[18]

## Acupressure
Scientists have mainly studied the effects of acupuncture on allergy and sensitivity symptoms, but some experts claim acupressure relieves the pain, inflammation, and discomfort of these symptoms as well. The acupuncture and acupressure acupoints for each condition are the

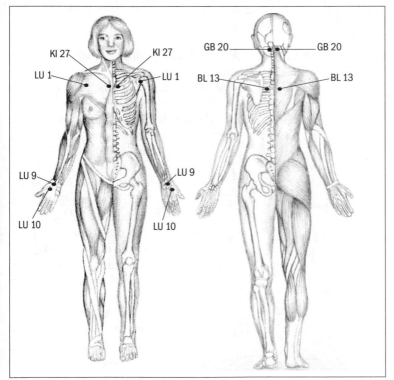

**Acupressure points helpful for allergy and asthma.**

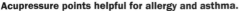

same. The major difference, obviously, is the method of stimulating the *qi*—through hand and finger pressure as opposed to needles. Acupressure techniques are excellent therapies for self-administered symptom control. However, for best results, seek the care of learned practitioners of either shiatsu or *Jin Shin Do*, two forms of acupressure.

*Shiatsu* means "finger pressure" in Japanese and was originally developed from ancient Chinese acupressure techniques. Shiatsu uses a sequence of firm, rhythmic pressure applied to specific points for 3-10 seconds and, like acupuncture, is designed to awaken, calm, and harmonize the meridians. Shiatsu affects not only the acupressure point but the entire mind and body. *Jin Shin Do* is another Japanese bodywork technique based on the original *Jin Shin Jyutu* founded by Jiro Murai. Master Murai based his system on moving the *qi* through the meridians by using certain combinations of acupressure points in a special sequence. Pressure is held for a minute or more until the practitioner can feel the flow of blood and *qi* through the point. Opening the releasing sequences is important to move the *qi* in the proper directions.

For **acupressure techniques and referrals**, contact: American Oriental Bodywork Association, 6801 Jericho Turnpike, Syosset, NY 11791; tel: 516-364-5533.

## Acupressure for Asthma Relief—

Sitting up in a comfortable position, follow these simple steps.

■ Firmly press acupoint Bladder 13 (BL 13, between the tip of the shoulder blade and spine) on your left side with your right fingers. Take five deep breathes as you press on these points. Then do the same on your right-side acupoint BL 13.

■ Then, make a fist with both hands, thumbs extended. Use your thumbs to firmly press the Kidney 27 (KI 27) acupoints on both sides of your chest. Exert pressure for five deep breaths.

■ Again make a fist with both hands, thumbs extended and pointing up. Use your thumbs to firmly press the Lung 1 (LU 1) acupoints on

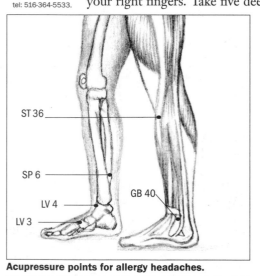

**Acupressure points for allergy headaches.**

both sides of your chest (you'll know you've found LU 1 when you find a knot or sensitive spot on the muscles that run horizontally below your collarbone). Hang your head forward toward your chest and relax while you hold pressure on these points for two minutes, breathing deeply.

■ Now find acupoints Lung 9 (LU 9) and Lung 10 (LU 10) on your left hand. First press LU 9 with your right thumb for a few breaths, then move to LU 10 for a few more breaths. Hold both points with your right thumb and index finger, lightly rubbing them for about a minute. Then switch hands.

### Acupressure for Allergic Rhinitis Relief—

■ For sinus headaches and other hay fever pain symptoms, try this point. Hold your left hand palm down, with fingers straight, and with your right hand apply pressure with our thumb to acupoint Large Intestine 4 (LI 4), which is in the middle of the fleshy part of your hand between the thumb and index finger. Hold for one minute and then switch hands. This is also effective for ear infections, arthritis pain, and headaches. Pregnant women should not use this point because it may stimulate uterine contractions.

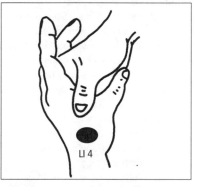

■ For stuffy nose and sinus headaches, place your index or middle fingers on each side of your nostril at acupoint Large Intestine 20 (LI 20, in the groove next to the nostril). Press on this point, putting pressure in an upward direction, building pressure gradually for one minute.

### Allergy/Sensitivity Headache Relief—These are the most common self-acupressure techniques for allergy headaches.

■ Follow the directions above for acupoint LI 4 for quick headache relief.

■ Press Gallbladder 20 (GB 20) for two minutes, building up pressure then releasing gradually. Afterwards, feel for tender spots within an inch of this point and massage them with circular motions.

■ For maximum relief from migraine headaches, apply pressure to Stomach 36 (ST 36), Spleen 6 (SP 6), Liver 3 (LV 3), Liver 4 (LV 4), and Gallbladder 40 (GB 40).

## Success Story: Acupressure Relieves an Allergy Headache

Chris, a traveling salesman in his early forties, had such uncomfortable allergy headaches that he was forced to quit working and go on disability for two years. His condition had progressed to the point where there were few things he could eat or drink, and his life was becoming limited. A friend sent him to see bodyworker Janiece Piper, M.S.W., C.A.M.T.

After giving Chris a 90-minute, full-body acupressure treatment, she taught him specific acupuncture points that he could stimulate on his own to help detoxify his system and relieve pain. These included Gall Bladder 20 (GB 20) on the back of his skull, Large Intestine 4 (LI 4), and Liver 3 (LV 3). Chris was highly motivated, and since Piper's treatment had brought him relief, he faithfully practiced self-acupressure four to fives times a day. Within two weeks of self-acupressure, plus four complete treatment sessions with Piper, Chris felt 80% better—good enough to return to work. Once back out on the road, he continued to stimulate the acupressure points and, within two months, his headaches disappeared entirely.

# Osseous Manipulation

Osseous manipulation is the repositioning of bones, including the bones of the spinal column, cranium, and other moveable joints. Chiropractors as well as naturopathic or qualified osteopathic physicians are trained and licensed to practice this type of therapy. Chiropractic is concerned with the relationship of the spinal column and the muscoskeletal structures of the body to the nervous system. The nervous system holds the key to the body's incredible potential to heal itself, because it controls the functions of all other systems of the body. The spinal column acts as a "switchboard" for the nervous system—when there is interference caused by slight misalignments of the spine (called subluxations), the transmission of the nervous system can be altered, like an electrical wire that has been impinged. This not only causes localized pain in the spine but can interfere with neurological information being transmitted to the major organs and cause dysfunction or disease. By adjusting the spine to remove subluxations, normal nerve function can be restored. Manipulation can help allergy and sensitivity patients with arthritis or symptomatic headaches and other muscle and joint inflammation.

**Craniosacral Therapy—**Another form of osseous manipulation is craniosacral therapy, a light touch alignment that corrects imbalances found among the breathing apparatus, the sacrum (base of the backbone attached to the pelvis), and the bones of the skull (cranium).

Contrary to common belief, the bones of the skull are not rigid and static, but move to accommodate pressure exerted by cerebrospinal fluid, and then return to their original position when the fluid is reabsorbed into the bloodstream. This cycle occurs from six to ten times per minute; however, stress, injury or dysfunction in other parts of the body can interfere with this movement, causing both physiological and psychological effects.

For more on **chiropractic**, contact: American Chiropractic Association, 1701 Clarendon Blvd., Arlington, VA 22209; tel: 703-276-8800; website: www.acatoday.com.

# Special Therapies for Asthma

Not being able to breathe normally may be the most frightening symptom of any allergy. Here are two physical therapies—one that must be administered by a trained practitioner, the other you can learn for yourself—that help alleviate the respiratory difficulties of reactive airway disease and asthma.

## Infraspinatus Respiratory Response (I.R.R.) Therapy

The Infraspinatus Respiratory Response (I.R.R.), sometimes also called the Infrascapula Respiratory Reflex, is a neuromuscular response that has a direct connection to the sympathetic branch of the autonomic nervous system (SEE QUICK DEFINITION). A nerve reflex prompts bronchial spasm, making the bronchioles constrict and produce phlegm, causing an asthma attack. The I.R.R. is also implicated in the onset of pneumonia and bronchitis. Manipulating this muscular response can relieve, even reverse, asthma symptoms, among other respiratory ailments, according to Harry H. Philibert, M.D., of Metairie, Louisiana.

Dr. Philibert has helped more than 5,000 patients experience immediate remission from respiratory disorders using a special protocol that treats the I.R.R. He developed this therapy after he discovered that palpating (SEE QUICK DEFINITION) the infraspinatus muscle caused pain in patients with asthma and other respiratory diseases but not in others. Recognizing a dysfunction in the neuromuscular reflex, Dr. Philibert developed a type of neural therapy whereby he injects the muscle with lidocaine (an anesthetic).

## QUICK DEFINITION

The **autonomic nervous system (ANS)** can be likened to your body's automatic pilot. It keeps you alive through breathing, heart rate, and digestion, without your being aware of it or participating in its activities. The ANS has two divisions: the sympathetic nervous system, which expends body energy, is associated with arousal and stress—it prepares us physically when we perceive a threat or challenge by increasing our heart rate, blood pressure, and muscle tension; the parasympathetic nervous system, which conserves body energy, slows heart rate and increases intestinal and most gland activity.

**Palpation** is a physical examination using the pressure of the hand or fingers on the surface of the body to determine the size, shape, consistency, and placement of the internal parts of the body.

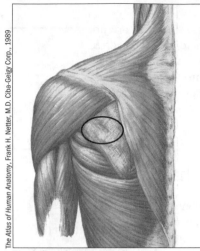

The Atlas of Human Anatomy, Frank H. Netter, M.D. Ciba-Geigy Corp., 1989

**The infraspinatus muscle.**

Dr. Philibert has taught his **I.R.R. technique** to approximately 3,000 doctors and offers periodic seminars. For more information, contact: Harry H. Philibert, M.D., 213 Live Oak, Metairie, LA 70005; tel: 504-837-2727.

This simple technique has demonstrated consistent results with medication-depended chronic asthmatics. While chronic asthma takes at least a few treatments to respond, there is usually an immediate reversal of the acute symptoms. Interestingly, the pain in the muscle also disappears.

During the I.R.R. treatment, the patient lies prone with arms hanging over the sides of the exam table; a cushion can be placed under the chest. The infraspinatus muscle is palpated and, if pain is present, the muscle is injected with 0.5% lidocaine hydrochloride solution sometimes diluted with 1 cc of a steroid called celestone. A few minutes after administering the lidocaine, the practitioner palpates the muscle again and repeats lidocaine injections if pain persists. This procedure is repeated until the patient is free of pain. Typically, each scapula is injected two or three times in a session until all tenderness is gone. Patients with a chronic disease such as asthma are seen every two weeks until the respiratory symptoms and muscular pain subside. Some individuals with an acute problem, such as reactive airway disease, require only a single session or one follow-up.

As part of the treatment, Dr. Philibert uses an oximeter to measure the patients' ability to breathe to capacity. He reports that one patient with moderate asthma had an oximeter reading of 94, indicating the percent of normal breathing and oxygen intake. After lidocaine injection, the patient reached a reading of 99% in less than two minutes. In other cases, he reports, the results are even more dramatic, with the numbers rising from the severely debilitated range to the normal range during a single treatment. Some chronically ill patients with readings in the 60s and 70s develop normal range readings in the high 90s by the end of one session and maintain that level by the end of several treatments. Steroid-dependent asthmatics who have suffered for decades have experienced remission of their symptoms, sometimes for months or years at a time, after a few treatments. Dr. Philibert reports that in a study of 25 asthmatics over a six-month period, all but one reported feeling better after I.R.R. treatment.

# I.R.R. Treatment Points

D r. Philibert's I.R.R. treatment protocol correlates roughly to the acupuncture point Small Intestine 11 (SI 11). This acupoint is known as "Celestial Gathering" in traditional Chinese medicine, because this is the gathering point of *qi* in the body. The suggested pressure point on the chest is nearly parallel (front to back) to SI 11 and corresponds to Lung 1 (LU 1). Called "Central Treasure," it is the intersection of the lung and spleen meridians and is the first point where *qi*—stored in the spleen—circulates in the body. Both points are likely to be painful or sensitive to touch for people with respiratory distress.

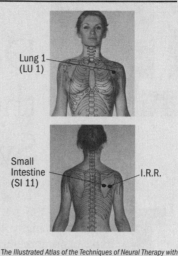

Lung 1 (LU 1)

Small Intestine (SI 11)

I.R.R.

The Illustrated Atlas of the Techniques of Neural Therapy with Local Anesthetics Karl F. Haug Publishers, FDR

## Buteyko Method

The Buteyko Breathing Reconditioning Technique can help asthmatics breathe normally again. Designed by Russian-born scientist Konstantin Pavlovich Buteyko, Ph.D., the technique consists of easy-to-learn shallow breathing exercises, usually taught in a 6-14 day program. Butekyo's theory is that asthmatics tend to hyperventilate, lowering their carbon dioxide levels, which in turn causes blood vessels to spasm, depriving the tissues of oxygen. In moderate amounts, carbon dioxide is a smooth muscle dilator.

Most conventional breathing techniques for asthma work on expanding the lung's capacity to inhale and to thereby take in larger and deeper breaths. Yet, despite a seeming contradiction of clinical thinking, the Buteyko method has been validated in research trials. In one study of 35 asthma sufferers who attended a workshop on the technique in Australia, 27 reported a decrease in symptoms after 4½ months; seven were able to overcome all attacks, 15 to overcome most; 12 totally reduced their use of bronchodilators; 14 reduced their steroid use. Twenty-three of the 35 stated that the technique was superior to conventional medicine's asthma treatment.[19]

For more about the **Buteyko Breathing Reconditioning Technique**, contact: Buteyko Asthma Management, P.O. Box 1458, Hastings, New Zealand 4215; tel: 646-878-0101; fax: 646-878-0103; website: www.buteyko.co.nz. For **practitioner referrals and workshops in the United States**, contact: Rosalba Courtney, D.O., N.D., C.A., Alive & Well Institute of Conscious Bodywork, 100 Shaw Drive, San Anselmo, CA 94960; tel: 415-258-0402 or 888-259-5961; fax: 415-258-0635.

# Desensitizing the Immune System

**T**HE PATH TO ALLERGY FREEDOM is one of many steps. Reducing your exposure to allergens and toxins, implementing therapeutic diets, and restoring barrier functions are major leaps toward health. Nevertheless, you may still be sensitized to allergens despite rigorous application of these therapies. Many allergy and sensitivity patients will find that they require desensitization treatments to experience complete and possibly permanent remission of their symptoms.

Desensitization is accomplished by the conventional allergist by convincing the immune system to quit attacking the offending substance (immunotherapy). This happens by administration of a progressively higher dose of the antigen via injections or sublingual drops, until the patient stops reacting. Unfortunately, this system has about a 40% rate of non-responders to the treatment. The treatment is costly, may have to be continued for three to five years, and results in approximately 20 deaths each year in the United States.

Some alternative forms of desensitization, such as Nambudripad's Allergy Elimination Technique (NAET) and Natural Elimination of Allergy Therapy (NEAT), convince the brain instead of the immune system to stop attacking the offending substances. This is accomplished on an energetic level by balancing the energy of the system while the

## In This Chapter

- Immunotherapy
- Serial Endpoint Titration (SET)
- Enzyme-Potentiated Desensitization (EPD)
- Homeopathic Antigens
- Autoimmune Urine Therapy (AIU)
- Nambudripad's Allergy Elimination Technique (NAET)
- Natural Elimination of Allergy Therapy (NEAT)

allergens are disturbing the electromagnetic circuit of the body.

Other alternative therapies, such as homeopathic antigens and autoimmune urine therapy, are based upon homeopathy's (SEE QUICK DEFINITION) main principle of "like cures like," meaning that a substance that causes particular symptoms in large doses can cure those symptoms when given in small doses. In the treatment of allergies, minute levels of the suspected allergy-provoking substance are given to bolster the body's tolerance of the allergen. When treating allergy and sensitivity, the body's immune response can be modulated through therapies drawing upon these homeopathic principles.

# QUICK
## DEFINITION

**Homeopathy** was founded in the early 1800s by German physician Samuel Hahnemann. Today, an estimated 500 million people worldwide receive homeopathic treatment; in Britain, homeopathy enjoys royal patronage. Homeopathy is now practiced according to two differing concepts. In classical homeopathy, only one single-component remedy is prescribed at a time, in a potency specifically adjusted to the patient; the physician waits to see the results before prescribing anything further. In complex homeopathy, typified by *Hepar compositum*, a prescription involves multiple substances given at the same time, usually in low potencies.

# Immunotherapy

Immunotherapy, or allergy shots, requires that patients receive injections containing extracts (minute amounts) of the allergy-inducing substance. The shots may be given as often as daily in the beginning of the program, decreasing to once or twice a month. With each shot, the allergen is administered in progressively stronger doses until reaching the "maintenance level," the point at which the allergen is "neutralized"—that is, it no longer provokes an allergic reaction. It can take between one and five years to reach this level. In some cases, sublingual drops of allergen extracts are used instead of subdermal injections.

Exactly how immunotherapy desensitizes an individual is presently unknown. It's theorized that immunotherapy somehow reorients the profile of T cells that trigger allergic reactions. Supporting this claim are reports that conventional immunotherapy diminishes the activity of eosinophils upon allergen challenge and reduces the amount of histamine released from mast cells and basophils. Immunoglobulin E production is also decreased following allergy shots.[1] Research has also shown that immunotherapy improves the integrity of nasal mucosa, reduces nasal inflammation, and reduces mast cell accumulation in nasal mucosa.[2]

## How Effective is Immunotherapy?

Clinical studies have found that immunotherapy is most effective for long-term relief from allergic rhinitis, particularly cases sparked by pol-

# Acupoints in Immunotherapy

Research has proven the efficacy of acupuncture in reducing and even preventing symptoms of allergy and sensitivity. A 1991 study also found that administering allergy shots in acupoints is effective in desensitizing allergy patients. In this study, conducted in China, researchers injected two courses of allergen extracts in acupoints on the heads of 102 patients with allergic rhinitis. After two years, 72.2% (74) of the treated patients were found to be mostly free of allergy symptoms, while 23.6% (24) experienced significant improvements.[6]

lens, dust mites, cockroaches, and other biological pollutants. In a 1997 report published in the *Journal of Allergy and Clinical Immunology*, researchers tested the effects of conventional immunotherapy on 20 hay fever patients who were allergic to ragweed pollen. All of these subjects had undergone immunotherapy with ragweed extract for a minimum of three years with good results. Half of the group was then randomly selected to receive placebo injections while the rest continued getting allergy shots. After one year, the researchers examined the subjects for biochemical markers (histamine and antibody levels) of ragweed allergy. They also reviewed the subjects' symptom diaries. Neither group experienced a relapse of allergy symptoms during pollen season, although the placebo group did show increased levels of inflammatory mediators.[3]

Another study, conducted at the Imperial College School of Medicine at the National Heart and Lung Institute in London, England, showed that immunotherapy has long-term, perhaps permanent, beneficial effects. This randomized, double-blind trial tested 32 hay fever patients with allergies to grass pollen. Each of the subjects had undergone at least three years of immunotherapy with favorable results. The researchers then randomly assigned the subjects into two groups—those who continued receiving allergy shots and those who received placebo shots; 15 untreated hay fever subjects served as controls. During three years of follow-up, the researchers found no significant differences in symptom relapse in the placebo or immunotherapy groups; however, the untreated control group experienced considerably more symptoms than the test groups. The researchers concluded that immunotherapy for at least three years can induce long-term remission of allergic rhinitis symptoms.[4]

Allergy shots have also been effective for asthma induced by pollens, dust mites, and other aeroallergens, and sublingual immunotherapy has proven effective for allergic rhinitis but not asthma.[5] Allergies to food and other environmental and chemical agents cannot be effectively treated with immunotherapy.

# Serial Endpoint Titration

Serial endpoint titration (SET) is both a diagnostic tool and a desensitization therapy that is uniquely tailored to each allergy patient. Here, you expose the patient's skin (usually on the upper arm) to a minute amount of the allergen, such as dust mite, then watch the reaction. If a skin wheal (reddish blotch) forms, then you dilute the mixture and apply it again; eventually you reach the endpoint dilution to which their system does not react allergically. You repeat the procedure for each of the individual's known allergens. The maximally tolerated dose (no skin wheal forms) becomes the amount of allergen extract administered either sublingually or intradermally to coax the patient's immune system into desensitizing itself to the offending substance.

For more about **serial endpoint titration (SET)**, see Chapter 3: Allergy/Sensitivity Testing, pp. 70-105.

Patients often receive SET shots or drops once or twice a week, depending on the severity of the allergy. It takes from two months to two years for a person to become desensitized to allergens in this way, says Albert Robbins, D.O., an osteopath practicing in Boca Raton, Florida. "Generally, you will see positive responses in three to six months." SET immunotherapy does not entirely prevent the individual from reacting to certain allergens, but it significantly raises the reaction threshold, such that a large exposure is required to provoke the allergic reaction.

# Enzyme-Potentiated Desensitization (EPD)

In 1967, British immunologist Leonard M. McEwen, M.D., discovered a technique that trains the immune system to be nonreactive to substances that usually provoke allergic symptoms. Dr. McEwen named his technique enzyme-potentiated desensitization (EPD) and described it as a form of applied immunotherapy.

EPD is now used by physicians in at least 12 countries (70 physicians in North America alone), while more than 7,200 patients are participating in a formal clinical trial of EPD, which began in 1994 under the auspices of the Food and Drug Adminstration. Stephen B. Edelson, M.D., medical director of the Edelson Center for Environmental and Preventive Medicine in Atlanta, Georgia, calls EDP "the most effective therapy for allergies ever developed. This is a vaccine that can, over time, cure allergies."

In EPD, an allergic patient is given a series of tiny standardized injections (usually in the forearm) of a wide variety of allergens from a single category, even though some of the items in the category may not be allergens for them. These injections, which are given over a period of weeks, differ from conventional allergy shots in at least three ways: first, with EPD, multiple related allergens (e.g., inhalants) are given whereas allergy shots focus on only a few or individual allergens; second, EPD injects doses that are much weaker than allergy shots; and third, given along with the allergens in an EPD injection is an enzyme called beta-glucuronidase.

This last component is very important because beta-glucuronidase, injected at a level comparable to that present in the body, acts as a catalyst to make the vaccine more potent—that is, it potentiates it. The allergens themselves, when given in such low doses, produce an immunity that eventually leads to desensitization, according to Dr. McEwen.

It is believed that EPD triggers a specific T cell (white blood cell) in the immune system, but researchers are not certain which one. It is likely an activated suppressor T cell, possibly a CD8+ cytotoxic cell. "EDP appears to cause a cloning of certain T cells in the immune system so that they become resistant cells," Dr. Edelson explains. "Then they start protecting against the production of T4 cells, which are the ones that lead to allergy symptoms."

The way that suppressor T cells start retraining the immune system to not react to the allergens in the injections is by disabling helper T cells that have been inappropriately coded to produce an allergic reaction. In any event, once the suppressor T cells are activated (it takes about three to four weeks for them to mature), they remain potent for about 24 weeks. This is a major reason why the injections are eventually spaced many weeks apart.

EPD has been used successfully to treat about 50 health conditions, mostly of an immune or autoimmune nature. (The latter is when the body attacks its own tissue as if it were an allergen, such as lupus or some forms of arthritis.) It has an overall success rate of between 75% and 80%, with an average decrease in use of medication of about 50%, according to W. A. Schrader, Jr., M.D., a physician based in Santa Fe, New Mexico, and the principal investigator for the EPD study. Research also suggests that about 60% of patients experience favorable results after the first injection.

In addition to its effectiveness with hay fever and allergic rhinitis, asthma, hives, eczema, and anaphylaxis, EDP can also improve allergy-related conditions, such as attention deficit hyperactivity disorder, autism, irritable bowel syndrome, ulcerative colitis, migraine headaches, and rheumatoid arthritis.

EPD treatments are generally given six to eight times, every two to three months; then the injections decrease to once every three to six months. They continue to decrease until they are given annually and, ideally, culminate in a booster being received once every nine years. According to Dr. McEwen's research, after 16 to 18 treatments, the therapy can be permanently discontinued for half of the patients without further recurrence of allergic symptoms. Out of the estimated 160,000 doses of EPD given since the late 1960s, no serious side effects have been reported.

Patients take a prescribed list of nutritional supplements in the weeks between shots and follow a circumscribed diet, avoiding all foods to which they are reactive. While EPD significantly reduces one's intolerance to allergenic foods, it does not necessarily eliminate all possibility of reacting to them. Known allergenic foods must be avoided in the early stages of the program, then consumed sparingly after completion of an EPD regimen.

## Success Story: EDP Eliminates Severe Allergies

Jane, 34, had a distressing list of debilitating allergy-associated symptoms. She had severe eczema on her face, arms, and hands, asthma, multiple chemical sensitivity, facial herpes, seasonal allergies, sinus infections, and autoimmune symptoms. Prior to consulting Dr. Stephen Edelson, M.D., Jane had been treated by seven physicians (three allergists, two internists, and two dermatologists) but had not improved at all.

At the time of seeing Dr. Edelson, she was taking prednisone (cortisone), three inhalants, and several antihistamines. "She was given drugs, antihistamines, steroids, and inhalants for her asthma—in other words, Band-Aids for all of her symptoms," comments Dr. Edelson.

Jane had nasal surgery for a deviated septum, hoping it would stop her sinus infections, against which antibiotics were only somewhat helpful. Instead, in the year after surgery, she had eight more infections—and her doctor proposed still more surgery for the problem. More ominous was the fact that the last conventional allergy shot Jane received had produced anaphylaxis, a severe, life-threatening allergic reaction. She ceased the shots after this near-disaster.

Before developing a treatment plan for Jane, Dr. Edelson ran a series of laboratory tests to get more information about her biochemical status. "I consider him somewhat of a detective, because he used every means at his disposal to find hidden problems that could be the cause of my condition," Jane comments. Over the course of two "intense" days, Jane went through a battery of customized allergy testing. These tests proved that multiple food allergies were at the root of most of her discomfort.

Dr. Edelson also found that Jane had a low level of natural killer cell activity (meaning her immune system was not effective in disposing of disease agents); that she had high levels of two indicators of allergy activity (immunoglobulins IgA and IgG); that she was deficient in zinc, magnesium, and selenium; and that she had a positive ANA reading (antinuclear antibody, indicating autoimmune antibodies in her system).

**Stephen B. Edelson, M.D.:** Edelson Center for Environmental and Preventive Medicine, 3833 Roswell Road, Suite 110, Atlanta, GA 30342; tel: 404-841-0088; fax: 404-841-6416; website www.ephca.com. For a list of **EPD practitioners**, contact: American EPD Society, 141 Paseo de Peralta, Santa Fe, NM 87501; tel: 505-984-0004; website: www. epdallergy.com.

Dr. Edelson started Jane on a series of EPD injections, spacing them ever farther apart, so that after three years she was getting one injection every six months. He also put Jane on a daily nutritional program including vitamin C (12,000 mg) to bolster her immune response and the amino acid lysine (5,000 mg) to reverse her herpes.

Within one year on this program, Jane was able to discontinue all her conventional drugs. Today, nearly four years after starting treatment, "Jane is greatly improved," states Dr. Edelson. Of her improvement, Jane notes: "The EPD treatment had a tremendous impact on my quality of life. Although I am still not able to eat some foods and still have slight problems with my asthma when I am overexposed [such as in a smoke-filled room], I feel I am doing at least 90% better."

## Homeopathic Antigens

As discussed in Chapter 12: Homeopathic and Physical Therapies, homeopathic medicine is based on three principles: like cures like (Law of Similars); the more a remedy is diluted, the greater its potency (Law of Infinitesimal Dose); and an illness is specific to the individual (a holistic medical model). The Law of Similars is the basis for using homeopathy as a desensitization therapy. Much like a vaccine or allergy shot, homeopathic desensitization uses low doses of antigens to reprogram the immune system to accept the offending substances. For example, if a patient is allergic to ragweed pollen, a homeopathic preparation containing a dilution of ragweed may be administered sublingually or intravenously. Over time, the immune system will no longer recognize the antigen as a dangerous substance, putting an end to allergic reactions. Unlike allergy shots or serial endpoint titration, patients can learn how to treat themselves with homeopathic antigens. The following case study illustrates how this form of desensitization therapy helped a woman overcome her debilitating allergies.

**Success Story: Ending Years of Allergies with Homeopathy**

When Jennifer, a 44-year-old teacher, first consulted with James W. Forsythe, M.D., H.M.D., Director of the Century Wellness Center in Reno, Nevada, she presented with a complex set of symptoms that had plagued her since she was a young teenager. She reported severe fatigue, headaches, facial swelling, blurred vision, sharp chest pains, abdominal cramps, diarrhea, earaches, memory loss and serious bouts with depression. Jennifer told Dr. Forsythe that she had almost begun to accept pain as a necessary part of life since previous physical examinations and blood tests had not revealed anything her physicians felt could account for her condition.

In 1975, after moving from Utah to Idaho, she was even tested for a brain tumor and Bell's Palsy, having developing neurological symptoms (some drooling and weakness of facial muscles) as well as pain in the ear, nose, and throat area. To her relief, both conditions were ruled out and, insightfully, her neurologist suggested that she be tested for allergies.

**Homeopathic antigens reprogram the immune system to accept the offending substances.**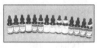

Traditional skin tests were performed (which can detect most airborne allergens and immediate-reaction food sensitivities) and it was found that Jennifer was highly allergic to many foods, molds, and pollens. Desensitization through conventional allergy shots was not very effective, Jennifer remembers, but her new awareness of allergies as a root cause of her problems was a breakthrough for her. Jennifer began to educate herself about allergies. She became acquainted with the concept of environmental illness and tried to keep her surroundings as free from adverse substances as possible. Avoidance, however, can be a tough task when you are allergic to as many things as Jennifer was.

Dr. Forsythe recalls her first visit. "She told me that all of her social plans were arranged around her health problems. If she wanted to attend some future function, she would have to plan far ahead and rest up for several days in order to have the energy to attend a special event. If she was invited to someone's home for dinner, she had to inquire about the menu beforehand and, if it contained foods to which she was highly allergic, she would accept the invitation but tell them she would eat before she came."

Additionally, she could not live in conventional housing. Most building materials and many indoor products contain significant amounts of formaldehyde and other chemicals that outgas and are a common source of reactivity. In order to avoid household triggers, when Jennifer moved to Nevada, she had a home specially constructed with allergy-free building materials, hardwood floors, tile, and all electric appliances. There was no fiberglass wallpaper, live plants, carpeting, or gas. Curtains were washable so that she did not come in contact with dry cleaning chemicals.

"She created an environment as clean and pure as it could possibly be," says Dr. Forsythe, "and she told me that, in her new home, she felt much better than she had as a child. Yet, she was far from living a normal life. She had not been able to eat lettuce for over ten years. She could not travel in the normal fashion and she had had to purchase a motor home so that she could control the kinds of food she ate on a daily basis when traveling. Everything revolved around her allergies and she knew that life had to be better than it was."

In 1989, Jennifer made a decision that she now considers was the most significant part of her journey toward a new and healthy life—she sought treatment at the Wellness Center. There, Dr. Forsythe and the staff worked with her for the next 2½ years, where she was treated homeopathically.

Dr. Forsythe's evaluation of Jennifer began with a thorough history and physical examination. "Her physical examination was remarkably unremarkable," he recalls. Laboratory tests, however, revealed that she played host to the herpes 6 virus, which is associated with chronic fatigue, and possessed antibodies to herpes 1, herpes 2, the Varicelli Zoster virus (connected to shingles) and the Epstein Barr virus, also associated with chronic fatigue. Additionally, she tested positive for Lyme disease. Mild anemia with low serum iron added to her energy drain, and additional chemical allergies were found to organophosphates, chloroform, and 2-4D (an herbicide), as well as soaps, phenol-based compounds (which are components of most conventional allergy shots), glycerin, and certain food additives.

Between fighting viruses and allergies, Jennifer's immune system had been severely weakened. "We try to find what has been impinging on the patient's immune system," Dr. Forsythe explains. "Then we go after it using homeopathic remedies to desensitize the patient's system. Very small doses of homeopathic preparations are given intravenously over a number of days [in Jennifer case, five days per week over a three-week period] to make the immune system recognize the virus or allergy and respond to it."

The specific homeopathic remedies Dr. Forsythe selected for

Jennifer contained a combination of immune enhancers. Specifically, *Chalcedonium*, to build up the immune system; *Gelsemium, Crataegis*, and *hepar* as immune stimulants especially effective for patients with allergies. In addition, Jennifer was given *Calcarea*, a constitutional remedy that fit her individual combination of symptoms. To reverse her iron deficiency, she received intramuscular iron shots. The dosages and appropriateness of Jennifer's remedies were checked by applied kinesiology (muscle testing) and electrodermal screening.

After leaving the Century Wellness Center, Jennifer continued her desensitization treatments to viruses and chemical allergies at home, where she self-injected the dilute homeopathic remedies Dr. Forsythe had given her and continued to watch her diet.

"With food allergies, you have to avoid the ones you are allergic to for a six-month period," states Dr. Forsythe. "Hopefully, by then, your immune system will be strong enough to tolerate them and you can add them back one at a time." As for the homeopathic treatment of viruses, Dr. Forsythe explains, "Viruses are one element which bring down the immune system and weaken the body's defenses. In almost all allergy patients, there's some viral insult, usually in the herpes family of viruses." When a patient receives a homeopathic remedy for a specific virus, according to Dr. Forsythe, "we feel it builds up the immune system and causes the body to suppress the virus. A lot of these viruses are dormant. They stay with us but only come to life when our immune systems are run down, or if there's stress or grief or trauma in our lives."

For the next 2$\frac{1}{2}$ years, Jennifer worked extensively with Dr. Forsythe and the staff at the center, and then had periodic check-ups to monitor her progress. At her last visit, she had very few symptoms, reports Dr. Forsythe. There were no signs of asthma, no lymph node swelling, no allergic rashes. A re-study of her viral titers showed improvement in comparison with prior studies. "She's had a very nice result," says Dr. Forsythe.

Jennifer is ecstatic about her improved health. As she tells it: "After the initial series of IV treatments, for the very first time in my life I felt good!" In contrast with prior traveling night-mares, where she had to prepare special food in her motor home, she recalls, "Recently, I took my mother on a nine-week trip to Arkansas to visit our relatives, and I was able to make the trip virtually trouble free. I was able to eat normal foods and lead a normal life. Nothing in my life had been normal before; it was truly a new beginning."

James Forsythe, M.D., H.M.D.: Century Wellness Center, 380 Brinkby Avenue, Reno, NV 89509; tel: 702-826-9500; fax: 702-329-6219.

Jennifer still has to be cautious about plants, flowers, and some foods, "but my reactions even to those are much milder now than in the past."

# Autoimmune Urine Therapy (AIU)

It may seem a hard fact to swallow, but urine has a broad spectrum of health benefits. We normally think of it only as a waste product that is unhealthy and unclean. But in actuality, healthy urine is completely sterile and rich in nutrients when it is first passed from the body. Modern drug manufacturers long ago discovered that many important chemical compounds are contained in urine. Urine is routinely collected from humans, horses, and other animals for the purpose of isolating and condensing desirable components. Premarin®, for instance, a type of estrogen used for hormone replacement therapy, is derived from the urine of pregnant mares. Urokinase, a drug commonly used to treat patients with advanced atherosclerosis (fatty calcified deposits on the arterial walls), is manufactured from urine collected from portable toilets. Most shampoos and cosmetics contain a component of urine, urea, or its synthetic counterpart known as carbamide.

Urine is composed of water, urea (a breakdown product of proteins and amino acids), hormones, enzymes, minerals, and salts, which are specific to the individual. The chemical components of a person's urine reflect the individual's health profile. This physiological "fingerprint" contains evidence of infectious agents, specific types of antibodies used to combat them, circulating immune complexes (antibodies that have attached themselves to antigens or foreign bodies), substances that have initiated an immune response, hormones and other natural chemicals used to regulate and control the body's functions, and synthesized vitamins and other nutritive substances.[7]

In the case of autoimmune and allergic diseases, in which the immune system is overactive, urine's precise mechanism of action is still not completely clear, but researchers hypothesize that the person's urine contains antibodies involved in the aggressive allergic response, along with the offending allergens. The antibody-antigen complexes that are residues of allergic reaction are obtained intact from sterile urine. The urine is then filtered through kidney dialysis filters in a sterile fashion so that only urea and antibodies remain. The urine is injected into the donor's buttocks, which distends the skin, activating immune responses. The chemicals responding to the immune activation recognize the antigen-antibody complexes in the urine as foreign and attack them by making antibodies to the antibodies of the donor's allergies. These new antibodies attack the initial antibodies and block the allergic reaction. This is a targeted blocking antibody therapy.

Doctors have used urine therapy as an injection because it works far better than drinking urine, but it can also be effective if taken orally. People with an aversion to drinking their own urine can start off very slowly following this procedure: in the morning, catch a small amount of urine in a clean cup, have another cup of filtered water available. Then, use a clean glass eyedropper and add just two drops of urine to the cup of water. Every few days, increase the amount of urine by one drop; go slowly, adding a little bit more urine each morning. The ideal dosage is ten drops of urine to one glass of water. Once this amount is reached, maintain it indefinitely. Urine tastes like salty water, but you can add a drop of peppermint oil to disguise the taste, if needed. Research has suggested that a person's ability to taste their own urine decreases as the therapeutic dose is reached.[8]

# Nambudripad's Allergy Elimination Technique (NAET)

Nambudripad's Allergy Elimination Technique (NAET) is a desensitization therapy developed by Devi S. Nambudripad, D.C., O.M.D., Ph.D., of Buena Park, California. It relies on altering energy flow through the body to treat symptoms of allergy and sensitivity. By examining the energy pathways, also called acupuncture meridians (SEE QUICK DEFINITION), practitioners are able to diagnose allergy/sensitivity triggers. Applied kinesiology (SEE QUICK DEFINITION), acupressure, acupuncture, and chiropractic are then used to alter the energy flow in an allergic body.

The secret to NAET, according to Dr. Nambudripad, is to retrain your brain and nervous system to no longer react to the offending substance. "We can reprogram our brains to perceive unsuitable energies as suitable ones and use them for our benefit rather than allow them to cause energy blockages and imbalances," she explains.

According to Dr. Nambudripad, your energy system and brain interpret a particular substance as potentially harmful to your body. For other people this item—a diamond ring, a carob-coated cherry, a

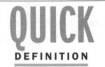

## QUICK
### DEFINITION

**Acupuncture meridians** are specific pathways in the human body for the flow of life force or subtle energy, known as *qi* (pronounced CHEE). In most cases, these energy pathways run up and down both sides of the body, and correspond to individual organs or organ systems, designated as Lung, Small Intestine, Heart, and others. There are 12 principal meridians and eight secondary channels. Numerous points of heightened energy, or *qi*, exist on the body's surface along the meridians and are called acupoints. There are more than 1,000 acupoints, each of which is potentially a place for acupuncture treatment.

**Applied kinesiology**, first developed by George Goodheart, D.C., of Detroit, Michigan, is the study of the relationship between muscle dysfunction (weak muscles) and related organ or gland dysfunction. Applied kinesiology employs a simple strength resistance test on a specific indicator muscle that is related to the organ or part of the body that is being tested. If the muscle tests strong (maintaining its resistance), it indicates health. If it tests weak, it can mean infection or dysfunction.

peanut—is a harmless, everyday item; but for your system, it's toxic. Your energy pathways freeze up as a way of defending the body against this unsuitable substance. This, in turn, blocks your energy meridians, and if the condition never changes, the overall functioning of your body suffers. In the past 15 years, Dr. Nambudripad reports that NAET alone has entirely relieved allergy symptoms or produced satisfactory improvements in 80%-90% of her patients.

## Success Story: NAET Eliminates Allergy Symptoms

Susan was a 19-year-old woman who came to Dr. Nambudripad complaining of severe lower back pain. She'd suffered with this for five days and was now having fever, chills, and severe headaches. A urine test suggested a possible kidney infection. Aspirin and a light antibiotic helped reduce her symptoms. Then she had a cup of fenugreek herbal tea—within 10 minutes she had an intense reaction: chills, muscular stiffness, and high fever. Dr. Nambudripad tested her at once for sensitivity to fenugreek tea using applied kinesiology.

The principle behind applied kinesiology is simple: the patient holds a substance that you think produces allergies while the physician tests the strength of certain muscles. You extend your arm and resist as the practitioner gently tries to push it down. Allergenic substances weaken your muscles, so if your arm goes down, you're probably allergic to the substance you're holding in your other hand. This is something you can do with a partner at home whenever you suspect an allergy or sensitivity. This method revealed that Susan was sensitive to fenugreek. Dr. Nambudripad also uses electrodermal screening to verify allergens.

Dr. Nambudripad found that Susan's kidney meridian got blocked by the fenugreek tea and kept generating the allergic symptoms of fever, chills, headaches, and kidney infection. "The sudden blocking of the meridians is one of the quickest defense mechanisms of the brain to stop the allergen from entering deeper into the body."

After discovering this information, the next step is to actually reprogram the patient's nervous system not to react anymore to the allergenic substance. Dr. Nambudripad used acupressure (she'll also use needle-based acupuncture when appropriate) to treat Susan's kidney meridian and organ imbalance at the same time that Susan held some fenugreek tea in her hand. The effect is to reorganize the body's way of reacting to a substance. Because the energy pathways are unblocked, your body does not have to defensively recoil every time it comes in contact with an allergenic substance. Using NAET, you undo your body's conditioned response and allow it to co-exist again with everyday items. You only have to stay away from the substance for 24 hours as your energy meridians "reset" themselves.

For a **list of NAET practitioners**, contact: Nambudripad's Allergy Research Foundation, 6714 Beach Blvd., Buena Park, CA 90621.

Within 30 minutes of applying NAET, Susan's temperature became normal. After the NAET session, Susan was able to resume drinking fenugreek tea without a relapse of symptoms.

# Natural Elimination of Allergy Therapy (NEAT)

The allergic response—sneezing, coughing, stuffed-up or runny noses, flushed cheeks, watery eyes, headaches—is a kind of learned behavior. Once your body recognizes a food, chemical, or plant pollen as dangerous, it stages an inflammatory response as an immune system defense. Eventually, if the exposure is not prolonged, the allergy symptoms subside, but the next time you have contact with the allergen, you will probably get the same package of unpleasant symptoms—unless you take steps to profoundly change the way your body reacts to these allergens.

Allergy reversal can be achieved by changing the energy dynamics of the nervous system using acupuncture, detoxification, and nutrient support. My approach is called Natural Elimination of Allergy Therapy, or NEAT. Eighty-seven percent of my allergy patients get good to excellent results in an average of ten NEAT sessions. The NEAT protocol is an adaptation of and progression from NAET. I studied with Dr. Nambudripad, then adapted the method, based on my knowledge of nutrition, acupuncture, and energy dynamics. I dropped the chiropractic component and systematized the treatment points, delivering them by hand through acupressure rather than acupuncture needles.

With NEAT, allergens are treated in large groups, each treatment spaced one week apart (NAET treats allergens individually or in small groups and in a very particular order); the treatment points are the same for all patients (NAET uses varying points); the functional integrity of the body's barrier functions is assessed and treated before desensitization; computerized electrodermal screening analyzes sensitivities (NAET uses manual muscle testing, although some practitioners use electrodermal screening and other techniques of antigen identification); and samples of suspected allergens are collected from the patient's living environment.

The key to success with NEAT lies in getting a great deal of information about the clinical status of allergy patients before prescribing a program. I emphasize the word program—NEAT is a protocol for the diagnosis and treatment of allergy/sensitivity disease and follows the principles outlined in this book. It is not just a desensitization technique. While standard laboratory tests and stool, urine, and immune profiles are used to assess barrier functions, immune, and endocrine status, NEAT primarily relies on electrodermal screening (EDS) for collecting precise data on a patient's sensitivities.

Nutrient deficiencies and barrier defaults are corrected before starting with the NEAT desensitization. Dealing with barrier functions is a key factor in successful allergy elimination. You must have mucous membranes that are moist and effective, skin that is intact and free of lesions, digestion that works. If not, you will resensitize to allergenic foods, despite treatment. In other words, if your barrier function is not working properly, you will become sensitive (allergic) to foods and substances. Damaged barriers "leak" large molecules of a substance into the blood and this causes sensitization.

In many cases, a two-week detoxification fast and internal cleansing program helps clean out the system and get the bowels moving more frequently and more fully. The periodic elimination of digestive, metabolic, and toxic environmental waste material is an extremely important process for achieving and maintaining optimal health. Among the highlights of this program are the following: drinking diluted fruit and vegetable juices, herbal teas, bottled water with fresh lemon juice, and fresh vegetable broths; the use of castor oil packs placed on the abdomen (to stimulate liver cleansing); herbal fiber supplements (psyllium seed, apple pectin, oat bran, bentonite clay); herbal laxatives (*Cascara sagrada*, senna, barberry, ginger, cayenne); alfalfa tablets (to provide chlorophyll which aids cleansing); garlic (to help rid the body of unwanted strains of bacteria); *L. acidophilus* (to repopulate the intestines with "friendly" bacteria); and enemas (coffee for five days, then goldenseal for five days).

A patient's potential allergic reaction to up to 2,000 different substances (even supplements and medications), retained as computerized energy (virtual) imprints, can be tested with the EDS device. Patients bring in samples of suspected allergens from their living environment: contents of a vacuum cleaner bag; dirt and lawn samples from their yard; samples from their bedroom vent, perfumes, cosmetics, toothpastes, soaps, household detergents, disinfectants, cleaning agents, and other high-exposure items (pillow and case, etc). EDS can test the patient's sensitivity (compatibility) to these everyday items.

There are two visits to gather data and repair barrier functions and support basic biochemistry. On the third visit, the patient is screened for inhalant sensitivities; on the fourth visit, for chemicals; on the fifth, for food allergies; and on the sixth, there is a "clean-up" session in which the patient is retested for sensitivity to all 2,000 items.

During the diagnostic phase, EDS determines energies to which the patient is reacting. A homeopathic remedy of all reacting (antigenic) energies is prepared in a vial. Energy is a field, not a thing—when a person holds on to the thing (vial), they are interacting with the energy field. The patient is tested with a muscle test (kinesiology) not holding the vial and will be "strong." Then, the patient holds the vial containing the adverse energies (antigens). The patient's energy responds to this adverse energy and starts to react to these imprints.

When you hold this vial, your brain—as it were, the head of your immune system—identifies the vial's component energies as foreign invaders so it can attack them. This interaction causes muscular weakness and the muscle test is repeated on the patient while they are holding the vial to show weakness. This indicates that the interaction is happening and that the patient's brain has identified the offending energies. While the patient is still holding the vial, an acupressure treatment is performed on the patient to specific Bladder meridian acupoints that are associated with the lungs, spleen and stomach energies, to the *huatuo jiagi* acupoints, and to extra-meridian points in a standardized sequence.

This balances the patient's energy while the offending energies are in the patient's field (holding the vial). This balanced energy gives the brain a new message: "My energy is normal, I don't have to attack these substances any more." This results in changing the default setting in your brain, so that now it carries out the new message. Because the treatment creates an adverse response in order to

## Highlights from the NEAT Patient Database

Over the years, since developing NEAT, I've tracked and tabulated outcomes on close to 2,000 patients. According to my self-compiled statistics, 87% of patients receiving NEAT had "good to excellent" results.

It takes an average of ten visits per patient for full relief of symptoms (two treatments before partial relief) and three annual visits thereafter for maintenance. Regarding success rate, 46% rate the treatment as excellent and 42% as good. The average cost for a successful treatment is $822 (including supplements, laboratory work, and office visits). These figures have been slightly modified since review by a statistician. The results are pending publication in a peer-reviewed journal.

correct it, patients get an aggravation of their symptoms in about 50% of cases while holding the vial or within the first 24 hours after treatment.

During the next 24 hours, the patient avoids any contact with all identified allergens for which they have been cleared, and avoids any energy upsets, such as anger, fright, or other strong stimulation, or any energy-based medicines, such as homeopathic remedies. These could distort or even cancel the new energy state in the process of being established.

The 24-hour excitement curfew is based on the traditional Chinese medicine precept that it takes that long for the body's basic life force energy, or $qi$, to pass through the 12 major meridians or energy channels (two hours for each meridian). After 24 hours, each meridian has "tasted" the new configuration of $qi$ and made appropriate adjustments. Energy treatment can alter physiologic response. In other words, by changing the way $qi$ flows through the energy channels, you can affect the way the body, nervous system, and organs function.

### The Advantages of NEAT

Since NEAT works by persuading the brain, rather than the immune system, to quit attacking offending substances, it has several advantages over conventional immunotherapy. First, although the immune system is difficult to change and takes a relatively long time to influence, the brain, because it is an organ that controls everything in the body, changes quickly. Since the brain controls the immune system, if the brain's message is "Don't attack," then the immune system cannot attack. Instead of taking months, possibly years, for immunotherapy to work, NEAT creates change within 24 hours.

Furthermore, this is a noninvasive technique that requires only minimal financial resources, compared with the cost of conventional therapy, which can run into several thousands of dollars. After the initial treatment, other than maintenance of barrier functions, symptoms are controlled with one to two NEAT sessions per year and minimal anthistamine/decongestant therapy. Also, although an aggravation of previously existing symptoms is commonly seen after each NEAT treatment, there are virtually no adverse effects.

## Success Story: Infantile Eczema Reversed with NEAT

Adam had endured eczema for seven of his ten months of life. He had not responded to conventional or herbal and nutritional treatment and the red blotches so dominated his face, his mother stopped taking baby pictures of him. His cheeks looked like raw hamburger patties with a thin coat of mustard.

Based on the information obtained from EDS, I concluded that Adam had sensitivities to numerous chemicals and that his rash was allergic in nature with a secondary complication of impetigo. This is a skin infection, marked by vesicles that rupture, forming yellow crusts; it is believed to be caused by a strain of either *Streptococcus* or *Staphylococcus* bacteria. I also learned that both of Adam's parents had allergies, thereby creating a strong predisposition that Adam too would be susceptible to allergies.

Using the NEAT protocol, I was able to completely clear up the facial rash within the first 24 hours. However, over the next week, the rash slowly returned. Further EDS testing revealed that Adam was allergic to a variety of inhalants, to which he was then desensitized through NEAT. This time his rash receded over the course of seven days.

At the next treatment, I found Adam to be allergic to many foods. Prominent among these were dairy, wheat, corn, soybean, peanut, chocolate, strawberry, and food additivies, but there were nearly one hundred in all. I desensitized him to these foods so he would not react allergically. Adam by this point had evidence of the eczematous rash only on his neck.

In the fourth treatment, I tested him again for sensitivities in the 2,000-item EDS repertory and found Adam still reacting to 37 items. At the four-month follow-up, he was allergic to only five items and subject to only occasional rashes, which flared then disappeared within hours.

For more on **electrodermal screening (EDS)**, see Chapter 3: Allergy/Sensitivity Testing, pp. 70-105.

The progression of healing in this case shows how allergies can exist in layers in the body. Some stronger energies

For more on **Natural Elimination of Allergy Therapy (NEAT)**, contact: Konrad Kail, N.D., U.S. Complementary Health, Inc. 3441 E. Tierra Buena Lane, Phoenix, AZ, 85032; tel: 602-493-1637; e-mail: kkail@home.com.

associated with allergenic substances can "cover up" weaker energies also associated with allergic reactions. Electrodermal testing assesses one layer or category of allergens at a time, starting with inhalants, then chemicals and foods, followed by the "clean-up" to retest for all 2,000 items. Findings on the clean-up session are "leftovers" that were recently uncovered—weaker, covered-up energies— or items the patient has resensitized to since their last visit. After two years of treatment—he had 12 desensitization sessions in all—Adam was symptom free.

Stress becomes harmful to the body when

it is prolonged or chronic, by influencing

the immune and hormonal systems.

For allergy sufferers, this can mean

an exacerbation of their allergic symptoms.

Stress can also lead to the

onset of allergy and sensitivity.

# CHAPTER 14

# Mind/Body Approaches to Allergy

**S**TRESS IS A COMMON PART of everyday life, but it can become harmful to the body when it is prolonged or chronic. It affects the body in very real, physical ways by influencing the immune and hormonal systems. For allergy sufferers, this can mean an exacerbation of allergic symptoms; stress can also lead to the onset of allergy and sensitivity. A basic premise of mind/body medicine is that chronic stress contributes to illness and that relaxation techniques and learning positive ways of coping with stress will improve your health. In this chapter, we examine how stress, suppressed emotions, and lifestyle choices can contribute to allergy and sensitivity. We also explore a number of therapies that can help you reprogram negative thought patterns into more healthful ones, deal with stress in a positive way, and incorporate habits for relaxation into your life.

## In This Chapter

- Stressed Out—A Pervasive Problem
- The Role of Stress in Allergic Conditions
- Success Story: Hypnotherapy Stops Stress-Induced Asthma
- Mind/Body Therapies for Healing Allergy and Sensitivity

## Stressed Out— A Pervasive Problem

Although the concept of stress—being "stressed out" or "under constant stress"—may be commonly discussed today, its role as a contributing factor in many diseases is underappreciated. Estimates suggest that as many as 70% to 80% of all visits to physicians' offices are for stress-related problems.[1] Chronic stress directly affects the immune system, and if not effectively dealt with, can seriously compromise health.

Stress is a pervasive problem among Americans, according to a poll of corporate executives. For example, 44% of employees polled said their work load is excessive; 43% are bothered by excessive job pressure; and 55% worry considerably about their company's future; 25% of both men and women feel stressed out at work every day, another 12% feel it almost every day, and another 38% feel it once to several days a week.[2]

Stress can be defined as a reaction (to any stimulus or interference) that upsets normal functioning and disturbs mental or physical health. It can be brought on by internal conditions such as illness, pain, emotional conflict, or psychological problems, or by external circumstances, such as bereavement, financial problems, loss of job or spouse, relocation, allergies, and electromagnetic fields. Stress can be positive or negative. Winning the lottery is probably as physically upsetting as the death of a close family member. Stress, when it becomes chronic, is often unrecognized by the person whose body is experiencing it; one begins to accept it as a fact of life, without being aware of how it is actually compromising body functions and preparing the foundation for illness.

More specifically, research confirms that high levels of emotional stress increase one's susceptibility to illness. Unrelieved, chronic stress begins taxing and eventually weakening or even suppressing the immune system. Stress can also lead to hormonal imbalances; which, in turn, interfere with immune function. Of all the body's systems, stress damages endocrine function the most. It does so by overly activating the sympathetic part of the autonomic nervous system, the part that controls the "fight-or-flight" response and initiates adrenaline and cortisol release.

Research in psychoneuroimmunology has shown that the immune and nervous systems are linked by extensive networks of nerve endings in the spleen, bone marrow, lymph nodes, and thymus gland (a primary source of T cells). At the same time, receptors for a variety of chemical messengers—catecholamines, prostaglandins, thyroid hormone, growth hormone, sex hormones, serotonin, and endorphins—have been found on the surfaces of white blood cells.

Such connections serve to integrate the activities of the immune, hormonal, and nervous systems, enabling the mind and emotional states to influence the body's resistance to disease,[3] potentially leading to infection and allergy.[4]

Pioneering stress researcher Hans Selye, M.D., a Canadian physiologist, noted a consistent pattern of response to stress and termed these the general adaptation syndrome (GAS), commonly referred to as the "fight-or-flight" response. The GAS occurs in three stages: the alarm reaction, the stage of resistance, and the stage of exhaustion.

## Common Causes of Stress

- Illness
- Pain
- Emotional Conflict
- Financial Problems
- Death in the Family
- Job/Career Pressures
- Allergies
- Poor Diet
- Substance Abuse
- Fatigue
- Environmental Pollution

Initially, the body's biochemistry tends to react to stress in an orderly fashion. Stimulation of the sympathetic nervous system (part of the autonomic nervous system) activates the secretion of hormones from the endocrine glands and constricts both the blood vessels and the involuntary muscles of the body. When the endocrine glands (pancreas, thyroid, thymus, pituitary, sex glands, and particularly the adrenals) are stimulated, heart rate, glucose metabolism, and oxygen consumption increase. The parasympathetic nervous system is also stimulated, which begins a process of relaxation. The pituitary gland responds by releasing a variety of hormones throughout the body, which influence the defensive and adaptive mechanisms. Endorphins, the body's own natural painkillers, are also released.

Dr. Selye points out, however, that eventually chronic stress depletes the body's resources and its ability to adapt. If stress continues and remains unattended for a long period, coping functions will be compromised and illness will result.[5]

## Symptoms Associated with Stress

- Anxiety
- Indigestion
- Weight Loss or Gain
- Depression
- Premenstrual Syndrome (PMS)
- Bad Breath or Body Odors
- Muscle Spasms

# Stress, the Adrenal Glands, and Allergy

The adrenal glands, part of the body's endocrine system, are located atop the kidneys. The glands are composed of two types of tissue: the adrenal medulla and the adrenal cortex. The adrenal medulla, comprising 10%-20% of the gland, is located in the interior portion and is responsible for the production of the hormones epinephrine (adrenaline) and norepinephrine (noradrenaline). These hormones are released in direct response to the sympathetic nervous system (the fight-or-flight response). The adrenal cortex, the outer layer, surrounds the medulla and accounts for 80%-90% of the gland. It is responsible for the production of corticosteroids (also called adrenal steroids). More than 30 different steroids have been isolated from the adrenal cortex, including cortisol and cortisone.

Cortisol secretion (as well as the adrenal gland's other steroids, DHEA, adrenaline, and aldosterone) occurs in daily cycles, peaking in the morning and having the lowest values at night. Cortisol promotes protein building, regulates insulin and glycogen synthesis, and helps produce prostaglandins (hormone-like fatty acids involved in inflammatory processes). Under conditions of stress, high amounts of cortisol are released. Imbalances in cortisol secretion are linked with low energy, inflammation, muscle dysfunction, impaired bone repair, thyroid dysfunction, immune system depression, sleep disorders, and poor skin regeneration. The adrenal glands also produce precursors to sex hormones, so hyperadrenal response increases sex hormones and hypoadrenal response decreases sex hormones.

During a stress response, the adrenal glands release high amounts of the hormone cortisol, which shuts off any allergic reactions. Adrenaline (or epinephrine), another hormone, is also released if you are frightened or angry, which is why during a severely stressful situation, such as on a battlefield, people with asthma are generally free of symptoms.[6]

If stress becomes chronic, however, the adrenals can become exhausted and depleted

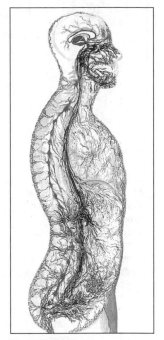

The autonomic nervous system (ANS) can be likened to your body's automatic pilot. It keeps you alive through breathing, heart rate, and digestion, without your being aware of it or participating in its activities. The ANS has two divisions: the sympathetic, which expends body energy; and the parasympathetic, which conserves body energy. The sympathetic nervous system is associated with arousal and stress; it prepares us physically when we perceive a threat or challenge by increasing our heart rate, blood pressure, and muscle tension. The parasympathetic nervous system slows heart rate and increases intestinal and most gland activity. It controls salivation, lacrimation (tears), urination, defecation, and glandular secretion.

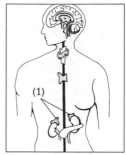

The adrenal glands (1) are two triangular-shaped glands above the kidneys. They release adrenaline and other hormones in the fight-or-flight response to stress.

For more on the **dangers of conventional allergy medicine**, see Chapter 11: Supplements for Symptom Control, pp. 278-303.

of their natural cortisol. If you have allergies, inflammation during allergic responses will worsen as your adrenal glands stop producing cortisol. This is not uncommon in people with persistent allergies, and, since allergies themselves are stressful, there is often a vicious cycle of allergies leading to weakened adrenals leading to more allergies. Additionally, the adrenal glands play a central role in maintaining the body's energy levels. When these glands are functioning poorly, the result can be allergic fatigue, muscle weakness, depression, and, in cases of allergy-induced arthritis, a magnification of arthritic symptoms.

For a patient in this situation, conventional medicine typically prescribes pharmaceutical drugs similar to cortisol (corticosteroids) for the pain and inflammation; prednisone, for example, is 30 times as potent as endogenous cortisol.[7] Adrenaline is also administered in cases of anaphylactic shock. Many practitioners of natural medicine feel that, while the judicious use of corticosteroids may be necessary for a short period of time to stabilize the patient, the long-term use and reliance on these powerful drugs is devastating. These drugs can suppress immunity, interfere with sleep cycles, and increase bone and collagen breakdown as well as suppress the proper function and production of the adrenal hormones and further diminish the functioning of the adrenal glands. When used topically, these drugs increases skin permeability, possibly leading to further sensitization.

## Asthma and Stress: A Vicious Cycle

Many asthma patients believe that stress triggers their asthma attacks. As mentioned above, short periods of acute stress boost production of important immune chemicals and cells in anticipation of an attack on the body. Acute stress also triggers the release of a stress protein into the lungs that has been shown to protect against lung injury in asthmatics.[9] When combined with the release of adrenaline during the stress response, this protective protein may provide a clue as to why asthmatics do not experience attacks during acute periods of stress. However, acute as well as chronic stress can lead to airway obstruction and other asthma symptoms, supporting many patients' view that stress is detrimental to their condition.

In a 1999 study, 30 adolescents with asthma and 20 controls were subjected to a stressful situation—a frustrating computer task. Heart rate, blood pressure, respiratory rate, deep inhalations, and sighs were measured as were asthma-specific processes such as lung function, wheezing, coughing, and breathlessness. The subjects also recorded their emotions during the task. All measurements indicated that the subjects were undergoing high levels of negative emotions and stress. None of the asthma participants experienced airway obstruction, wheezing, significant periods of coughing, or reduction in lung function. However, all of the asthmatic subjects suffered from breathlessness, many of them severely. In fact, the breathlessness experienced was higher than the breathlessness provoked by irritating substances before the test. The researchers confirmed that while stress may not trigger a full-blown asthma attack, it can induce breathlessness in patients with asthma.[10]

## Panic Disorder May Be an Allergic Disease

We know that some cases of schizophrenia, autism, and other mental disorders are linked to allergies, but what about anxiety disorders? In a 1992 study, researchers compared various physiological factors (vasomotor reactions, heart rate, and hyperventilation) in 23 patients with panic disorder and/or agoraphobia (fear of public places) and 50 patients with IgE-mediated allergy. The researchers found that 74% of the panic disorder subjects also tested positive for allergies; however there were no more anxiety disorders in the allergic patients in comparison with the general population. These findings suggest that panic disorder and agoraphobia may actually be allergic diseases, rather than merely psychological events.[8]

In another experiment, more than 130 adults with asthma documented, three times a day for three weeks, their stressors, frequency of asthma symptoms, peak flow readings (a measure of how much air the lungs expel), and use of beta-agonist bronchodilators. Stress was positively correlated with lowered breathing ability, as measured by peak flow rates, and increased symptoms of asthma and use of bronchodilators.[11] Researchers suggest that stress provokes breathing problems because it appears to promote the adhesion of leukocytes to bronchial ciliary cells, accelerating allergic inflammatory reactions and asthma.[12]

Asthma is also a major source of stress, especially for children and their parents. Asthmatic children, in particular, appear to be bound in a vicious cycle, whereby stress contributes to asthma attacks, which cause more stress, leading to more attacks as well as stress-related psychological problems. Studies have shown that in severely asthmatic children, those who are plagued by depression as well as persistent family conflict are at a greater risk than others for suffering a fatal asthma attack.[13] Moreover, in a study comparing asthmatic children with non-asthmatic controls, the asthma group had significantly more total anxiety disorders, school problems, psychiatric illnesses, and family stress.[14]

## When Stress is Skin Deep

Many allergic people notice that their skin disorders worsen during stress. Confirming these observations was a Japanese survey that measured cases of atopic dermatitis following the Great Hanshin Earthquake in Kobe, Japan, in 1995. In this survey, 1,457 people with atopic dermatitis were divided into three geographic groups—area A, an area that experienced severe damage during the earthquake; area B, mild damage; and the control area, no damage. Researchers found that 38% of area A and 34% of area B patients suffered flare-ups of their symptoms following the earthquake, while only 7% of the control group experienced exacerbation of their skin condition. Sixty-three percent of area A patients and 48% of area B patients reported suffering from stress due to the earthquake, while only 19% of the controls did. The researchers concluded that the stress directly exacerbated atopic dermatitis symptoms in a significant number of the population affected by the quake.[15]

How does stress wreak such havoc on the skin? Scientists have discovered that stress is associated with an increased number and activation of mast cells, which release vasoactive (dilating) and pro-inflammatory mediators.[16] However, it appears that cortisol is released in lower amounts or somehow blunted in patients with skin allergy.

For example, in a 1997 study, 15 children with atopic dermatitis and 15 controls were assigned to perform stressful tasks, consisting mainly of public speaking and mental arithmetic tasks in front of an audience.[17] The subjects with eczema were in remission and off medication for at least three weeks. Researchers tested salivary cortisol release and heart rates of all children to measure their stress response to these tasks. All subjects showed high levels of stress; however, the children with atopic dermatitis showed a significantly blunted cortisol response compared to that of the controls. The researchers did not follow up to see whether the children experienced eczema flare-ups, but the cortisol response indicated that atopic children may have an underfunctioning endocrine system. Researchers hypothesized that the endocrine system plays a regulatory role in immune function, and endocrine dysfunction could explain why atopic individuals experience stress-induced flare-ups of symptoms.

It appears that skin allergies may also occur due to a stress-triggered redistribution of leukocytes, immune cells involved in allergic reactions. A recent study found that acute stress induces a large-magnitude, rapid, and reversible dispersal of leukocytes from the blood (where they normally circulate) to other areas of the body. This change in leukocyte distribution is mediated by adrenal stress hormones. The skin is one of the target organs of this redistribution of leukocytes, perhaps in anticipation of physical injury. Experiments show that acute stress significantly enhances delayed (cell-mediated) skin reactions.[18]

### The Psychology of Chemical Sensitivity

Conventional medicine often dismisses chemical sensitivity as a psychosomatic condition. Although many clinical ecologists and alternative medicine practitioners have made efforts to dispel this thinking—backed by clinical research that proves chemical sensitivity has a physiological and medical basis—it is important to recognize that chemical sensitivity arises from psychological stress.

In a 1998 study, researchers compared the early-life stress ratings, parental relationships, and health status of three groups of middle-aged women: those afflicted with low-level chemical sensitivity and depressive symptoms; depressed women with no signs of chemical intolerance; and controls.[19] The researchers found that both chemically sensitive women and depressed women had higher incidences of early-life difficulties and childhood abuse than controls, but chemically sensitive women had an added stressor—poor relationships with their fathers. These findings suggest that women who experienced many stressful situations are more at risk to develop chemical sensitivities.

Another study surveyed 2,160 employees in 67 office buildings with no recognized environmental problems. The researchers found that there was a prevalence of sick building syndrome among office workers who reported high levels of physical and mental stress and poor work cooperation.[20] It's likely that work-related stress makes people more prone to becoming sensitized to ordinary office chemicals.

For more on **chemical sensitivity**, see Chapter 2: Causes of Allergy and Sensitivity, pp. 38-69, and Chapter 5: Environmental Control, pp. 128-157

## Success Story: Hypnotherapy Stops Stress-Induced Asthma

Some physicians believe there is often a strong emotional underpinning to asthma, but it isn't always easy to help a patient identify and

# Are You Stressed Out?

If you answer "yes" to more than five of the questions below, it indicates that you have too much stress in your life. In parentheses after each question are some potential underlying causes for the problem. Your doctor may also recommend tests to measure the adrenal health and hormone levels to determine the effects of stress on your body.

- Do you often grind your teeth? (digestive dysfunction, parasites)
- Is your breath shallow and irregular? (low metabolic energy, food allergies)
- Are your hands and feet cold? (hormonal imbalance, adrenal/thyroid weakness)
- Do you have trouble sleeping or tend to wake up tired? (liver dysfunction, food allergies)
- Do you often have an upset stomach? (food allergies)

- Do you get mad or irritated easily? (liver dysfunction)
- Do you feel worthless? (low metabolic energy, chronic fatigue)
- Do you constantly worry? (hormonal imbalance)
- Do you have problems concentrating and articulating your thoughts? (low metabolic energy, digestive or hormonal imbalance)
- Do you frequently fidget, chew your fingers, or bite your nails? (food allergies, digestive disturbances)
- Do you have high blood pressure? (food allergies, digestive disturbances)
- Do you eat, drink, or smoke excessively? (low metabolic energy, poor diet)
- Do you sometimes turn to recreational drugs just to get away? (low metabolic energy, poor diet)

**Adrenal hormone function tests** are discussed in Chapter 3: Allergy/Sensitivity Testing, pp. 70-105.

then clear that emotion. In such cases, hypnotherapy has a role, according to clinical hypnotherapist Joseph Riccioli, C.Ht., NBCDCH, director of the Hypnosis Healing Center in Totowa, New Jersey.

Rosie, 28, had lived with asthma for 20 years. She had a history of stress-related problems, including insomnia, and had several times consulted a psychiatrist for relief of her anxiety. Rosie wasn't happy with the outcome of these consultations because she was reluctant to take the powerful conventional drugs these doctors had prescribed. She thought she'd try a different tack—hypnosis.

When Rosie told Dr. Riccioli that she had officially been diagnosed as having anxiety disorder, he replied, "In hypnotherapy, we do not diagnose; we directly communicate with and probe the subconscious mind to find a probable cause for a person's unhealthy state, be it physical and/or emotional."

Hypnotherapy helps patients understand that emotional states are linked to illness. "When an unresolved issue is held onto for a period of time," explains Dr. Riccioli, "it can create a conflict between the subconscious and conscious minds. If it remains unresolved, it may manifest itself emotionally, as depression or anxiety, for example. If this persists, it may eventually internalize and manifest itself physically as symptoms."

Dr. Riccioli's clinical interest was in discovering Rosie's feelings about her condition. "The subconscious mind remembers everything. It's just a question of getting to that information," he says. During regression hypnosis, Rosie's memory took her back to her childhood, when she was eight years old. This was the first time she experienced feelings of anxiety, say Dr. Riccioli. She remembered that her parents fought continuously; on one occasion, they had a particularly vigorous altercation that so upset Rosie that she began crying. Her parents paid no attention to her distress and made no effort to comfort her.

"This experience is what we call the initial synthesizing event," says Dr. Riccioli. Soon after this argument, Rosie developed asthmatic symptoms. "The primary causes of her bronchial constriction and spasm were her nerves acting on her lungs," he explains. During the regression therapy, Rosie appeared to relive this painful experience—she cried, became nervous, and began showing signs of breathing difficulty, says Dr. Riccioli.

These were positive signs, as the pall of childhood emotional trauma was about to be lifted from Rosie's lungs. Using a combination of psychological techniques—such as "working with the inner child, love, forgiveness, and reframing"—Dr. Riccioli helped Rosie understand and resolve the cause of her anxiety and simultaneously release the cause of her asthma.

Joseph Riccioli, C.Ht., NBCDCH: Hypnosis Healing Center, 205 Route 46W, Totowa, NJ 07512; tel: 973-837-9599; website: www.healinghypnosis.com.

"When she left my office after that single 2½-hour session, Rosie was like a new person," says Dr. Riccioli. Shortly thereafter, her asthma improved so much that she was able to finally discontinue all of her conventional asthma drugs after two decades of suffering.

# Mind/Body Therapies for Healing Allergy and Sensitivity

According to Hans Selye, M.D., whether a person experiences stress as a positive motivational force or as a negative detrimental one depends on their perception of the stress.[21] People who perceive that they are in control of their lives and generally feel good about themselves (referred to as an "inner locus of control") will use life's stressors in a positive fashion. However, those who feel that their life circumstances are controlled by outside forces and other people ("outer locus of control") tend to react negatively to stress. There are some that control the flow and some that are controlled by it. For example, according to one study, the severity of skin reactions during times of stress is associated with coping style and other cognitive responses to stress, not with the actual cause of stress.[22] Perception of stress can make skin reactions better or worse.

The locus of control can be consciously shifted by deliberately "reprogramming" the mind, with positive instead of negative thoughts, through meditation, cognitive therapy, Neuro-Linguistic Programming, and HeartMath techniques. Relaxation therapies such as biofeedback, hypnotherapy, guided imagery, flower remedies, and aromatherapy, among others, can help reduce your stress levels and prevent allergy flare-ups. In fact, clinical research confirms that combating anxiety-provoking thoughts and using progressive relaxation and diaphragmatic breathing can be beneficial for patients who suffer stress-induced asthma symptoms.[23]

## Meditation

Meditation is a safe and simple way to balance a person's physical, emotional, and mental states. It is easy to learn and can be useful both for treating stress and in pain management. Meditation, in the broadest sense, is any activity that keeps the attention focused in the present. When the mind is calm and focused in the present, it is neither reacting to past events or preoccupied with future plans, two major sources of chronic stress. There are many forms of meditation, but they can be categorized into two main approaches, concentration meditation and mindfulness meditation.

Concentration meditation focuses the "lens of the mind" on one object, sound (mantra), the breath, an image, or thought, to still the mind and allow greater awareness or clarity to emerge. The breath is one of the most popular objects of focus in this type of meditation. As the person focuses on the ebb and flow of their breath, the mind is absorbed in the rhythm and becomes more placid, tranquil, and still. Mindfulness-based meditation entails bringing the mind to a still point, tuning out the world and bringing the mind to a halt as much as possible. Mindfulness meditation helps us practice non-judgment. The meditator sits quietly and simply witnesses whatever goes through the mind, not reacting or becoming involved with thoughts, memories, worries, or images. This helps the person gain a more calm, clear, and non-reactive state of mind.

Transcendental Meditation™ (TM), a popular form of concentration meditation, is the most well-documented regarding the physiological effects of meditation, with more than 500 clinical studies conducted to date.[25] Research shows that, during TM practice, the body gains a deeper state of relaxation than during ordinary rest or sleep.[26] Brain wave changes indicate a state of enhanced awareness and coherence and TM has been found to increase intelligence, creativity, and perceptual ability and reduce blood pressure and rates of illness by 50%.[27] TM also causes decreased blood levels of cortisol, a hormone responsible for many of the deleterious physiological changes seen with stress.[28] By reducing cortisol levels, the adrenal glands are allowed to heal, which positively influences allergic inflammation.

## Cognitive Therapy

It has been estimated the average human being has around 50,000 thoughts per day, according to Richard Carlson, author of *Don't Sweat The Small Stuff...And It's All Small Stuff*. Unfortunately, he reminds us, many of them are going to be negative—angry, fearful, pessimistic, or worrisome. Up to 85% of the thinking we regularly engage in is negative and self-defeating.[29]

The basis of cognitive therapy is to identify—through maintaining a journal and by introspection—the negative, self-defeating inner dialogue of thoughts (what cognitive therapists refer to as "automatic thoughts"). Positive, coping thoughts can then be used to counter the negative thoughts. The goal is to pull yourself out of reflexive self-destructive mental behavior that may be

## Write Your Way to Allergy-Free Health

According to a study published in the *Journal of the American Medical Association*, writing about traumatic life experiences helps alleviate asthma and rheumatoid arthritis, a condition often caused by allergy. In this study, 39 patients with asthma and 32 with rheumatoid arthritis were assigned to write about the most stressful event in their lives; 22 other asthma subjects and 19 arthritis patients, serving as controls, were asked to write about emotionally neutral topics. All subjects were measured for severity of symptoms before the writing project, at two weeks, two months, and four months following the assignment. Four months after the treatment, the asthma patients in the writing groups experienced a lung function improvement of 12.5%, while the arthritis patient experienced a 28% reduction in disease severity. None of the control patients showed any change. The researchers concluded that patients with mild to moderately severe asthma or rheumatoid arthritis who write about stressful life events may experience significant improvements in their conditions that could not be attributed to medical care.[24]

## A Simple Meditation Exercise

The first step to practicing meditation is learning to breathe in a manner that facilitates a state of calmness and awareness. Jon Kabat-Zinn, Ph.D., founder and director of the Stress Reduction Clinic at the University of Massachusetts Medical Center, recommends the following exercise for achieving a sense of calmness—find a quiet place where you will not be disturbed and practice for several minutes each day:

■ Assume a comfortable posture lying on your back or sitting. If you are sitting, keep the spine straight and let your shoulders drop.

■ Close your eyes if it feels comfortable.

■ Bring your attention to your belly, feeling it rise or expand gently on the in-breath and fall or recede on the out-breath. Keep the focus on your breathing.

■ When your mind wanders off the breath, notice what it was that took you away and then gently bring your attention back to your belly and the feeling of the breath moving in and out. If your mind wanders away from the breath, your "job" is simply to bring it back to the breath every time, no matter what it has become preoccupied with.

Practice this exercise for 15 minutes every day, whether you feel like it or not, for one week and see how it feels to incorporate a disciplined meditation practice into your life.

---

For more on **cognitive therapy**, contact: University of Pennsylvania Center for Cognitive Therapy, 3600 Market Street, 8th Floor, Philadelphia, PA 19104, tel: 215-898-4100; fax: 215-898-1865. The American Institute for Cognitive Therapy, 136 E. 57th Street, Suite 1101, New York, NY 10022; tel: 212-308-2440.

exacerbating your illness and to bolster the positive, self-reliant aspect of your personality.

Cognitive therapy does not focus on the root causes of psychological problems, rather it seeks to support health by interrupting the flow of negative thoughts. Countering each negative thought on paper with a list of positive responses to the same problem enables the mind to reframe the situation. For allergy sufferers, replacing negative thoughts with positive ones can help facilitate healing. Cognitive therapy may also be helpful for dealing with pain. The intensity of your condition is partly determined by how you perceive it—if you "catastrophize" the reaction or sensitivity, you may actually make it worse. Cognitive therapy can be used to gain control of your thought processes and allow you to alter your perception of pain.

### Neuro-Linguistic Programming

A technique similar to cognitive therapy, Neuro-Linguistic Programming (NLP) helps people detect unconscious patterns of thought, behavior, and attitudes that contribute to their illness. These unconscious patterns are then reprogrammed in order to alter psychological responses and facilitate the healing process. *Neuro* refers to the way the brain works and how thinking demonstrates consistent and detectable patterns; *linguistic* refers to the verbal and nonverbal expressions of thinking patterns; *programming* refers to how these patterns are recognized and understood by the mind and how they can be altered.

NLP was developed in the early 1970s by a professor of linguistics and a student of psychology and mathematics, both at the University of California at Santa Cruz. They studied the thinking processes, language patterns, and behavioral patterns of several accomplished individuals. They found that body cues—eye movement, posture, voice tone, and breathing patterns—coincided with certain unconscious patterns of a person's emotional state. Based on their findings, they developed the NLP technique to help people with emotional problems.

People who have difficulty recovering from physical illness have often adopted negative beliefs about their recovery. They perceive themselves as helpless, hopeless, or worthless, expressed in statements like "I can't get healthy" or "There's no hope." NLP tries to move the person from their present state of discomfort to a desired state of health by helping reprogram these beliefs about healing.

NLP practitioners ask questions to discover how the person relates to issues of identity, personal beliefs, life goals, and their health, then observe the person's language patterns, eye movements, postures, muscle tension, and gestures. These relay information about how the person relates to their condition in both conscious and unconscious ways, revealing what limiting beliefs may exist.

These belief structures can then be altered using NLP. The practitioner will ask the person to see herself in a state of health. By doing so, an outcome is set that facilitates the healing process. The brain's natural response is to duplicate whatever images or beliefs are created about getting better.[30] The brain then triggers the necessary immunological responses to guide the body toward health.

NLP has proved successful in treating people with chronic illnesses, such as AIDs, cancer, allergies, and arthritis. Once a chronically ill patient adopts new patterns of thought and behavior, an outcome is set that triggers the necessary immunological responses to guide the body toward its goal of health and well-being.

For more on **Neuro-Linguistic Programming**, contact: NLP University/Dynamic Learning Center, P.O. Box 1112, Ben Lomond, CA 95005; tel: 831-336-3457; fax: 831-336-5854; website: www.nlpu.com. NLP Comprehensive, 12567 West Cedar Drive, Suite 102, Lakewood, CO 80228; tel: 800-233-1657 or 303-987-2224; website: www.nlpcomprehensive.com. NLP Seminars Group International, P.O. Box 424, Hopatcong, NJ 07843; tel: 973-770-1084; website: www.purenlp.com.

## Biofeedback

Biofeedback training is a method of learning how to consciously regulate normally unconscious bodily functions (such as breathing, heart rate, and blood pressure) through the use of simple electronic devices. Biofeedback is particularly useful for learning to reduce stress, eliminate headaches, reduce muscle spasms, and relieve pain, all components of allergy and sensitivity reactions. It can also intercept a chronic fight-or-flight response and aid in revitalizing adrenal gland functions. By teaching patients both relaxation techniques and control over their muscle spasms, biofeedback helps them reduce or eliminate pain associated with allergy.[31]

For information on **biofeedback** or for referrals, contact: Association for Applied Physiopsychology and Biofeedback, 10200 West 44th Avenue, Suite 304, Wheat Ridge, CO 80033; tel: 303-422-8436; fax: 303-422-8894; website: www.aapb.org.

Biofeedback devices give immediate "feedback" or information about the biological system of the person being monitored, so that he or she can learn to consciously influence that system. For example, a person seeking to regulate their heart rate would train with a biofeedback device set up to transmit one blinking light or one audible beep per heartbeat. Electrodes are placed on the patient's skin (a simple, painless process). The patient is then instructed to use various techniques such as meditation, relaxation, and visualization to effect the desired response (muscle relaxation, lowered heart rate, or lowered temperature). The biofeedback device reports the patient's progress by a change in the speed of the beeps or flashes. By learning to alter the rate of the flashes or beeps, the person would be subtly programmed to control the heart rate.

"Central for a person in pain is the need to begin to take some degree of control of the situation, to feel empowered to influence the processes at work and not to feel himself or herself to be a mere object. When a person suffering pain understands the causes, natures, mechanisms, and role of the pain or illness, a vital step has been taken in the successful handling of the problem," according to Leon Chaitow, N.D., D.O.[32] Biofeedback helps the patient take this critical step in controlling allergy-related pain.

## Hypnotherapy

Hypnotherapy has therapeutic applications for both psychological and physical disorders. A skilled hypnotherapist can facilitate profound changes in respiration and relaxation to create positive shifts in behavior and an enhanced sense of well-being. A physiological shift can be observed in a hypnotic state, as can greater control of autonomic nervous system functions normally considered to be beyond one's ability to control. Stress reduction is a common occurrence as is a lowering of blood pressure.

Hypnosis can be used to alleviate many varieties of pain, headaches and migraines, and various allergies. It works by accessing the unconscious mind and training it to react in a positive way to the experience of pain and discomfort, such as inducing an immediate sense of relaxation. Hypnotherapy can be a nurturing and highly relaxing experience. Certified hypnotherapists do not attempt to control your mind or take you into a state so deep that you do not have control over yourself. Most people are aware of everything that transpires during a hypnotherapy session, yet they are able to mobilize deeper levels of their mind to facilitate healing.

For more about **hypnotherapy**, contact: Bryan Knight, The International Registry of Professional Hypnotherapists, 7306 Sherbrooke Street West, Montreal, Quebec, Canada H4B 1R7; tel: 514-489-6733; fax: 514-485-3828; website: www.hypnosis.org.

In one study, 38 patients with skin allergy underwent three sessions in the laboratory—the first in which skin allergic reactions were provoked, another that served as a control, and a third during which the subjects underwent a cognitive-hypnotic procedure involving imagery and visualization. After hypnosis, the subjects' skin wheals significantly decreased compare to the control session. The researchers concluded that hypnosis instilled a sense of peacefulness and lowered blood pressure, which contributed to the reduction in skin symptoms.[33]

Hypnotherapy is currently taught in several allopathic medical programs and has been approved by the American Medical Association as a clinical adjunct in the management of chronic pain.[34] Some states certify the profession of hypnotherapy by requiring a certain level of training. Other types of practitioners, such as psychotherapists and body workers, may also use hypnosis as a tool to help their patients relax.

Some hypnotherapists can train you to hypnotize yourself. Self-hypnosis has been found to be beneficial to allergy sufferers. In a 1995 study, 34 allergy patients were taught self-hypnosis and practiced this therapy for two months. At the end of the period, 76% of the subjects reported an improvement in their symptoms, while 86% of patients on medication said they decreased their usage of these medicines.[35]

## Guided Imagery/Visualization

Using the power of the mind to evoke a positive physical response, guided imagery and visualization can modulate the immune system and reduce pain. The patient uses the imagination to elicit positive physiological responses. By directly accessing emotions, imagery can help an individual understand the needs that may be represented by an

# 14 Steps to Less Stress

Although stressful situations are unavoidable, the following guidelines can help you avoid the emotional strain of stress:

- Plan regular diversions and cultivate interests outside of work.
- Get enough sleep—establish a regular bedtime hour and avoid sleeping pills.
- Do exercises that you enjoy, appropriate for your age and physical condition, on a daily basis.
- Avoid hurry and worry—these are learned behaviors that can interfere with your patterns of eating, sleeping, working, and recreation; they can be unlearned.
- Don't be afraid of compromise. In a stressful situation, you can either fight back, back off, or compromise. Seldom are the ideal circumstances available.
- Love more—learn to use things and love people rather than vice versa.
- Identify your fears. You can even list them. Fears add to paralysis.
- Make a decision, right or wrong, and then act on it. Anxiety results when you sit in the middle, allowing your fears to tug at you from opposite directions.
- Laugh more—laughter is a good tension breaker.
- Try to remain calm in the face of stressful situations. After unavoidable upsets, reestablish serenity.
- Avoid self-pity.
- Avoid loneliness—reach out and take the initiative in friendship.
- Avoid coping solutions that involve alcohol or drugs. This also applies to stimulants such as tobacco, caffeine, and sugar.
- Consider alleviating stress and achieving a state of relaxed awareness through techniques such as meditation, yoga, *qigong*, biofeedback, prayer, or self-hypnosis.

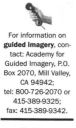

For information on **guided imagery**, contact: Academy for Guided Imagery, P.O. Box 2070, Mill Valley, CA 94942; tel: 800-726-2070 or 415-389-9325; fax: 415-389-9342.

illness and can help develop ways to meet those needs. Imagery is also one of the quickest and most direct ways to become aware of emotions and their effects on health, both positive and negative.

Imagery is simply a flow of thoughts that one can see, hear, feel, smell, taste, or experience. According to Martin L. Rossman, M.D., of the Academy for Guided Imagery, in Mill Valley, California, while the sensory phenomenon that is being experienced in the mind may not represent external reality, it always depicts internal reality. What Dr. Rossman means is that the sensations in the body that imagery creates are very real phenomena that can be measured via laboratory devices. Research using brain scans indicates that imagery activates parts of the cerebral cortex and centers of the primitive brain. During visualization, the visual (optic) cortex is active, and when sounds are imagined, the auditory cortex is active. It appears that the cortex can create imaginary realities and the lower centers (and perhaps every cell in the body) respond to this information.

"If you are a good worrier," states Dr., Rossman, "and especially if you ever 'worry yourself sick,' you may be an especially good candidate for learning how to positively affect your health with imagery, as the internal process involved in worrying yourself sick and 'imagining yourself well' are quite similar."[36] Imagery is a proven method for pain relief, helps people tolerate medical procedures, reduces side effects of treatments, and stimulates the body to heal.

**Allergy Elimination Imagery**—Mental health author and visualization expert Patrick Fanning includes several allergy visualizations in his book *Visualization for Change*.[37] The following, a brief synopsis based on one of his allergy visualizations, illustrates the role of metaphor in creating vivid images to facilitate the desired outcome—an elimination of your allergies:

Visualize a police SWAT team. Imagine them storming through the neighborhood (your body) as they mistakenly pursue innocent allergens whom they believe are terrorists (antibodies attacking harmless substances). When they learn that they have made a mistake and that there are no criminals in the area, they quietly retreat (you are now imagining the allergic reaction being turned off).

An affirmation, such as "Everything is under control" or "My body responds appropriately," can accompany such a visualization. To be most effective, the imagery should be vivid and detailed as in watching a movie.

### HeartMath

It's no secret that the heart is directly involved in our experience of emotions. Most people are aware that fright, anxiety, and stress, among other feelings, rev up the heart rate—a pounding heart is a common sign of strong emotions. Indeed, scientists have found that even the slightest emotional change immediately shifts heart rate variability (HRV).

Heart rate variability is the measurement of beat-to-beat changes in the heart rate; it is also called heart rhythm. Contrary to some commonly held beliefs, a healthy heart does not beat at steady intervals throughout the day. In fact, the intervals between heartbeats vary, even while we're asleep. Scientists at the Institute of HeartMath, in Boulder Creek, California, have found that the HRV serves as a communication tool among the heart, brain, and body. A sudden, rapid, erratic heartbeat pattern signals the brain and body via the nervous system that an emotionally charged situation is at hand.

# Herbal Allies for Stress Management

Several herbs can help you relax and avoid being overwhelmed by stress. Below are some of the most popular and widely available calming herbs.[38] As with all herbs, pregnant or nursing women or people on medications should consult their doctors before taking remedies. Also, make sure you're not allergic to the herbs; some people may be allergic to chamomile or hops. These herbs function as mild sedatives, so use with caution.

■ Chamomile (*Matricaria recutita*): A calming herb good for insomnia and nervousness, it also reduces inflammation of the skin and mucous membranes. German chamomile is stronger than Roman chamomile. Typical dose: up to six 300-400 mg capsules daily; 1/2-1 tsp dried flowers in one cup of hot water three to four time daily; 10-40 drops of tincture three times daily.

■ Hops (*Humulus lupulus*): Good for nervous tension, excitability, restlessness, anxiety, and sleep problems. Typical dose: 1 tsp. dried hops in one cup hot water daily; 10-40 drops of tincture three times daily.

■ Passionflower (*Passiflora incarnata*): Good for anxiety and attendant insomnia. Typical dose: 1/2 tsp dried herb in one cup hot water daily; 20-40 drops of tincture up to four times daily.

■ Skullcap (*Scutellaria lateriflora*): A mild sedative good for frazzled nerves. Typical dose: up to six 425 mg capsules daily; 1-2 tsp dried herb one cup hot water daily; 20-40 drops of tincture up to four times daily.

■ Valerian (*Valeriana officinalis*): Excellent for anxiety and insomnia. Typical dose: 10-30 drops tincture daily; one 300-400 mg capsule daily as needed. May cause temporary stomach upset in some people.

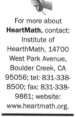

For more about **HeartMath**, contact: Institute of HearthMath, 14700 West Park Avenue, Boulder Creek, CA 95056; tel: 831-338-8500; fax: 831-338-9861; website: www.heartmath.org.

For more on **using magnesium for reducing allergy symptoms**, see Chapter 11: Supplements for Symptom Control, pp. 278-303.

Learning to modulate heart rate variability can effectively reduce negative responses to stressful situations, and improve your health. The Institute of HeartMath has developed special techniques, under the name HeartMath, that are clinically proven to turn off the stress response and lower cortisol release,[39] improve cognitive performance and mood,[40] and reduce hypertension and the risk of dying from congestive heart failure and coronary heart disease.[41] These techniques employ strategies similar to cognitive therapy, biofeedback, visualization, transcendental meditation, and other established mind/body protocols.

One technique, called Freeze-Frame, is an effective stress-management strategy for dealing with daily stresses. It enables patients to arrest the stress response to difficult situations by replacing negative perceptions with positive feelings, such as feelings of appreciation, love, or fun. These feelings restore calm and control to the heart rate variability. This technique also encourages individuals to let the "higher" heart (the source of compassion) instead of the intellect (logical impartiality) guide them in appropriately responding to emotional situations in the future. The higher heart acts in a way that benefits both you and other people; for instance, avoiding an argument by finding common ground. The "lower" heart reacts sympathetically and with excessive sensitivity to other people's problems as well as to stressful situations; it isn't conducive to stress management. The intellect sometimes contradicts the higher heart, due to its tendency to simplify matters into black and white, right and wrong, and to exacerbate stressful situations.

## Restricted Environmental Stimulation Therapy (R.E.S.T.)

Restricted Environmental Stimulation Therapy (R.E.S.T.), a therapeutic tool that has been researched for more than 35 years, is known to aid individuals in relaxation. The principle behind this therapy is the isolation of the individual from sensory input from the external environment, accomplished by using a flotation tank.

Patients customarily float for one hour in a small, shallow flotation tank or pool. The water is 18 inches deep and supersaturated with 1,000-1,500 pounds of Epsom salts (magnesium sulfate). This makes the water so buoyant that it is impossible to sink. One just floats effortlessly on the surface and experiences something that only astronauts usually experience—the feeling of weightlessness. In addition, the environment of the flotation tank is specifically designed to reduce the perception of all external stimuli ("sensory deprivation"), which can lead to powerful healing effects on the body and mind. The water and air temperature is kept constant at 93°-94° F; this allows the person to lose the ability to dis-

## The Five Steps of Freeze-Frame

Here are the five steps of the Freeze-Frame stress management technique, as developed by scientists at the Institute of HeartMath and included in the book *The HeartMath Solution*.[42]

1. Recognize the stressful feeling and Freeze-Frame it. Take a time-out.

2. Make a sincere effort to shift your focus away from the racing mind or disturbed emotions to the area around your heart. Pretend you're breathing through your heart to help focus your energy in this area. Keep your focus there for ten seconds or more.

3. Recall a positive, fun feeling or time you've had in life and try to re-experience it.

4. Using your intuition, common sense, and sincerity, ask your heart, "What would be a more efficient response to the situation, one that would minimize future stress?"

5. Listen to what your heart says in answer to your question. It's an effective way to put your mind and emotions in check and find an "in-house," common-sense solution.

For more information on **flotation tanks**, contact: The Floatation Tank Association, P.O. Box 1396, Grass Valley, CA 95945-1396; tel: 916-432-4502; fax: 916-432-3794.

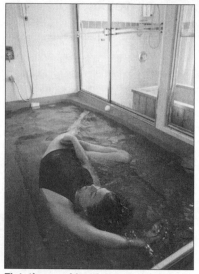

Flotation provides the most reliable induction of deep relaxation attainable without medication or years of training in meditation or biofeedback.

cern where the body ends and the outer environment begins.

Flotation provides the most reliable induction of deep relaxation attainable without medication or years of training in meditation or biofeedback. R.E.S.T. has been scientifically documented to produce a myriad of psychological and physiological responses that are conducive to relaxation. The following are particularly beneficial to the allergy patient: a decrease in pain,[43] diminished response to stress,[44] a decline in plasma cortisol levels,[45] and an increase in magnesium levels.[46] Magnesium is important because it helps muscles to relax and low levels can contribute to muscle spasms; asthma patients often have a deficiency of magnesium.

## Flower Essence Remedies

Flower essence remedies directly address a person's emotional state in order to facilitate both psychological and physiological well-being. By balancing negative feelings and stress, flower remedies can effectively remove the emotional barriers to health and recovery. Flower remedies comprise subtle liquid preparations made from the fresh blossoms of flowers, plants, bushes, even trees, to address emotional, psychological, and spiritual issues underlying physical and medical problems. The approach was pioneered by British physician Edward Bach in the 1930s, when he introduced the 38 Bach Flower Remedies, based on English plants.

For more about **flower essences**, contact: Flower Essence Society, P.O. Box 459, Nevada City, CA 95959; tel: 800-736-9222 or 530-265-9163; fax: 530-265-0584; website: www.flowersociety.org.

Today, an estimated 20 different brands of flower remedies, based on plants native to many landscapes, from Australia to India to Alaska, offer about 1,500 different blends for a diverse range of psychological conditions. The flower remedies each address a particular emotional issue: Lavender is recommended for overwhelming nervousness; Pink Yarrow is for those who are excessively susceptible to absorbing the emotional stress and psychic negativity from others; Elm is for those who feel overwhelmed and stressed out from assuming too many responsibilities. Five-Flower Formula (Rescue Remedy) is suggested as a first-line of defense after an episode of extreme stress, such as an accident. An individual formula can be made by combining four to six of the remedies and taking them orally or rubbing them into the skin. They can be taken for a short time to cope with a crisis or for a period of months.

## Aromatherapy

Aromatherapy is a unique branch of herbal medicine that utilizes the medicinal properties found in the essential oils of various plants. Through a process of steam distillation or cold-pressing, the volatile constituents of the plant's oil (its essence) are extracted from its flowers, leaves, branches, or roots. The immediate and often profound effect that essential oils have on the central nervous system also makes aromatherapy an excellent method for stress management.[48] The term *aromatherapy* was coined in 1937 by the French chemist Rene-Maurice Gattefosse, who observed the healing effect of lavender oil on burns.

Essential oils have a number of pharmacological properties—antibacterial, antiviral, antispasmodic, as diuretics (promoting production and excretion of urine), and as vasodilators (widening blood vessels). They are able to energize or pacify, detoxify, and help digestion. The oils' therapeutic properties also make them effective for treating infection, interacting with the various branches of the nervous system, modifying

## How to Use Aromatherapy

Aromatherapy uses essential oils to affect the body in several ways. The benefits of essential oils can be obtained through inhalation, external application, or ingestion.

■ Through a diffusor: Diffusors disperse microparticles of the essential oil into the air. They can be used to achieve beneficial results in respiratory conditions, or to simply change the air with the mood-lifting or calming qualities of the fragrance.

■ External application: Oils are readily absorbed through the skin. Convenient applications are baths, massages, hot and cold compresses, or a simple topical application of diluted oils.[47] Essential oils in a hot bath can stimulate the skin, induce relaxation, and energize the body. In massage, the oils can be worked into the skin and depending on the oil and the massage technique, can either calm or stimulate an individual. When used in compresses, essential oils soothe minor aches and pains, reduce swelling, and treat sprains.

■ Floral waters: These can be sprayed into the air or sprayed on skin that is too sensitive to the touch.

■ Internal application: For certain conditions (such as organ dysfunction), it can be advantageous to take oils internally. It is essential to receive proper medical guidance for internal use of oils.

For information about **aromatherapy oils**, contact:

PhytoMedicine Company, 6701 Sunset Drive, Suite 100, Miami, FL 33143; tel: 305-662-6396; fax: 305-667-5619.

Many essential oils come from plants that are weeds or used as highway barriers. Many people are sensitized to them and will have reactions when they are applied. Especially be careful of melaleuca (tea tree oil), sage, rosemary, juniper, and cedar. In their pure state, certain oils, such as clove and cinnamon, can cause irritation or skin burns. These oils require careful and expert application. It is recommended that they be diluted with a less irritating oil before being applied to the skin. Essential oils can cause toxic reactions if ingested. Consult a physician before taking any oils internally.

immune response, and harmonizing moods and emotions. Aromatic molecules that interact with the nasal cavity give off signals that travel to the limbic system, the emotional switchboard of the brain.[49] There, they create impressions associated with previous experiences and emotions. The limbic system is directly connected to those parts of the brain that control heart rate, blood pressure, breathing, memory, stress levels, and hormone balance.

John Steele, Ph.D., of Sherman Oaks, California, and Robert Tisserand, of London, England, leading researchers in the field of aromatherapy, have studied the effects on brain-wave patterns when essential oils are inhaled or smelled. Their findings show that oils such as orange, jasmine, and rose have a tranquilizing effect and work by altering the brain waves into a rhythm that produces calmness and a sense of well-being.[50] Essential oils like citronella and *Eucalyptus citriodora* can be diffused in the air or rubbed on the wrists, solar plexus, and temples for quick and effective relaxation. Lavender oil added to the bath or sprayed on the bed sheets reduces tension and enhances relaxation.[51] Roman chamomile (*Anthemis nobilis*) is also recommended to calm an upset mind or body. A drop rubbed on the solar plexus can bring rapid relief of mental or physical stress.

## Qigong

*Qigong* (also referred to as chi-kung) is an ancient exercise that stimulates and balances the flow of *qi* along acupuncture meridians (energy pathways). *Qigong* cultivates inner strength, calms the mind, and restores the body to its natural state of health. *Qigong* is fairly easy to learn and can be done by the severely disabled as well as the healthy. *Qigong* practice can range from simple calisthenics-type movements with breath coordination to complex exercises that direct brain-wave frequencies, deep relaxation, and breathing to improve strength and flexibility and reverse damage caused by prior injuries and disease.

*Qigong* can be especially helpful to allergy patients because it initiates relaxation, moderates pain and depression, and regulates the immune system. It also enhances the lymphatic flow, which improves the ability of the body to detoxify and deliver vital, replenishing nutrients to target tissues. *Qigong* can also balance the function of hormone-producing glands, which mediate pain and mood.

*Qigong* has also been found to stabilize and improve immune function, an important benefit for allergy patients who are suffering from overwhelmed, hyperactive immune systems. In a 1995 study, healthy male volunteers between the ages of 20 and 50 were trained in *qigong* for five months. At the end of that time, their white blood cell levels were measured. Researchers showed that levels of important T cells (called CD4) were elevated, indicating a stronger immune system.[52]

See "Qigong,"
pp. 422-433, and
"Yoga," pp. 469-481.

## Yoga

Yoga is one of the most ancient systems of self-healing practiced today. Yoga teaches a basic principle of mind/body unity: if the mind is chronically restless and agitated, the health of the body will be compromised. Similarly, if the body is in poor health, mental strength and clarity will be adversely affected. The art of yoga can bring about harmony and oneness of mind, body, and spirit.

Classical yoga is divided into eight branches that give guidance as to the proper diet, hygiene, detoxification regimes, and physical/psychological practices to help the individual integrate their personal, psychological, and spiritual awareness. The most well-known and popular of the yogic branches is Hatha yoga, which teaches certain *asanas* (postures) and breathing techniques to create profound changes in the body and mind. According to Ameni Harris, a nutritionist and yoga teacher trained at the Integral Yoga Ashram in Buckingham, Virginia, yoga can benefit most illnesses if done on a regular basis. One goal of yoga is to harness and stimulate the flow of *prana*, or life energy (similar to *qi* in the Chinese system). The blockage of *prana*, through improper diet, lifestyle stressors, or imbalance in one's physical, emotional, or spiritual health, can lead to illness.

For **Ameni Harris'** yoga and stress management instructional guide or video, contact: Ameni Harris, 37 Geraldine Circle, Trumbull, CT 06611; tel: 203-261-6256.

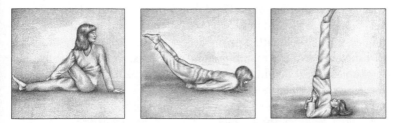

Yoga postures or *asanas*: half spinal twist, locust, and shoulder stand.

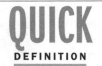

## QUICK
### DEFINITION

The **lymphatic system** consists of lymph fluid and the structures (vessels, ducts, and nodes) involved in transporting it from tissues to the bloodstream. Lymph fluid occupies the space between the body's cells and contains plasma proteins, foreign particles, and cellular wastes. Lymph nodes are clusters of immune tissue that work as filters or "inspection stations" for detecting and removing foreign and potentially harmful substances in the lymph fluid. While the body has hundreds of lymph nodes (more than 500), they are mostly clustered in the neck, armpits, chest, groin, and abdomen. The lymphatic system is the body's master drain, collecting and filtering the lymph fluid and conveying it to the bloodstream, thereby clearing waste products and cellular debris from the tissues.

Breathing techniques and duration of holding certain postures remove barriers to the flow of *prana* and can improve oxygen intake by as much as seven times over a normal breath, according to Harris.[53]

In addition to improving circulation of blood, lymph, and *prana*, yoga corrects imbalances of hormones by regulating chakras (the energy centers that correspond to hormone-producing glands). The lymphatic system (SEE QUICK DEFINITION) doesn't have a pump of its own, instead it depends on movement of the body to transport fluid in and out of tissues. When a person is inactive or motion is imbalanced, the lymphatic fluid can become stagnant and create disease. Through yoga's stretches and postures, lymphatic fluid is pumped throughout the body, removing toxins and waste products from cells and delivering fresh nutrients.

"Anyone can do yoga, no matter what age or shape you are in," states Harris. "Even if you are very ill, you can begin with gentle, modified postures, using props, pillows, or the wall to buttress you in weakened areas. Before pursuing a yoga practice, one should discuss it with a physician and should seek out a qualified yoga teacher for proper instruction. Videos are also excellent tools for the beginner, as it is important to see the postures being performed." The safest and most reliable way to use yoga therapeutically is to follow a balanced program of postures to achieve an overall normalizing and health-inducing effect. It is best for the beginner to start with a simple program of basic postures. A structured course can teach the fundamental breathing techniques and postures for exercises later practiced on one's own.

Scientists have also found that yoga can be therapeutic for people with asthma.[54] In one study, 17 adult asthmatics ranging from 19 to 52 years old, were divided into two groups—nine were taught yoga techniques, including breath-slowing exercises, physical posture exercises, and mediation; the remaining eight patients served as controls. The test subjects were taught yoga three times a week for 16 weeks. During the 16 weeks, all subjects maintained logs of symptoms and medication use; the researchers also took samples of morning and evening peak flow readings (how amount of air they can expire—low levels indicate airway obstruction). By the end of the test period, researchers found that the test group reported a significant degree of relaxation and positive attitude compared to the control group. They also tended to use inhalers less than the controls did. Pulmonary function did not vary significantly between groups, but the yoga techniques did prove to prevent exacerbation of asthma attacks.[55]

# Endnotes

## Chapter I

### Understanding Allergy and Sensitivity

1 American Academy of Allergy, Asthma & Immunology. *The Allergy Report* 1 (Milwaukee, WI: American Academy of Allergy, Asthma & Immunology, 2000), 1.

2 Ibid., 2.

3 A. Schapowal. "Do Allergic Diseases Increase?" *Allergologie* 20:11 (1997), S560-S564.

4 Marshall Plaut, M.D. "New Directions in Food Allergy Research." *Journal of Allergy and Clinical Immunology* 100:1 (July 1997), 7-10.

5 "Multiple Chemical Sensitivity: A 1999 Consensus." *Archives of Environmental Health* 54:3 (May/June 1999), 147-149.

6 Ibid., 147-149.

7 Jonathan Brostoff, M.D., and Linda Gamlin. *The Complete Guide to Food Allergy and Intolerance* (New York: Crown Publishers, 1989), 1-9.

8 Theron G. Randolph, M.D. *Human Ecology and Susceptibility to the Chemical Environment* (Springfield, IL: C.C. Thomas, 1962).

9 Hugh A. Sampson, M.D. "Food Allergy." *Journal of the American Medical Association* 278:22 (1997), 1888-1894.

10 M. Turner-Warwick. "Epidemiology of Nocturnal Asthma." *American Journal of Medicine* 85:1B (1988), 6-8. See also: D.J. Pincus, W.R. Beam, and R.J. Martin. "Chronobiology and Chronotherapy of Asthma." *Clinics in Chest Medicine* 16 (1995), 699-713. A DiStefano et al. "Nocturnal Asthma: Mechanisms and Therapy." *Lung* 175 (1997), 53-61.

11 National Jewish Center for Immunology and Respiratory Medicine. *New Directions* 25:2 (Spring 1996), 1-2.

12 M.H. Chandler et al. "Premenstrual Asthma: The Effect of Estrogen on Symptoms, Pulmonary Function, and Beta 2 Receptors." *Pharmacotherapy* 17:2 (March/April 1997), 224-234.

13 M.H. Smolensky, A. Reinberg, and G. Labrecque. "Twenty-Four Hour Pattern in Symptom Intensity of Viral and Allergic Rhinitis: Treatment Implications." *Journal of Allergy and Clinical Immunology* 95:5 Part 2 (May 1995), 1084-1096.

14 American Academy of Allergy, Asthma & Immunology. *The Allergy Report* 2 (Milwaukee, WI: American Academy of Allergy, Asthma & Immunology, 2000), 69.

15 Edward Edelson. *The Encyclopedia of Health: Allergies* (New York: Chelsea House Publishers, 1989), 53.

16 U.S. Centers for Disease Control and Prevention. *Fastats A to Z: Allergies/Hay Fever* (May 1998). Available on the Internet at web page: www.cdc.gov/nchswww/fastats/allergys.htm

17 American Academy of Allergy, Asthma & Immunology. *The Allergy Report* 1 (Milwaukee, WI: American Academy of Allergy, Asthma & Immunology, 2000), 1.

18 Jonathan Corren, M.D. "The Impact of Allergic Rhinitis on Bronchial Asthma." *Journal of Allergy and Clinical Immunology* 101:2 Part 2 (February 1998), S352-S356.

19 American Academy of Allergy, Asthma & Immunology. *The Allergy Report* 2 (Milwaukee, WI: American Academy of Allergy, Asthma & Immunology, 2000), 156.

20 American Academy of Allergy, Asthma & Immunology. *The Allergy Report* 1 (Milwaukee, WI: American Academy of Allergy, Asthma & Immunology, 2000), 2.

21 Michael Murray, N.D., and Joseph Pizzorno, N.D. *Encyclopedia of Natural Medicine*, Revised 2nd Edition (Rocklin, CA: Prima Publishing, 1998), 261.

22 U.S. Centers for Disease Control and Prevention. *Vital and Health Statistics, Current Estimates from the National Health Interview Survey*, 1994 DHHS Publication

No. PHS96-1521 (Washington, DC: U.S. Department of Health and Human Services, Public Health Services, National Center for Health Statistics, 1995).

23 U.S. Department of Health and Human Services. "Table 10: Number of Deaths from 72 Selected Causes, Human Immunodeficiency Virus Infection, and Alzheimer's Disease by Age, U.S., 1997." *National Vital Statistics Report* 47:19 (June 30, 1999).

24 American Academy of Allergy, Asthma & Immunology. *Asthma and Allergy Management News* (June 1997), 3.

25 S. Quirce and J. Sastre. "Occupational Asthma." *Allergy* 53 (1998), 633-641.

26 U.S. Centers for Disease Control and Prevention. *Vital and Health Statistics, Current Estimates from the National Health Interview Survey*, 1994 DHHS Publication No. PHS96-1521 (Washington, DC: U.S. Department of Health and Human Services, Public Health Services, National Center for Health Statistics, I995).

27 Claudia Glenn Dowling and Anne Hollister. "An Epidemic of Sneezing and Wheezing." *Life* (May 1997), 78-92.

28 R. Evans. "Asthma Among Minority Children: A Growing Problem." *Chest* 101:6 (1992), 3668-3671.

29 American Academy of Allergy, Asthma & Immunology. *The Allergy Report* 1 (Milwaukee, WI: American Academy of Allergy, Asthma & Immunology, 2000), 3.

30 Jonathan Corren, M.D. "The Impact of Allergic Rhinitis on Bronchial Asthma." *Journal of Allergy and Clinical Immunology* 101:2 Part 2 (February 1998), S352-S356.

31 American Academy of Allergy, Asthma & Immunology. *The Allergy Report* 1 (Milwaukee, WI: American Academy of Allergy, Asthma & Immunology, 2000), 3.

32 American Academy of Allergy, Asthma & Immunology. *The Allergy Report* 2 (Milwaukee, WI: American Academy of Allergy, Asthma & Immunology, 2000), 111.

33 Ibid.

34 American Academy of Allergy, Asthma &

Immunology. *The Allergy Report* 3 (Milwaukee, WI: American Academy of Allergy, Asthma & Immunology, 2000), 17.

35 Ibid., 71.

36 "Hotline." *American Family Physician* (June I997).

37 American Academy of Allergy, Asthma & Immunology. *Fast Facts: Statistics on Asthma & Allergic Diseases* ((Milwaukee, WI: American Academy of Allergy, Asthma & Immunology, October 1999). Available at website: www.aaaai.org.

38 Michael Murray, N.D. and Joseph Pizzorno, N.D. *Encyclopedia of Natural Medicine*, Revised 2nd Edition (Rocklin, CA: Prima Publishing, 1998), 468.

39 Ibid., 468.

40 American Academy of Allergy, Asthma & Immunology. *Allergic Disorders: Promoting Best Practice—Executive Summary Report* (Milwaukee, WI: American Academy of Allergy, Asthma & Immunology, November 1998), 3.

41 Jacqueline Krohn, M.D., Frances A. Taylor, M.A., and Erla Mae Larson, R.N. *The Whole Way to Allergy Relief and Prevention, Revised Edition* (Vancouver, B.C.: Hartley & Marks Publishers, 1996), 125.

42 Sherry A. Rogers, M.D. *The E.I. Syndrome: An Rx For Environmental Illness* (Syracuse, NY: Prestige Publishing, 1986), 325.

43 W. J. Meggs. "Mechanisms of Allergy and Chemical Sensitivity." *Toxicology and Industrial Health* 15:3-4 (April-June 1999), 331-338.

44 Cynthia Wilson. "MCS: A World-Wide Problem." *Our Toxic Times* (August 1995), 1-5.

45 National Foundation for the Chemically Hypersensitive. *Cheers* 1 (1989), 6.

## Chapter 2

### Causes of Allergy and Sensitivity

1 P. Parronchi et al. "Genetic and Environmental Factors Contributing to the Onset of Allergic Disorders." *International Archives of Allergy and Immunology* 121:1 (January 2000), 2-9.

See also: C. Ober et al. "Variation in the Interleukin 4–Receptor Alpha Gene Confers Asthma and Atopy in Ethnically Diverse Populations." *American Journal of Human Genetics* 66:2 (February 2000), 517-526.

2 T.D. Howard, D.A. Meyers, and E.R. Bleecker. "Mapping Susceptibility Genes for Asthma and Allergy." *Journal of Allergy and Clinical Immunology* 10:2 Part 2 (February 2000), 477-481.

3 P.S. Gao et al. "Variants of NOS1, NOS2, and NOS3 Genes in Asthmatics." *Biochemical and Biophysical Research Communications* 267:3 (January 2000), 761-763. See also: H. Grasemann, C.N. Yandava, and J.M. Drazen. "Neuronal NO Synthase (NOS1) is a Major Candidate Gene for Asthma." *Clinical and Experimental Allergy* 29:Suppl 4 (December 1999), 39-41.

4 J.W. Gerrard et al. "The Familial Incidence of Allergy Disease." *Annals of Allergy* 36 (1976), 10.

5 F. Haschke et al. "Does Breast Feeding Protect from Atopic Diseases?" *Padiatrie und Padologie* 25:6 (1990), 415-420.

6 D. de Boissieu, C. Dupont, and J. Badoual. "Allergy to Nondairy Proteins in Mother's Milk as Assessed by Intestinal Permeability Tests." *Allergy* 49:10 (December 1994), 882-884.

7 K. Van Duren-Schmidt et al. "Prenatal Contact with Inhalant Allergens." *Pediatric Research* 41:1 (January 1997), 128-131.

8 J.A. Warner et al. "Prenatal Origins of Allergic Disease." *Journal of Allergy and Clinical Immunology* 105:2 Part 2 (February 2000), 493-498.

9 V. Singh and V. Yang. "Serological Association of Measles Virus and Human Herpes Virus-6 with Brain Autoantibodies in Autism." *Clinical Immunology and Immunopathology* 88:1 (1988), 105-108.

10 A. Assa'ad and M. Lierl. "Effect of Acellular Pertussis Vaccine on the Development of Allergic Sensitization to Environmental Allergens in Adults." *Journal of Allergy and Clinical Immunology* 105:1 Part 1 (January 2000), 170-175.

11 P.M. Matricardi et al. "Exposure to Foodborne and Orofecal Microbes Versus Airborne Viruses in Relation to Atopy and Allergic Asthma: Epidemiological Study." *British Medical Journal* 320 (February 12, 2000), 412-407.

12 P. Ernst and Y. Cormier. "Relative Scarcity of Asthma and Atopy among Rural Adolescents Raised on a Farm." *American Journal of Respiratory and Clinical Care Medicine* 161:5 (May 1, 2000), 1563-1566.

13 Erika Isolauri, M.D. "Intestinal Involvement in Atopic Disease." *Journal of the Royal Society of Medicine* 90:Supplement 30 (1997), 15-20.

14 P. V. Kirjavainen and G.R. Givson. "Healthy Gut Microflora and Allergy: Factors Influencing Development of the Microbiota." *Annals of Medicine* 31:4 (August 1999), 288-292.

15 D.M. Fergussen, J.L. Horwood, and F.T. Shannon. "Early Solid Feeding and Recurrent Childhood Eczema: A 10-Year Longitudinal Study." *Pediatrics* 86:4 (October 1990), 541-546.

16 Leo Galland, M.D. *The Four Pillars of Healing* (New York: Random House, 1997), 188-191.

17 Humbart Santillo. *Food Enzymes: The Missing Link to Radiant Health* (Prescott, AZ: Holm Press, 1987), 19-22. See also: Carolee Bateson-Koch, D.C., N.D. *Allergies: Disease in Disguise* (Burnaby, BC, Canada: Alive Books, 1994), 97.

18 Jonathan Brostoff, M.D., and Linda Gamlin. *The Complete Guide to Food Allergy and Intolerance* (New York: Crown, 1989), 264-265.

19 James Braly M.D. *Dr. Braly's Food Allergy & Nutrition Revolution* (New Canaan, CT: Keats Publishing, 1992), 241.

20 B. Salah et al. "Nasal Mucociliary Transport in Healthy Subjects Slower When Breathing Dry Air." *European Respiratory Journal* 1:9 (October 1988), 852-855.

21 D. Passali et al. "Nasal Allergy and Atmospheric Pollution." *International Journal of Pediatric Otorhinolaryngology* 49:Suppl 1 (October 5, 1999), S257-S260. See also: N. Keles, C. Ilicali, and K. Deger. "The Effects of Different Levels of Air Pollution on Atopy and

Symptoms of Allergic Rhinitis." *American Journal of Rhinology* 13:3 (May/June 1999), 185-190.

22 National Air Quality and Emissions Trend Report, 1997. (Washington, DC: U.S. Environmental Protection Agency, Office of Air Quality Planning and Standards, December 1998).

23 J.O. Crawford and S.M. Bolas. "Sick Building Syndrome, Work Factors and Occupational Stress." *Scandinavian Journal of Work and Environmental Health* 22:4 (August 1996), 243-250.

24 William J. Rea, M.D. *Chemical Sensitivity*, Vol. 3 (Boca Raton, FL: CRC Lewis, 1996), 1555-1579.

25 G.E. Hatch. "Asthma, Inhaled Oxidants, and Dietary Antioxidants." *American Journal of Clinical Nutrition* 61:3 Suppl (March 1995), 625S-630S.

26 William Lee Cowden, M.D. "Is Your Shower Toxic? Some Pollution Solutions." *Alternative Medicine* 29 (April/May 1999), 69.

27 Aristo Vojdani, Ph.D., M.T. "Evidence for the Mechanisms Behind Immunotherapy: Current Applications and Promising Potential Use for the Future." Presentation at American Academy of Environmental Medicine 33rd Annual Meeting, Baltimore, MD (November 1998).

28 William Lee Cowden, M.D. "Is Your Shower Toxic? Some Pollution Solutions." *Alternative Medicine* 29 (April/May 1999), 69.

29 I. Skare and A. Engqvist. "Human Exposure to Mercury and Silver Released from Dental Amalgam Restorations." *Archives of Environmental Health* 49 (1994), 384-394.

30 W. Melillo. "How Safe is Mercury in Dentistry?" The Washington Post Weekly *Journal of Medicine, Science and Society* (September 1991), 4.

31 Agency for Toxic Substances and Disease Registry, 1993. Division of Toxicology Chart.

32 World Health Organization. *Environmental Health Criteria for Inorganic Mercury* 118 (Geneva, Switzerland: World Health Organization, 1991).

33 David W. Quig. "Metal Binding Proteins and Heavy Metal Detoxification." Presentation at American Academy of Environmental Medicine 33rd Annual Meeting, Baltimore, MD (November 1998).

34 William J. Rea, M.D. *Chemical Sensitivity*, Vol. 3 (Boca Raton, FL: CRC Lewis, 1996), 1555-1579.

35 "Copper Toxicity Paper 5." Available from: Eck Institute of Applied Nutrition and Bioenergetics, Ltd., 8650 North 22nd Avenue, Phoenix, AZ 85021; tel: 602-995-1580.

36 D.N. Taylor et al. "Effects of Trichloroethylene in the Exploratory and Locomotor Activity in Rats Exposed During Development." *Science of the Total Environment* 47 (1985), 415-420. See also: H.N. Arito et al. "Partial Insomnia, Hyperactivity and Hyperdipsia Induced by Repeated Administration of Toluene in Rats: Their Relation to Brain Monoamine Metabolism." *Toxicology* 37:1-2 (1985), 99-110.

37 Kenneth Bock, M.D., and Nellie Sabin. *The Road to Immunity* (New York: Pocket Books, 1997), 38.

38 G. Mann. "Hypothesis: The Role of Vitamin C in Diabetic Angiopathy." *Perspectives in Biology and Medicine* 17 (1974), 210-217. See also: G. Mann and P. Newton. "The Membrane Support of Ascorbic Acid." *Annals of the New York Academy of Sciences* 258 (1975), 243-251.

39 A. Sanchez et al. "Role of Sugars in Human Neutrophilic Phagocytosis." *American Journal of Clinical Nutrition* 26 (1973), 1180-1184. See also: W. Rindsdorf, E. Cherskin, and R. Ramsay. "Sucrose, Neutrophi Phagocytosis, and Resistance to Disease." *Dental Survey* 52 (1976), 46-48. J. Bernstein et al. "Depression of Lymphocyte Transformation Following Oral Glucose Ingestion." *American Journal of Clinical Nutrition* 30 (1977), 613.

40 Jon D. Kaiser. *Immune Power* (New York: St. Martin's Press, 1993), 29.

## Chapter 3

### Allergy/Sensitivity Testing

1 Jaqueline Krohn, M.D., Frances A. Taylor, M.A., and Erla Mae Larson, R.N. *The Whole Way to Allergy Relief & Prevention* (Vancouver, BC, Canada: Hartley & Marks Publishers, 1996), 55.

2 J. Krop et al. "A Double-Blind, Randomized, Controlled Investigation of Electrodermal Testing in the Diagnosis of Allergies." *Journal of Alternative and Complementary Medicine* 3:3 (Fall 1997), 241-248.

3 Will Block and John Morgenthaler, "Food Allergies More Common Than You Think: Interview with Michael Rosenbaum, M.D." *Life Enhancement* 34 (June 1997), 3-7.

4 Elson Haas, M.D. *Staying Healthy with Nutrition* (Berkeley, CA: Celestial Arts, I992), 879.

5 Ralph Golan, M.D. *Optimal Wellness* (New York: Ballantine Books, 1995).

6 Stephen Langer, M.D., with James F. Scheer. *Solved: The Riddle of Weight Loss* (Rochester, VT: Healing Arts Press, 1989), 52.

7 Ralph Golan, M.D. *Optimal Wellness* (New York: Ballantine Books, 1995).

8 Phillip Shinnick. "An Introduction to the Basic Technique and Theory of Omura's Bi-Digital O-Ring Test." *American Journal of Acupuncture* 24:2/3 (1996), 195-204.

9 Doris J. Rapp, M.D., F.A.A.A., F.A.A.P. "Make the Connection." Available from: Practical Allergy Research Foundation. P.O. Box 60, Buffalo, NY 14223; tel: 800-787-8780.

10 F.J. Kelly et al. "Altered Lung Antioxidant Status in Patients with Mild Asthma." *The Lancet* 354:9177 (August 7, 1999), 482-483.

11 David Casemore, M.D. "Foodborne Protozoal Infection." *The Lancet* 336 (December 1990), 1427-1432.

12 D.W. Bendig, M.D. "Diagnosis of Giardiasis in Infants and Children by Endoscopic Brush Cytology." *Journal of Pediatric Gastroenteroloogy and Nutrition* 8:2 (1989), 204-206.

## Chapter 4

### Prevention of Sensitization

1 Saul Pilar, M.D. "Help for Allergies." *Townsend Letter for Doctors & Patients* (April 1997).

2 R.K. Chandra. "Food Hypersensitivity and Allergic Disease: A Selective Review." *American Journal of Clinical Nutrition* 66 (1997), 526S-529S.

3 W.H. Oddy, et al. "Association between Breast Feeding and Asthma in 6-Year-Old Children: Findings of a Prospective Birth Cohort Study." *British Medical Journal* 319 (September 25, 1999), 815-819.

4 Martin C. Harmsen et al. "Antiviral Effects of Plasma and Milk Proteins: Lactoferrin Shows Potent Acitivity Against Both Human Immunodeficiency Virus and Human Cytomegalovirus Replication in Vitro." *Journal of Infectious Disease* 172 (1995), 380-388.

5 D. Dai and W.A. Walker. "Protective Nutrients and Bacterial Colonization in the Immature Human Gut." *Advances in Pediatrics* 46 (1999), 353-382

6 F. Haschke et al. "Does Breast Feeding Protect from Atopic Diseases?" *Padiatrie und Padologie* 25:6 (1990), 415-420.

7 Ranjit Kumar Chandra. "Food Hypersensitivity and Allergic Disease: A Selective Review." *American Journal of Clinical Nutrition* 66 (1997), 526S-529S.

8 D. de Boissieu et al. "Multiple Food Allergy: A Possible Diagnosis in Breastfed Infants." *Acta Paediatrica* 86:1 (October 1997), 1042-1046.

9 Ranjit Kumar Chandra. "Food Hypersensitivity and Allergic Disease: A Selective Review." *American Journal of Clinical Nutrition* 66 (I997), 526S-529S.

10 D.M. Fergussen, J.L. Horwood, and F.T. Shannon. "Early Solid Feeding and Recurrent Childhood Eczema: A I0-Year Longitudinal Study." *Pediatrics* 86:4 (October 1990), 541-546.

11 Ranjit Kumar Chandra. "Food Hypersensitivity and Allergic Disease: A Selective Review." *American Journal of Clinical Nutrition* 66 (1997), 526S-529S.

12 J. Raloff. "Family Allergies? Keep Nuts Away from Baby." *Science News* 149 (May 4, 1996), 279.

13 Ibid., 279.

14 Peggy O'Mara, ed. *Vaccination: The Issue of Our Times* (Santa Fe, NM: Mothering Resource Library, 1997), 58, 68.

15 J.S. Alm et al. "Atopy in Children of Families with an Anthroposophic Lifestyle." *The Lancet* 353:163 (May 1, 1999), 1485-1488.

16 Zoltan P. Rona, M.D. *Childhood Illness and Allergy Connection* (Rocklin, CA: Prima Publishing, 1997), 111.

17 "The First International Public Conference on Vaccination." *Mothering* 86 (January 1998), 44.

18 E.L. Hurwitz and H. Morgenstern. "Effects of Diphtheria-Tetanus-Pertussis or Tetanus Vaccination on Allergies and Allergy-Related Respiratory Symptoms among Children and Adolescents in the United States." *Journal of Manipulative and Physiological Therapeutics* 23:2 (February 2000), 81-90.

19 M. Paunio et al. "Measles History and Atopic Diseases?: A Population-Based Cross-Sectional Study." *Journal of the American Medical Association* 283:3 (January 19, 2000), 343-346.

20 E.L. Hurwitz and H. Morgenstern. "Effects of Diptheria-Tetanus-Pertussis or Tetanus Vaccination on Allergies and Allergy-Related Respiratory Symptoms Among Children and Adolescents in the United States." *Journal of Manipulative and Physiological Therapeutics* 23:2 (February 2000), 81-90.

21 M.R. Odent et al. "Pertussis Vaccination and Asthma: Is There a Link?" *Journal of the American Medical Association* 272 (August 24-31, 1994), 592-593.

22 S.O. Shaheen et al. "Measles and Atopy in Guinea-Bissau." *The Lancet* 347:9018 (June 29, 1996), 1792-1796.

23 S.A. Lewis and J.R. Britton. "Measles Infection, Measles Vaccination and the Effect of Birth Order in the Aetiology of Hay Fever." *Clinical and Experimental Allergy* 28:12 (December 1998), 1493-1500.

24 Zoltan P. Rona, M.D. *Childhood Illness and Allergy Connection* (Rocklin, CA: Prima Publishing, 1997), 109.

25 Robert S. Ivker, D.O. *Sinus Survival* (New York: Jerermy P. Tarcher, 1995), 139.

26 Zoltan P. Rona, M.D. *Childhood Illness and the Allergy Connection* (Rocklin, CA: Prima Publishing, 1997), 31.

27 A. Custovic et al. "Indoor Allergens Are a Primary Cause of Asthma." *European Respiratory Review* 8:532 (1998), 155-158.

28 Robert S. Ivker, D.O. *Sinus Survival* (New York: Jerermy P. Tarcher, 1995), 123-124.

# Chapter 5

## Environmental Control

1 Lynn Lawson. *Staying Well in a Toxic World* (Chicago: The Noble Press, I993), 29.

2 William R. Kellas, M.D., and Andrea S. Dworkin, N.D. *Surviving the Toxic Crisis* (Olivenein, CA: Professional Preference, I996), 26.

3 The Burton Goldberg Group. *Alternative Medicine: The Definitive Guide* (Tiburon, CA: Future Medicine Publishing, 1995), 186, 211.

4 Margaret R. Becklake and Pierre Ernst. "Environmental Factors" *The Lancet* 350:Suppl 2 (October 1997), 10-13.

5 D. Passali et al. "Nasal Allergy and Atmospheric Pollution." *International Journal of Pediatric Otorhinolaryngology* 49:Suppl 1 (October 5, 1999), S257-S260.

6 J.Q. Koenig. "Air Pollution and Asthma." Journal of Allergy and Clinical *Immunology* 104:4 Part 1 (October 1999), 717-722.

7 M. Kryzyzanowski, J.J. Quackenboss, and M.D. Lebowitz. "Chronic Respiratory Effects of Indoor Formaldehyde Exposure." *Environmental Research* 52 (1990), 117-125.

8 Jacqueline Krohn, M.D., Frances A. Taylor, M.A., and Erla Mae Larson, R.N. *The Whole Way to Allergy Relief & Prevention* (Vancouver, BC, Canada: Hartley & Marks, 1996), 121.

9 Wei Yang et al. "Air Pollution and Asthma Emergency Room Visits in Reno, Nevada." *Inhalation Toxicology* 9 (1997), 15-29.

10 U. Kramer et al. "Traffic-Related Air Pollution is

Associated with Atopy in Children Living in Urban Areas." *Epidemiology* 11:1 (January 2000), 64-70.

11 N. Keles, C. Ilicali, and K. Deger. "The Effects of Different Levels of Air Pollution on Atopy and Symptoms of Allergic Rhinitis." *American Journal of Rhinology* 13:3 (May/June 1999), 185-190.

12 Jacqueline Krohn, M.D., Frances A. Taylor, M.A., and Erla Mae Larson, R.N. *The Whole Way to Allergy Relief & Prevention* (Vancouver, BC, Canada: Hartley & Marks, 1996), 116.

13 Walter J. Crinnion, N.D. "Environmental Medicine, Part 1: The Human Burden of Environmental Toxins and Their Common Health Effects." *Alternative Medicine Review* 5:1 (2000), 54.

14 Doris Rapp, M.D. *Is This Your Child?* (New York: William Morrow, 1991), 309-310.

15 H.S. Nelson. "Allergen and Irritant Control: Importance and Implementation." *Clinical Cornerstone* 1:2 (August/September 1998), 57-68.

16 "Lead May Provoke Allergic Reaction." *Medical Tribune* (May 4, 1995), 19.

17 Public Health Service. "Dental Amalgam: A Scientific Review and Recommended Public Health Service Strategy for Research, Education and Regulation." *Final Report of the Subcommittee on Risk Management of the Committee to Coordinate Environmental Health and Related Programs* (January 1993).

18 "Dental Mercury Hygiene: Summary of the Recommendations in 1990." *Journal of the American Dental Association* 122 (August 1991), 122.

19 Environmental Protection Agency. "819 Cities Exceed Lead Level for Drinking Water." *EPA Environmental News Publication* A-107 (May 11, 1993), R110.

20 J.H. Woltgens, E.J. Etty, and W.M. Nieuwland. "Prevalence of Mottled Enamel in Permanent Dentition of Children Participating in a Fluoride Programme at the Amsterdam Dental School" *Journal de Biologie Buccale* 17:1 (March 1989), 15-20.

21 C. Danielson et al. "Hip Fractures and Fluoridation in Utah's Elderly Population." *Journal of the American Medical Association* 268:6 (August 1992), 746-748.

22 Rosalind C. Anderson, Ph.D. "Toxic Emissions from Carpets." *Journal of Nutritional & Environmental Medicine* 5:4 (1995), 375-386.

23 Jacqueline Krohn, M.D., Frances A. Taylor, M.A., and Erla Mae Larson, R.N. *The Whole Way to Allergy Relief & Prevention* (Vancouver, BC, Canada: Hartley & Marks, 1996), 149.

24 The American Lung Association Asthma Advisory Group with Norman H. Edelman, M.D. *American Lung Association Family Guide to Asthma and Allergies* (New York: Little Brown, 1997), 82.

25 N.W. Wilson, N.P. Robinson, and M.B. Hogan. "Cockroach and other Inhalant Allergies in Infantile Asthma." *Annals of Allergy, Asthma and Immunology* 83:1 (July 1999), 27-30.

26 Frederic A. Schulaner, M.D. "Cockroach Allergen and Asthma." *New England Journal of Medicine* 337:11 (1997), 791.

27 N. A. Ashford. "Low-Level Chemical Sensitivity: Implication for Research and Social Policy." *Toxicology and Industrial Health* 15:3-4 (April-June 1999), 421-427.

28 G. H. Ross et al. "Neurotoxicity in Single Photon Emission Computer Tomography Brain Scans of Patients Reporting Chemical Sensitivities." *Toxicology and Industrial Health* 15:3-4 (April-June 1999), 415-420.

29 "Multiple Chemical Sensitivity: A 1999 Consensus." *Archives of Environmental Health* 54:3-4 (May/June 1999), 147-149.

30 H. Hu et al. "Development of a Brief Questionnaire for Screening for Multiple Chemical Sensitivity Syndrome." *Toxicology and Industrial Health* 15:6 (October 1999), 582-588. See also: C.S. Miller and T.J. Prihoda. "The Environmental Exposure and Sensitivity Inventory EESI): A Standardized Approach for Measuring Chemical Intolerances for Research and Clinical Applications." *Toxicology and Industrial Health* 15:3-4 (April-June 1999), 370-385.

31 R. Kreutzer, R.R. Neutra, and N. Lashauay. "Prevalence of People Reporting Sensitivities

to Chemicals in a Population-Based Survey." *American Journal of Epidemiology* 150:1 (July 1, 1999), 1-12.

32 R.C. Anderson and J.H. Anderson. "Sensory Irritation and Multiple Chemical Sensitivity." *Toxicology and Industrial Health* 15:3-4 (April-June 1999), 339-345.

33 W.J. Meggs. "Mechanisms of Allergy and Chemical Sensitivity." *Toxicology and Industrial Health* 15:3-4 (April-June 1999), 331-338.

34 C.M. Baldwin, I.R. Bell, and M.K. O'Rourke. "Odor Sensitivity and Respiratory Complaint Profiles in a Community-Based Sample with Asthma, Hay Fever, and Chemical Odor Intolerance." *Toxicology and Industrial Health* 15:3-4 (April-June 1999), 403-409.

35 R.H. Dunstan et al. "A Preliminary Investigation of Chlorinated Hydrocarbons and Chronic Fatigue Syndrome." *Medical Journal of Australia* 163:6 (September 18, 1995), 294-297.

36 C.S. Miller. "Are We on the Threshold of a New Theory of Disease? Toxicant-Induced Loss of Tolerance and Its Relationship to Addiction and Abdiction." *Toxicology and Industrial Health* 15:3-4 (April-June 1999), 285-294.

37 M.S. Jaakkola and J.J. Jaakkola. "Office Equipment and Supplies: A Modern Occupational Health Concern?" *American Journal of Epidemiology* 150:11 (December 1999), 1223-1238. See also: S.K. Brown. "Assessment of Pollutant Emissions from Dry-Process Photocopiers." *Indoor* Air 9:4 (December 1999), 259-267.

38 G.P. Pappas. "The Respiratory Effects of Volatile Organic Compounds" *International Journal of Occupational and Environmental Health* 6:1 (January-March 2000), 1-8.

39 Walter J. Crinnion, N.D. "Environmental Medicine, Part 2—Health Effects of and Protection from Ubiquitous Airborne Solvent Exposure." *Alternative Medicine Review* 5:2 (2000), 138.

40 Mark J. Mendell et al. "Elevated Symptom Prevalence Associated with Ventilation Type in Office Buildings." *Epidemiology* 7 (1996), 583-589.

41 A.P. Jones. "Asthma and Domestic Air Quality." *Social Science and Medicine* 47:6 (1998), 755-764.

42 G. Smedje et al. "Asthma among Secondary Schoolchildren in Relation to the School Environment." *Clinical and Experimental Allergy* 27 (1997), 1270-1278.

43 S. Quirce and J. Sastre. "Occupational Asthma." *Allergy* 53 (1998), 633-641.

44 Michael Hodgson, M.D., M.P.H. "The Medical Evaluation" and "The Sick Building Syndrome" in Effects of the Indoor Environment on Health. Cited in: *Occupational Medicine: State of the Art Reviews* 10:1 (January-March 1995), 167-194.

45 R.L. Bergmann et al. "Allergen Avoidance Should Be First Line Treatment for Asthma." *European Respiratory Review* 8:53 (1998), 161-163. See also: David J. Hill et al. "The Melbourne House Dust Mite Study: Eliminating House Dust Mites in the Domestic Environment." *Journal of Allergy and Clinical Immunology* 99 (March 1999), 323-329.

46 B.C. Wolverton, A. Johnson, and K. Bounds. "Interior Landscape Plants for Indoor Air Pollution Abatement." National Aeronautics and Space Administration: John C. Stennis Space Centers, Stennis Space Center, Missouri (1989).

47 Walter J. Crinnion, N.D. "Environmental Medicine, Part 2—Health Effects of and Protection from Ubiquitous Airborne Solvent Exposure." *Alternative Medicine Review* 5:2 (2000), 139.

48 Case studies presented at the 33rd Annual Meeting of the American Academy of Environmental Medicine, held in Baltimore, MD, November 6-8, 1998. For syllabus, contact: American Academy of Environmental Medicine, P.O. Box CN 1001-8001, New Hope, PA 18938; tel: 215-862-4544; fax: 215-862-4583.

# Chapter 6

## Therapeutic Diets

1 Alan S. Levin, M.D., and Merla Zellerbach. *The Type 1/Type 2 Allergy Relief Program* (Los Angeles: Jeremy P. Tarcher, 1983), 96-99.

2 K.A. Daly. "Epidemiology of Otitis Media." *Otolaryngologic Clinics of North America* 24 (1991), 775-786.

3 P.B. Van Cauwenberge. "The Role of Allergy in Otitis Media with Effusion." *Therapeutische Umschau* 39 (1982), 1011-1016. See also: P. Bellionin, A. Cantani, and F. Salvinelli. "Allergy: A Leading Role in Otitis Media with Effusion." *Allergologia et Immunopathologia* 15 (1987), 205-208. T.M. Nsouli et al. "Role of Food Allergy in Serous Otitis Media." *Annals of Allergy* 73 (1994), 215-219.

4 T.M. Nsouli et al. "Role of Food Allergy in Serous Otitis Media." *Annals of Allergy* 73 (1994), 215-219.

5 L.C. Kleinman et al. "The Medical Appropriateness of Tympanostomy Tubes Proposed for Children Younger Than 16 Years in the United States." *Journal of the American Medical Association* 271 (1994), 1250-1255.

6 U.M. Saarinin. "Prolonged Breast Feeding as Prophylaxis for Recurrent Otitis Media." *Acta Paediatrica Scandinavica* 71 (1982), 567-571.

7 T.M. Nsouli et al. "Role of Food Allergy in Serous Otitis Media." *Annals of Allergy* 73 (1994), 215-219.

8 M.A. Van de Laar et al. "Food Intolerance in Rheumatoid Arthritis II: Clinical and Histological Aspects." *Annals of Rheumatic Disease* 51:3 (1992), 303-306.

9 A.M. Denman et al. "Joint Complaints and Food Allergic Disorders." *Annals of Allergy* 51:2 Part 2 (1983), 260-263.

10 R.S. Panush et al. "Food-Induced (Allergic) Arthritis: Inflammatory Arthritis Exacerbated by Milk." *Arthritis and Rheumatism* 29:2 (February 1986), 220-226.

11 U. Bengtsson et al. "Survey of Gastrointestinal Reactions to Food in Adults in Relation to Atopy Presence of Mucus in the Stools, Swelling of Joints, and Arthralgia in Patients with Gastrointestinal Reactions to Foods." *Clinical and Experimental Allergy* 26:12 (December 1996), 1387-1394.

12 D. Beri et al. "Effect of Dietary Restrictions on Disease Activity in Rheumatoid Arthritis." *Annals of Rheumatic Disease* 47:1 (January 1988), 69-72.

13 Joseph Egger, M.D. et al. "Is Migraine Food Allergy?" *The Lancet* 2:8355 (October 15, 1983), 865-869.

14 S. Riestra, E. Fernandez, and L. Rodrigo. "Liver Involvement in Coeliac Disease." *Revista Espanola de Enfermedades Digestivas* 91:12 (December 1999), 846-852.

15 I. Hill et al. "The Prevalence of Celiac Disease in At-Risk Groups of Children in the United States." *Journal of Pediatrics* 136:1 (January 2000), 86-90.

16 F.J. Simoons. "Celiac Disease as a Geographic Problem." Cited in: D.N. Walker and N. Kretchmer, eds. Food, Nutrition, and Evolution (New York: Masson Publishers, 1981), 179-200.

17 S. Auricchio et al. "Does Breast-Feeding Protect Against the Development of Clinical Symptoms of Celiac Disease in Children?" *Journal of Pediatric Gastroenterology and Nutrition* 2 (1983), 428-433. See also: S.P. Fallstrom, J. Winberg, and H.J. Anderson. "Cow's Milk Malabsoption as a Precursor of Gluten Intolerance." *Acta Paediatrica Scandinavica* 54 (1965): 101-115.

18 U. Srinivasan et al. "Lactase Enzyme, Detected Immunohistochemically, is Lost in Active Celiac Disease, but Unaffected by Oats Challenge." *American Journal of Gastoenterology* 94:10 (October 1999), 2936-2941.

19 A. Galli-Tsinopoulou et al. "Autoantibodies pre-dicting Diabetes Mellitus Type 1 in Celiac Disease." *Hormonal Research* 52:3 (1999), 119-124.

20 S.G. Cole and M.F. Kagnoff. "Celiac Disease." *Annual Review of Nutrition* 5 (1985), 241-266.

21 G.F. Meloni et al. "The Prevalence of Celiac Disease in Infertility." *Human Reproduction* 14:11 (November 1999), 2759-2761.

22 C. Sategna-Guidetti et al. "The Effects of 1-Year Gluten Withdrawal on Bone Mass, Bone Metabolism and Nutritional status in Newly-Diagnosed Adult Coeliac Disease Patients." *Alimentary Pharmacology and Therapeutics* 14:1 (January 2000), 35-43.

23 S. Mishkin. "Dairy Sensitivity, Lactose Malabsorption, and Elimination Diets in Inflammatory Bowel Disease." *American Journal of Clinical Nutrition* 65:2 (February 1997), 564-567.

24 G. Joachim. "The Relationships Between Habits of Food Consumption and Reported Reactions to Food in People with Inflammatory Bowel Disease—Testing the Limits." *Nutrition and Health* 13:2 (1999), 69-83.

25 Michael Murray, N.D., and Joseph Pizzorno, N.D. *Encyclopedia of Natural Medicine Revised 2nd Edition* (Rocklin, CA: Prima Publishing, 1998), 589.

26 J. Eaden et al. "Colorectal Cancer Prevention in Ulcerative Colitis: A Case Study." *Alimentary Pharmacology and Therapeutics* 14:2 (February 2000), 145-153.

27 R.C. Knibb et al. "Psychological Characteristics of people with Perceived Food Intolerance in a Community Sample." *Journal of Psychosomatic Research* 47:6 (December 1999), 545-554.

28 Carl T. Hall. "Pediatricians' Group Issues Guide for ADD Diagnosis." *San Francisco Chronicle* (May2, 2000).

29 "Wrong Medical Approach." *San Francisco Chronicle* (March 22, 2000).

30 Erica Goode. "'Troubling' Rise in Preschoolers' Use of Psychiatric Drugs." *The New York Times (February 23,* 2000).

31 James Braly, M.D. *Dr. Braly's Food Allergy & Nutrition Revolution* (New Canaan, CT: Keats Publishing, 1992), 304.

32 T. Uhlig et al. "Topographic Mapping of Brain Electrical Activity in Children with Food-Induced Attention Deficit Hyperkinetic Disorder." *European Journal of Pediatrics* 156:7 (July 1997), 557-561.

33 M. Boris and F.S. Mandel. "Foods and Additives are Common Causes of the Attention Deficit Hyperactive Disorder in Children." *Annals of Allergy* 72:5 (May 1994), 462-468.

34 Diagnostic Classification Steering Committee, Michael J. Thorpy, ed. *The International Classification of Sleep Disorders: Diagnostic and Coding Manual* (Rochester, MN: American Sleep Disorders Association, 1990).

35 U.S. Dept. of Health and Human Services. *Sleep Disorders* Publication No. (ADM) 87-1541 (Washington, DC: U.S. Government Printing Office, 1987).

36 W.L. Robson et al. "Enuresis in Children with Attention-Deficit Hyperactivity Disorder." *Southern Medical Journal* 90:5 (May 1993), 503-505.

37 J. Egger et al. "Effect of Diet Treatment on Enuresis in Children with Migraine or Hyperkinetic Behavior." *Clinical Pediatrics* 31:5 (May 1992), 302-307.

38 R. Bussing, R.C. Burket, and E.T. Kellehen. "Prevalence of Anxiety Disorders in a Clinic-Based Sample of Pediatric Asthma Patients." *Psychosomatics* 37:2 (March/April 1996), 108-115.

39 M. Gauci et al. "A Minnesota Multiphasic Personality Inventory Profile of Women with Allergic Rhinitis." *Psychosomatic Medicine* 55:6 (November/December 1993), 533-540.

40 I.R. Bell et al. "Depression and Allergies: Survey of a Nonclinical Population." *Psychotherapy and Psychosomatics* 55:1 (1991), 24-31.

41 D.N. Vlissodes, A. Venulet, and F.A. Jenner. "A Double-Blind Gluten-Free/Gluten-Load Controlled Trial in a Secure Ward Population." *British Journal of Psychiatry* 148 (April 1986), 447-452.

42 S. Lucarelli et al. "Food Allergy and Infantile Autism." *Panminerva Medica* 37:3 (September 1995), 137-141.

43 A. Pelliccia et al. "Partial Cryptogenetic Epilepsy and Food Allergy/Intolerance. A Causal or a Chance Relationship?" Reflections on Three Clinical Cases." *Minerva Pediatrica* 51:5 (May 1999), 153-157.

44 J.C. Breneman. "Allergy Elimination Diet as the Most Effective Gallbladder Diet." *Annals of Allergy* 26 (1968), 83-87.

45 J. Siegel. "Gastointestinal Ulcer—Arthus Reaction!" *Annals of Allergy* 32 (1974), 127-130.

46 E.L. Hurwitz and H. Morgenstern. "Cross-Sectional Associations of Asthma, Hay Fever, and Other Allergies with Major Depression and Low-Back Pain Among Adults Aged 20-39 Year in the United States." *American Journal of Epidemiology* 150:10 (November 1999), 1107-1116.

47 James Braly M.D. *Dr. Braly's Food Allergy & Nutrition Revolution* (New Canaan, CT: Keats Publishing, 1992), 48.

48 H. Haas et al. "Dietary Lectins Can Induce In Vitro Release of IL-4 and IL-13 from Human Basophils Cells." *European Journal of Immunology* 29:3 (March 1999), 918-927.

49 Ann Louise Gittleman, M.D., with James Templeton and Candelora Versace. *Your Body Knows Best* (New York: Pocket Books, 1997), 37

50 Peter J. D'Adamo with Catherine Whitney. *Eat Right 4 Your Type* (New York: G.P. Putnam's Sons, 1996), 159.

51 Ibid., 25.

52 T. Caballero and M. Martin-Esteban. "Association Between Pollen Hypersensitivity and Edible Vegetable Allergy: A Review." *Journal of Investigational Allergology and Clinical Immunology* 8:1 (January/February 1998), 6-16.

53 J.H. Mikkola et al. "Hevein-like Protein Domains as Possible Cause of Allergen Cross-Reactivity Between Latex and Banana." *Journal of Allergy and Clinical Immunology* 102:6 Part 1 (December 1998), 1005-1012.

54 James Braly M.D. *Dr. Braly's Food Allergy & Nutrition Revolution* (New Canaan, CT: Keats Publishing, 1992), 61.

55 Denise Mann. "Genetically Engineered Foods May Be Allergenic." *Medical Tribune* (April 18, 1996), 2.

56 Marion Nestle, Ph.D., M.PH., "Allergies to Transgenic Foods—Questions of Policy." *New England Journal of Medicine* 334:11 (March 14, 1996), 688-692.

## Chapter 7

### Healing Leaky Gut Syndrome

1 P. Dupuy et al. "Low-Salt Water Reduces Intestinal Permeability in Atopic Patients." *Dermatology* 198:2 (1999), 153-155.

2 P. Braquet. Ginkgolides: Chemistry, Biology, Pharmacology and Clinical Perspectives, Vol. I (Barcelona, Spain: J. Prous Science Publishers, 1988). See also: P. Braquet, ed. *Ginkolides: Chemistry Biology, Pharmacology and Clinical Perspectives*, Vol. II (Barcelona, Spain: J. Prous Science Publishers, 1989). E. W. Fungfeld, ed. *Rokan: Ginkgo Biloba* (New York: Springer Verlag, 1988).

3 Walter H. Lewis and Memry Elvin Lewis. *Medical Botany: Plants Effecting Man's Health* (New York: John Wiley and Sons, 1977).

4 Kerry Bone. *Phytosynergistic Prescribing: A Professional Prescribers Reference Guide to Herbal Formulas* (Lake Oswego, OR: Communications Medicus), 17, Formula 5.

5 Simon Y. Mills, M.A. *The Dictionary of Modern Herbalism* (Rochester, VT: Healing Arts Press, 1988), 138.

6 David Hoffmann. *The Herb User's Guide* (Northamptonshire, England: Thorsens Publishers, 1987), 55.

7 Ibid.

8 John Lust. *The Herb Book* (New York: Bantam Books, 1974), 270.

9 Steven Foster. *Chamomile Botanical Series* 307 (Austin, TX: American Botanical Council, 1991).

10 David Hoffmann. *The New Holistic Herbal* (Rockport, MA: Element, 1991), 204.

11 V.P. Choundhry, M. Sabir, and V.N. Bhide. "Berberine in Giardiasis." *Indian Pediatrics* 9:3 (March 1972), 143-146.

12 Y. Kumazawa et al. "Activation of Peritoneal Macrophages by Berberine-Alkaloids in Terms of Induction of Cytostatic Activity." *International Journal of Immunopharmacology* 6 (1984), 587-592.

13 R.R. van der Hulst et al. "Glutamine and the

Preservation of Gut Integrity." *The Lancet* 334 (1993), 1363-1365.

14 H. Chun, M. Sasaki, Y. Fugiyama, and T. Bamba. "Effect of Anteral Glutamine on Intestinal Permeability and Bacterial Translocation after Abdominal Radiation Injury in Rats." *Journal of Gastroenterology* 32:2 (1997), 189-195.

15 R. Denno et al. "Glutamine-Enriched Total Parenteral Nutrition Enhances Plasma Glutathione in the Resting State." *Journal of Surgical Research* 61:1 (1996), 35-38.

16 C.J. Johnston, C.G. Meyer, and J.C. Srilakshmi. "Vitamin C Elevates Red Blood Cell Glutathione in Healthy Adults." *American Journal of Clinical Nutrition* 58 (1993), 103-105.

17 A. Witschi et al. "The Systemic Availability or Oral Glutathione." *European Journal of Clinical Pharmacology* 43 (1992), 667-669.

18 T.M. Hagen et al. "Bioavailability of Dietary Glutathione: Effect on Concentration." *American Journal of Physiology* 259:4 Pt 1 (1990):G524-G529. T.M. Hagen, T.Y. Aw, and D.P. Jones. "Glutathione Uptake And Protection Against Oxidative Injury in Isolated Kidney Cells." *Kidney International* 34:1 (1988), 74-81. T.M. Vincenzini, F. Favilli, and T. Iantomasi "Intestinal Uptake and Transmembrane Transport Systems of Intact GSH: Characteristics and Possible Biological Role." *Biochimica et Biophysica Acta* 1113:1 (1992), 13-23. B.M. Lomaestro and M. Malone. "Glutathione in Health and Disease: Pharmacotherapeutic Issues." *Annals of Pharmacotherapy* 29 (December 1995), 1263-1273.

19 A.F. Burton and F.H. Anderson. "Decreased Incorporation of 14C-Glucosamine Relative to 3H-N-Acetylglucosamine in the Intestinal Mucosa of Patients with Inflammatory Bowel Disease." *American Journal of Gastroenterology* 78 (1983), 19-22.

20 Michael A. Schmidt, D.C., C.N.S., and Jeffrey Bland, Ph.D. "Thyroid Gland as Sentinel: Interface Between Internal and External Environment." *Alternative Therapies* 3:1 (January 1997), 78-81.

21 Stephen Langer, M.D., and James F. Scheer. *Solved: The Riddle of Illness* (New Canaan, CT: Keats Publishing, 1995), 31.

22 Ibid., 32.

23 Ibid., 15-17.

24 Michael A. Schmidt, D.C., C.N.S., and Jeffrey Bland, Ph.D. "Thyroid Gland as Sentinel: Interface Between Internal and External Environment." *Alternative Therapies* 3:1 (January 1997), 78-81.

25 Y.B. Tripathi et al. "Thyroid-Stimulatory Action of Z-Guggulsterone: Mechanism of Action." *Planta Medica* 54 (1988), 271-277.

26 B. Saunier et al. "Cyclic AMP Regulation of Gs Protein: Thyrotropin and Forskolin Increase the Quantity of Stimulatory Guanine Nucleotide-Binding Proteins in Cultured Thyroid Follicles." *Journal of Biological Chemistry* 265 (1990), 19942-19946. P.P. Roger et al. "Regulation of Dog Thyroid Epithelial Cell Cycle by Forskolin: An Adenylate Cyclase Activator." *Experimental Cell Research* 172 (1990), 282-292. B. Haye et al. "Chronic and Acute Effects of Forskolin on Isolated Thyroid Cell Metabolism." *Molecular and Cellular Endocrinology* 43 (1990), 41-50.

27 David Hoffmann. *The Herb User's Guide* (Wellingborough, Northamptonshire, England: Thorsens Publishing, 1987), 44.

28 Ralph Golan, M.D. *Optimal Wellness* (New York: Ballantine, 1995), 149-150.

29 Edward Howell, M.D. *Food Enzymes for Health and Longevity* (Woodstock Valley, CT: Omangod Press, 1980).

30 G. Uhli and J. Seifert. "The Effect of Proteolytic Enzymes (Traumanase) on Post-Traumatic Edema." *Fortschritte der Medizin* 99 (1994), 554-556.

31 V. Balakrishnan, A, Hareendran, and C. Sukumaran Nair. "Double-Blind Cross-Over Trial of an Enzyme Preparation in Pancreatic Steatorrhea." *Journal of the Association of Physicians of India* 29 (1981), 207-209.

32 Gregory S. Kelly. "Bromelain: A Literature Review and Discussion of Its Therapeutic Applications." *Alternative Medicine Review* 1:4 (1996), 245.

33 V. Tretter V et al. "Fucose Alpha-1,3 Linked to the Core Region of Glycoprotein N-Glycans Creates an Important Epitope for IgE From Honeybee Venom Allergic Individuals." *International Archives of Allergy and Immunology* 102 (1993), 259-266. E. Batanero et al. "Cross-Reactivity Between the Major Allergen From Olive Pollen and Unrelated Glycoproteins: Evidence of an Epitope in the Glycan Moiety of the Allergen." *Journal of Allergy and Clinical Immunology* 97 (1996), 1264-1271.

34 A. Gutfreund, S. Taussig, and A. Morris. "Effect of Oral Bromelain on Blood Pressure and Heart Rate of Hypertensive Patients." *Harvard Medical Journal* 37 (1978), 143-146.

35 Diane Robertson. *Jamaican Herbs* (Montego Bay, Jamaica: DeSola Pinto, 1982).

36 Michael T. Murray, N.D. "Chronic Candidiasis: A Natural Approach." *American Journal of Natural Medicine* 4:4 (May 1997), 13.

37 J. Savolainen et al. "*Candida Albicans* Mannan- and Protein-Indiced Humoral, Cellular and Cytokine Responses in Atopic Dermatitis Patients." *Clinical Experiments in Allergy* 29:6 (June 1999), 824-831.

38 E. Morita et al. "An Assessment of the Role of Candida Albicans Antigen in Atopic Dermatitis." *Journal of Dermatology* 26:5 (May 1999), 282-287.

39 A. Adachi et al. "Role of *Candida* Allergen in Atopic Dermatitis and Efficacy of Oral Therapy With Variuos Antifungal Agents." *Arerugi* 48:7 (July 1999), 719-725.

40 P.S. Moraes. "Recurrent Vaginal Candidiasis and Allergic Rhinitis: A Common Association." *Annals of Allergy, Asthma, and Immunology* 81:2 (August 1998), 165-169.

41 Simon Martin. *Candida: The Natural Way* (Boston: Element Books, 1998), 10-11. This information is adapted from a *Candida* Questionnaire developed by William Crook, M.D., and included in his book *The Yeast Connection Handbook* (Jackson, TN: Professional Books, 1996), 15-19.

42 D. M. Blair, C. S. Hangee-Bauer, and C. Calabrese. "Intestinal Candidiasis, *Lactobacillus acidophilus* Supplementation and Crook's Questionnaire." *Journal of Naturopathic Medicine* 2 (1991), 33-37.

43 Tim Birdsall. "Gastrointestinal Candidiasis: Fact or Fiction?" *Alternative Medicine Review* 2:5 (1997), 346-348.

44 Erika Isolauri, M.D. "Intestinal Involvement in Atopic Disease." *Journal of the Royal Society of Medicine* 90:Supplement 30 (1997), 15-20.

45 Heli Majamaa, M.D., and Erika Isolauri, M.D. "Probiotics: A Novel Approach in the Management of Food Allergy." *Journal of Allergy and Clinical Immunology* 99 (1997), 179-185. See also: P.V. Kirjavainen and G.R. Gibson. "Health Gut Microflora and Allergy: Factors Influencing Development of the Microbiota." *Annals of Medicine* 31:4 (August 1999), 288-292.

46 Michael T. Murray, N.D. "Probiotics: Acidophilus, Bifidobacter, and FOS." *American Journal of Natural Medicine* 3:4 (1996), 11-14. Elizabeth Lipski, M.S., C.C.N. *Digestive Wellness* (New Canaan, CT: Keats, 1996). John A. Catanzaro, N.D., and Lisa Green, B.Sc., "Microbial Ecology and Dysbiosis in Human Medicine." *Alternative Medicine Review* 2:3 (1997), 202-209. John A. Catanzaro, N.D., and Lisa Green, B.Sc., "Microbial Ecology and Probiotics in Human Health (Part II)." *Alternative Medicine Review* 2:4 (1997), 296-305. P.S. Moshchich et al. "Prevention of Dysbacteriosis in the Early Neonatal Period Using a Pure Culture of Acidophilic Bacteria." *Pediatriia* (1989), 25-30. S.J. Bhatia et al. "*Lactobacillus acidophilus* Inhibits Growth of Campylobacter pylori in Vitro." *Journal of Clinical Microbiology* 27:10 (1989), 2328-2330.

47 Joseph Pizzorno, N.D. and Michael T. Murray, N.D., eds. *A Textbook of Natural Medicine* (Seattle, WA: John Bastyr College Publications, 1988-89).

48 W.J. Crinnion. "Clinical Trial Results on Neesby's Capricin." (Unpublished manuscript). Available from: Probiologic, Inc., 1803 132nd Avenue NE, Bellevue, WA 98005.

49 Paul Bergner. *The Healing Power of Garlic*

(Rocklin, CA: Prima Publishing, 1995), 98-100.

50 Heinrich P. Koch, Ph.D, M.Pharm., and Larry D. Lawson, Ph.D. *Garlic: The Science and Therapeutic Application of Allium sativum L. and Related Species* (Baltimore, MD: Williams & Wilkins, 1996), 168-172.

51 Cass Ingram, D.O. *The Cure Is in the Cupboard: How to Use Oregano for Better Health* (Buffalo Grove, IL: Knowledge House, 1997), 14-16, 34, 50.

## Chapter 8

### Intestinal Detoxification

1 William Mitchell, N.D. "Allergies: Immediate-type Hypersensitivity." *The Protocol Journal of Botanical Medicine* (Autumn 1995), 66.

2 Joseph Pizzorno, N.D. *Total Wellness* (Rocklin, CA: Prima Publishing, 1996), 105.

3 L.K.T. Lam et al. "Isolation and Identification of Kahweol Palmitate and Cafestol Palmitate as Active Constituents of Green Coffee Beans that Enhance Glutathione-S-Transferase Activity in the Mouse." *Cancer Research* 42 (1982), 1193-1198.

4 Howard Straus. "Coffee Corner." *Gerson Healing Newsletter* 11:5 (1996), 9-11.

5 Eugene Zampieron, N.D., A.H.G., and Ellen Kamhi, Ph.D., R.N. *The Natural Medicine Chest* (New York: M. Evans, 1999), 52-54.

6 C. J. Poutinen. *Herbs for Detoxification* (New Canaan, CT: Keats, 1977), 67.

7 M. World et al. "Cyanidanol-3 for Alcoholic Liver Disease: Result of a Six-Month Clinical Trial." *Alcoholism* 19 (1984), 23-29.

8 Maoshing Ni, Ph.D., C.A., with Cathy McNease, B.S., M.H. *The Tao of Nutrition* (Santa Monica, CA: SevenStar Communications, 1994), 11.

9 D. W. Bendig, M.D. "Diagnosis of Giardiasis in Infants and Children by Endoscopic Brush Cytology." *Journal of Pediatric Gastroenterology and Nutrition* 8:2 (1989), 204-206.

10 A. Daxhner et al. "Gastroallergic Anisakiasis: Borderline Between Food Allergy and Parasitic Disease—Clinical and Allergologic Evaluation of 20 Patients with Confirmed Acute Parasitism by Anisakis Simplex." *Journal of Allergy and Clinical Immunology* 105:1 Part 1 (January 2000), 176-181.

11 M.C. Di Prisco et al. "Association Between Giardiasis and Allergy." *Annals of Allergy, Asthma, and Immunology* 81:3 (September 1998), 261-265.

12 D.I. Pritchard. "The Pro-Allergic Influences of Helminth Parasites." *Memorias do Instituto Oswaldo Cruz* 92: Suppl 2 (1997), 15-18.

13 Dan Bensky et al. *Chinese Herbal Medicine: Materia Medica* (Seattle, WA: Eastland Press, 1986), 630.

14 D. Mirelman et al. "Inhibition of Growth of Entamoeba Histolitica by Allicin, the Active Principle of Garlic Extract (Allium sativum)." *Journal of Infectious Disease* 156:1 (1987), 243-244.

15 S. Gupte. "Use of Berberine in the Treatment of Giardiasis." *American Journal of Diseases of Children* 129 (1975), 866.

16 Joseph Pizzorno, N.D. *Total Wellness* (Rocklin, CA: Prima Publishing, 1996), 79.

17 Martha Windholz, ed. *Merck Index: An Encyclopedia of Chemicals and Drugs* 9th Edition (Rahway, NJ: Merck, 1976), 1214.

18 "Antibiotic Alternative Proven Effective." *The GSE Report* 1:1, 1.

19 Earl Mindell, R.Ph., Ph.D. *Earl Mindell's Supplement Bible* (New York: Simon and Schuster, 1998), 63.

20 The Burton Goldberg Group. *Alternative Medicine: The Definitive Guide* (Tiburon, CA: Future Medicine Publishing, 1995), 782-787.

## Chapter 9

### Supporting the Skin

1 V. Schriener et al. "Barrier Characteristics of Different Human Skin Types Investigated with X-Ray Diffractioin, Lipid Analysis, and Electron Microscopy Imaging." *Journal of Investigative Dermatology* 114:4 (April 2000), 654-660. See also: J.A. Bouwstra et al. "A Model Membrane Approach to the Epidermal Permeability Barrier: An X-Ray Diffraction Study." *Biochemistry* 36:25 (June

1997), 7717-7725.

2 G. Yosipovitch et al. "Time-Dependent Variations of the Skin Barrier Function in Humans: Transepidermal Water Loss, Stratum Corneum Hydration, Skin Surface pH, and Skin Temperature." *Journal of Investigative Dermatology* 110:1 (January 1998), 20-23.

3 E. Proksch and J. Brasch. "Influence of epidermal Permeability Barrier Disruption and Langerhans' Cells Density on Allergic Contact Dermatitis." *Acta Dermato-Venereologica* 77:2 (March 1977), 102-104.]

4 R. Ghadially. "Aging and the Epidermal Permeability Barrier: Implications for Contact Dermatitis." *American Journal of Contact Dermatitis* 9:3 (September 1998), 162-169.

5 B. Niggemann et al. "Outcome of Double-blind, Placebo-Controlled Food Challenge Test in 107 Children with Atopic Dermatitis." *Clinical and Experimental Allergy* 29:1 (January 1999), 91-96.

6 I. Hamilton et al. "Small Intestinal Permeability in Dermatological Disease." *Quarterly Journal of Medicine* 56:221 (September 1985), 559-567.

7 T. Schafer et al. "Association Between Severity of Atopic Eczema and Degree of Sensitization to Aeroallergens in Schoolchildren." *Journal of Allergy and Clinical Immunology* 104:6 (December 1999), 1280-1284.

8 M. Fartasch. "Epidermal Barrier in Disorders of the Skin." *Microscopy Research and Technique* 38:4 (August 1997), 361-372

9 American Academy of Allergy, Asthma & Immunology. *The Allergy Report* 2 (2000), 111.

10 P.S. Friedmann and B.B. Tan. "Mite Elimination—Clinical Effect on Eczema." *Allergy* 53:48 Supplement (1998), 97-100.

11 John O.A. Pagon, D.C. *Healing Psoriasis: The Natural Alternative* (Englewood Cliffs, NJ: The Pagano Organization, 1991), 22.

12 H.S. Capoore et al. "Does Psychological Intervention Help Chronic Skin Conditions." *Postgraduate Medical Journal* 74:877 (November 1998), 662-664.

13 L. Naldi et al. "Dietary Factors and Risk of Psoriasis: Results of an Italian Case-Control Study." *British Journal of Dermatology* 134:1 (January 1996), 858.

14 K. Kragballe and K. Fogh. "A Low-Fat Diet Supplemented with Dietary Fish Oil (Max-EPA) Results in Improvement of Psoriasis and in Formation of Leukotriene B5." *Acta Dermato-Venereologica* 69:1 (1989), 23-28.

15 S. Zamboni et al. "Dietary Behaviour in Psoriatic Patients." *Acta Dermato-Venereologica Supplementum* 146 (1989), 182-183.

16 V.A. Ziboh, C.C. Miller, and Y. Cho. "Metabolism of Polyunsaturated Fatty Acids by Skin Epidermal Enzymes: Generation of Antiinflammatory and Antiproliferative Metabolites." *American Journal of Clinical Nutrition* 71:1 Suppl (January 2000), 361S-366S.

17 Ibid.

18 D.F. Horrobin. "Essential Fatty Acid Metabolism and Its Modificatin in Atopic Eczema." *American Journal of Clinical Nutrition* 71:1 Suppl (January 2000), 367S-372S.

19 V. Willemaers et al. "Atopic Dermatitis." *Revue Medicale de Liege* 53:2 (February 1998), 67-70. See also: L. Galland. "Increased Requirements for Essential Fatty Acids in Atopic Individuals: A Review with Clinical Descriptions." *Journal of the American College of Nutrition* 5:2 (1986), 213-228.

20 M. Denda et al. "Low Humidity Stimulates Epidermal DNA Synthesis and Amplifies the Hyperproliferative Response to Barrier Disruption: Implication for Seasonal Exacerbations of Inflammatory Dermatoses." *Journal of Investigative Dermatology* 111:5 (November 1998), 873-888.

21 D. Abeck and M. Mempel. "Staphylococcus aureus Colonization in Atopic Dermatitis and Its Therapeutic Implications." *British Journal of Dermatology* 139: Supplement 53 (December 1998), 13-16.

22 K. Brockow et al. "Effect of Gentian Violet, Corticosteriod and Tar Preparations in Staphylococcus-aureus-colonized Atopic Eczema." *Dermatology* 199:3 (1999), 231-236.

23 R.R. Warner et al. "Water Disrupts Stratum Corneum Lipid Lamellae: Damage Is Similar to Surfactants." *Journal of Investigative Dermatology* 113:6 (December 1999), 960-966.

24 S. Meguro et al. "Stratum Corneum Lipid Abnormalities in UVB-Irradiated Skin." *Photochemistry and Photobiology* 69:3 (March 1999), 317-321.

25 W.M. Holleran et al. "Structural and Biochemical Basis for the UVB-Induced Alterations in Epidermal Barrier Function." *Photodermatology, Photoimmunology and Photomedicine* 13:4 (August 1997), 117-128. See also: A. Haratake et al. "UVB-Induced Alterations in Permeability Barrier Function: Roles for Epidermal Hyperproliferation and Thymocyte-Mediated Response." *Journal of Investigative Dermatology* 108:5 (May 1997), 769-775.

26 W. Wigger-Alberti et al. "Effects of Various Grit-Containing Cleansers on Skin Barrier Function." *Contact Dermatitis* 41:3 (September 1999), 136-140.

27 T. Shukuwa and A.M. Kligman. "Disaggregation of Corneocytes from Surfactant-Treated Sheets of Stratum Corneum in Hyperkeratosis on Psoriasis, Icthyosis Vulgaris and Atopic Dermatitis." *Journal of Dermatology* 24:6 (June 1997), 361-369.

28 Mary Ann Moon. "Powder-Free Gloves Reduce Allergic Reactions." *Medical Tribune* (December 29, 1997), 9.

29 X. Baur et al. "Results of Wearing Test with Two Different Latex Gloves with and Without the Use of Skin-Protection Cream." *Allergy* 53:4 (April 1998), 441-444.

30 Mary Ann Moon. "Powder-Free Gloves Reduce Allergic Reactions." *Medical Tribune* (December 29, 1997), 9.

31 M. Fartasch, E. Schnetz, and T.L. Diepgen. "Characterization of Detergent-Induced Barrier Alterations—Effect of Barrier Cream on Irritation." *Journal of Investigative Dermatology Symposium Proceedings* 3:2 (August 1998), 121-127.

32 P.G. van der Valk and H.I. Maibach. "Do Topical Corticosteriods Modulate Skin Irritation in Human Beings? Assessment by Transepidermal Water Loss and Visual Scoring." *Journal of the American Academy of Dermatology* 21:3 Part 1 (September 1989), 519-522.

33 P.M. Elias et al. "Retinoid Effects on Epidermal Structure, Differentiation, and Permeability." *Laboratory Investigation* 44:6 (June 1981), 531-540. See also: I. Effendy et al. "Differential Irritant Skin Response to Topical Retinoic Acid and Sodium Lauryl Sulphate: Alone and in Crossover Design." *British Journal of Dermatology* 134:3 (March 1996), 424-430.

34 J.W. Fluhr et al. "Tolerance Profile of Retinol, Retinaldehyde and Retinoic Acid under Maximized and Long-Term Clinical Conditions." *Dermatology* 199: Suppl 1 (1999), 57-60.

35 S.J. Moloney and J.J. Tea "Alkane–Induced Edema Formation and Cutaneous Barrier Dysfunction." *Archives for Dermatological Research* 280:6 (1998), 375-379.

36 William Regelson, M.D. and Carol Colman. *The Super-Hormone Promise* (New York: Simon & Schuster, 1996), 92.

37 F. Paquet et al. "Sensitive Skin at Menopause: Dew Point and Electrometric Properties of Stratum Corneum." *Maturitas* 28:3 (January 1998), 221-227.

38 C. Pierard et al. "Skin Water-Holding Capacity and Transdermal Estrogen Therapy for Menopause: A Pilot Study." *Maturitas* 22:2 (September 1995), 151-154.

39 J. Harvell, I. Hussona-Saeed, and H.I. Maibach. "Changes in Transepidermal Water Loss nad Cutaneous Blood Flow During the Menstrual Cycle." *Contact Dermatitis* 27:5 (November 1992), 294-301.

40 I.H. Ginsburg et al. "Role of Emotional Factors in Adults with Atopic Dermatitis." *International Journal of Dermatology* 32:9 (September 1993), 656-660.

41 M.A. Gupta et al. "Early Onset Psoriasis: A Study of 137 Patients." *Acta Dermato-Venereologica* 76:6 (November 1996), 464-466. See also: Betsy Bates. "Early-Onset Psoriasis Associated with Anger." *Clinical Psychiatry News* 25:10 (1997), 15.

42 M. Denda et al. "Stress Alerts Cutaneous Permeablity Barrier Homeostasis." *American Journal of Physiology* 278:2 (February 2000), R367-372.

43 M.L. Williams et al. "Ontogeny of the Epidermal Permeability Barrier." *Journal of Investigative Dermatology Symposium Proceedings* 3:2 (August 1998), 75-79.

44 K. Hanley et al. "Hypothyroidism Delays Fetal Stratum Corneum Development in Mice." *Pediatric Research* 42:5 (November 1997), 610-614.

45 P. Jensen. "Alternative Medicine and Chronic Skin Disease. Use of Alternative Treatments among Patients with Atopic Dermatitis and Psoriasis." *Tidsskrift For Den Norske Laegeforening* 110:22 (September 1990), 2869-2872.

46 M. Gfesser et al. "The Early Phase of Epidermal Barrier Regeneration is Faster in Patients with Atopic Eczema." *Dermatology* 195:4 (1997), 332-336.

47 E.M. Zettersten et al. "Optimal Ratios of Topical Stratum Corneum Lipids Improves Barrier Recovery in Chronologically Aged Skin." *Journal of the American Academy of Dermatology* 37:3 Part 1 (September 1997), 403-408.

48 P. Berbis, S. Hesse, and Y. Privat. "Essential Fatty Acids and the Skin." *Allergie et Immunologie* 22:6 (June 1990), 225-231.

49 H.M. Sheu et al. "Permeability Barrier Abnormality of Hairless Mouse Epidermis after Topical Corticosteriod: Characterization of Stratum Corneum Lipids by Ruthenium Tetroxide Staining and High-Performance Thin-Layer Chromatography." *Journal of Dermatology* 25:5 (May 1998), 281-289.

50 H.M. Sheu et al. "Depletion of Stratum Corneum Intercellular Lipid Lamellae and Barrier Function Abnormalities After Long-Term Topical Corticosteriods." *British Journal of Dermatology* 136:6 (June 1997), 884-890.

51 Hasnai Walji, Ph.D. *Evening Primrose Oil* (London: Thorsons, 1996), 28.

52 B.M. Henz et al. "Double-Blind, Multicentre Analysis of the Efficacy of Borage Oil in Patients with Atopic Eczema." *British Journal of Dermatology* 140:4 (April 1999), 685-688.

53 E. Soylan et al. "Dietary Supplementation with Very Long-Chain n-3 Fatty Acids in Patients with Atopic Dermatitis. A Double-Blind Multicentre Study." *British Journal of Dermatology* 130:6 (June 1994), 757-764.

54 E. Held, S. Sveinsdottir, and T. Agner. "Effect of Long-Term Use of Moisturizer on Skin Hydration, Barrier Function, and Susceptibility to Irritants." *Acta Dermato-Venerologica* 79:1 (January 1999), 49-51.

55 M. Loden, A.C. Andersson, and M. Lindberg. "Improvement in Skin Barrier Function in Patients with Atopic Dermatitis after Treatment with a Moisturizing Cream (Candoderm)." *British Journal of Dermatology* 140:2 (February 1999), 264-267.

56 D.W. Ramsing and T. Agner. "Preventative and Therapeutic Effects of a Moisturizer. An Experimental Study of Human Skin." *Acta Dermato-Venereologica* 77:5 (September 1997), 335-337.

57 E. Berardesca et al. "Alpha Hydroxyacids Modulate Stratum Corneum Barrier Function." *British Journal of Dermatology* 137:6 (December 1997), 934-938. See also: H.L. Hood et al. "The Effects of an Alpha Hydroxy Acid (Glycolic Acid) on Hairless Guinea Pig Skin Permeability." *Food and Chemical Toxicology* 37:11 (November 1999), 1105-1111.

58 J.W. Fluhr et al. "Glycerol Accelerates Recovery of Barrier Function in Vivo." *Acta Dermato-Venereologica* 79:6 (November 1999), 418-421.

59 E. Schopf, J.M. Mueller, and T. Ostermann. "Value of Adjuvant Basic Therapy in Chronic Recurrent Skin Diseases. Neurodermatitis Atopica/Psoriasis Vulgaris." *Hautarzt* 46:7 (July 1995), 451-454.]

60 H.S. Wolf et al. "Detection of Polycyclic Aromatic Hydrocarbons in Skin Oil Obtained from Roofing Workers." *Chemosphere* 11 (1982), 595.

61 D.W. Schnare et al. "Body Burden Reductions of PCBs, PBBs, and Chlorinated Pesticides in Human Subjects." *Ambio* 13 (1984), 5-6.

62 William J. Rea, M.D. Chemical Sensitivity, Vol. 4 (Boca Raton, FL: CRC Lewis, 1997), 2463.

## Chapter 10

### Supporting the Respiratory System

1 Robert S. Ivker, D.O. Sinus Survival (New York: Jeremy P. Tarcher/Putnam, 1995), 5-6.

2 Ibid., 20.

3 B. Salah et al. "Nasal Mucociliary Transport in Healthy Subjects Slower When Breathing Dry Air." European Respiratory Journal 1:9 (October 1988), 852-855.

4 J. Widdicombe. "Relationships Among the Composition of Mucus, Epithelial Lining Ligquid, and Adhesion of Microorgan-ism." American Journal of Respiratory and Critical Care Medicine 151:6 (June 1995), 2088-2092.

5 U.S. Environmental Protection Agency. National Air Quality and Emissions Trend Report, 1997. (Washington, DC: U.S. Environmental Protection Agency, Office of Air Quality Planning and Standards, December 1998).

6 F.J. Kelly. "Altered Lung Antioxidant Status in Patients with Mild Asthma." The Lancet 354:9177 (August 7, 1999), 482-483.

7 T.S. Hiura et al. "Chemicals in Diesel Exhaust Particles Generate Reactive Oxygen Radicals and Induce Apoptosis in Macrophages." Journal of Immunology 163:10 (November 15, 1999), 5582-5591.

8 D. Passali et al. "Nasal Allergy and Atmospheric Pollution." International Journal of Pediatric Otorhinolaryngology 49:Suppl 1 (October 5, 1999), S257-S260. See also: N. Keles, C. Ilicali, and K. Deger. "The Effects of Different Levels of Air Pollution on Atopy and Symptoms of Allergic Rhinitis." American Journal of Rhinology 13:3 (May/June 1999), 185-190.

9 C. Rusznak et al. "Cigarette Smoke Potentiates House Dust Mite Allergen-Induced Increase in the Permeability of Human Bronchial Cells in Vitro." American Journal of Respiratory Cell and Molecular Biology 20:6 (June 1999), 1238-1250.

10 E. Houtmeyers et al. "Effects of Drugs on Mucus Clearance." European Respiratory Journal 14:2 (August 1999), 452-467.

11 C.J. Johnston, C.G. Meyer, and J.C. Srilakshmi. "Vitamin C Elevates Red Blood Cell Glutathione in Healthy Adults." American Journal of Clinical Nutrition 58 (1993), 103-105.

12 L.S. Greene. "Asthma and Oxidative Stress: Nutritional, Environmental, and Genetic Risk Factors." Journal of the American College of Nutrition 14:4 (August 1995), 317-324.

13 F.J. Kelly. "Glutathione: In Defence of the Lung." Food and Chemical Toxicology 37:9-10 (September/October 1999), 963-966.

14 F.J. Kelly. "Altered Lung Antioxidant Status in Patients with Mild Asthma." The Lancet 354:9177 (August 7, 1999), 482-483.

15 A. Soutar, A. Seaton, and K. Brown. "Bronchial Reactivity and Dietary Antioxidants." Thorax 52:2 (February 1997), 166-170.

16 L.S. Greene. "Asthma and Oxidative Stress: Nutritional, Environmental, and Genetic Risk Factors." Journal of the American College of Nutrition 14:4 (August 1995), 317-324.

17 L. Galland. "Biochemical Abnormalities in Patients with Multiple Chemical Sensitivities." Occupational Medicine 2:4 (October-December 1987), 713-720.

18 A.M. Sustiel et al. "Asthmatic Patients Have Neutrophils That Exhibit Diminished Responsiveness to Adenosine." American Review of Respiratory Disease 140:6 (December 1989), 1556-1561.

19 N.N. Jarjour and W.J. Calhoun. "Enhanced Production of Oxygen Radicals in Asthma." Journal of Laboratory and Clinical Medicine 123:1 (January 1994), 131-136. See also: H. Kanazawa et al. "The Role of Free Radicals in Airway Obstruction in Asthmatic Patients." Chest 100:5 (November 1991), 1319-1322.

20 L. Vargas et al. "A Study of Granulocyte Respiratory Burst in Patients with Allergic Bronchial Asthma." Inflammation 22:1 (February 1998), 45-54.

21 A. Witschi et al. "The Systemic Availability or Oral Glutathione." European Journal of Clinical Pharmacology 43 (1992), 667-669.

22 T.M. Hagen et al. "Bioavailability of Dietary Glutathione: Effect on Concentration." *American Journal of Physiology* 259:4 Pt 1 (1990):G524-G529. T.M. Hagen, T.Y. Aw, and D.P. Jones. "Glutathione Uptake And Protection Against Oxidative Injury in Isolated Kidney Cells." *Kidney International* 34:1 (1988), 74-81. T.M. Vincenzini, F. Favilli, and T. Iantomasi "Intestinal Uptake and Transmembrane Transport Systems of Intact GSH: Characteristics and Possible Biological Role." *Biochimica et Biophysica Acta* 1113:1 (1992), 13-23. B.M. Lomaestro and M. Malone. "Glutathione in Health and Disease: Pharmacotherapeutic Issues." *Annals of Pharmacotherapy* 29 (December 1995), 1263-1273.

23 A. Gillissen and D. Nowak. "Characterization of N-acetylcysteine and Ambroxolin Anti-Oxidant Therapy." *Respiratory Medicine* 92:4 (April 1998), 609-623.

24 N. Banzet, D. Francois, and B.S. Polla. "Tobacco Smoke Induces Mitochondrial Depolarization Along with Cell Death: Effects of Antioxidants." *Redox Resp* 4:5 (1999), 229-236.

25 T.S. Hiura et al. "Chemicals in Diesel Exhaust Particles Generate Reactive Oxygen Radicals and Induce Apoptosis in Macrophages." *Journal of Immunology* 163:20 (November 15, 1999), 5582-5591.

26 A. Strapkova et al. "Mechanisms of the Effect of Oxidants on the Respiratory System." *Bratislavske Lekarske Listy* 100:10 (1999), 541-547.

27 J.A. Colome et al. "Effect of N-acetylcysteine on the Oxidative Burst Induced by Phagocytosis of Bacteria in the Human Leukocytes." *Methods and Findings in Experimental and Clinical Pharmacology* 20:4 (May 1998), 301-305.

28 G.S. Kelly. "Clinical Applications of N-acetylcys-teine." *Alternative Medicine Review* 3:2 (April 1998), 114-127.

29 O. Kalayci et al. "Serum Levels of Antioxidant Vitamins (Alpha Tocopherol, Beta Carotene, and Ascorbic Acid) in Children with Bronchial Asthma." *Turkish Journal of Pediatrics* 42:1 (January-March 2000), 17-21.

30 G.E. Hatch. "Asthma, Inhaled Oxidants, and Dietary Antioxidants." *American Journal of Clinical Nutrition* 61:3 Suppl (March 1995), 625S-630S.

31 O. Kalayci et al. "Serum Levels of Antioxidant Vitamins (Alpha Tocopherol, Beta Carotene, and Ascorbic Acid) in Children with Bronchial Asthma." *Turkish Journal of Pediatrics* 42:1 (January-March 2000), 17-21.

32 M. Kodama et al. "Autoimmune Disease and Allergy are Controlled by Vitamin C Treatment." *In Vivo* 8:2 (March/April 1994), 251-257.

33 O. Kalayci et al. "Serum Levels of Antioxidant Vitamins (Alpha Tocopherol, Beta Carotene, and Ascorbic Acid) in Children with Bronchial Asthma." *Turkish Journal of Pediatrics* 42:1 (January-March 2000), 17-21.

34 D.F.L. Money. "Vitamin E and Selenium Deficiencies and Their Possible Aetological Role in Sudden Infant Death Syndrome." *New Zealand Medical Journal* 71 (1970), 32-34.

35 O. Andersen and J.B. Nielsen. "Effects of Simultaneous Low-Level Dietary Supplementation with Inorganic and Organic Selenium on Whole-Body, Blood, and Organ Levels of Toxic Metals in Mice." *Environmental Health Perspectives* 102:Suppl. 3 (1994), 321-324.

36 M. Mutanen. "Bioavaliablity of Selenium." *Annals of Clinical Research* 18 (1986), 48-54.

37 Centers for Disease Control. "Selenium Intoxication." *Morbidity and Mortality Weekly Report* 33 (1984), 157.

38 L. Glick. "Deglycrrhizinated Liquorice in Peptic Ulcer." *The Lancet* ii (1982), 817. See also: Z.A. Kassir. "Endoscopic Controlled Trial of Four Drug Regimes in the Treatment of Chronic Duodenal Ulceration." *Irish Medical Journal* 78 (1985), 153-156.

39 J. van Marle et al. "Deglycyrrhizinised Liquorice (DGL) and the Renewal of Rat Stomach Epithelium." *European Journal of Pharmacology* 72 (1981), 219-225. See also: K.D. Bardhan et al. "Clinical Trial of Deglycyrrhizinised Liquorice in Gastric Ulcer." *Gut* 19 (1978), 779-782.

## Chapter 11

### Supplements for Symptom Control

1 "Office Emergencies: Strategies to Prevent—and Control—Anaphylaxis." *Consultant* (November 1998), 2640.

2 Gary E. Hatch. "Asthma, Inhaled Oxidants, and Dietary Antioxidants." *Journal of Clinical Nutrition* 61:3 (March 1995), 625S-630S. See also: F.J. Kelly et al. "Altered Lung Antioxidant Status in Patients with Mild Asthma." *The Lancet* 354:9177 (August 7, 1999), 482-483.

3 C.S. Johnston, L.J. Martin, and X. Cai. "Antihistamine Effect of Supplemental Ascorbic Acid and Neutrophil Chemotaxis." *Journal of the American College of Nutrition* 11:2 (April 1992), 172-174.]

4 M. Kodama et al. "Vitamin C Infusion Treatment Enhances Cortisol Production of the Adrenal via the Pituitary ACTH Route." *In Vivo* 8:6 (November/December 1994), 1079-1085.

5 H.A. A. Cohen, I. Neuman, and H. Nahum. "Blocking Effect of Vitamin C in Exercise-Induced Asthma." *Archives of Pediatric and Adolescent Medicine* 151:4 (April 1997), 367-370.

6 C. Bucca et al. "Effect of Vitamin C on Histamine Bronchial Responsiveness of Patients with Allergic Rhinitis." *Annals of Allergy* 65:4 (October 1990), 311-314.

7 C.S. Johnston and B. Luo. "Comparison of the Absorption and Excretion of Three Commercially Available Sources of Vitamin C." *Journal of the American Dietetic Association* 94 (1994), 779-781.

8 O. Kalayci et al. "Serum Levels of Antioxidant Vitamins (Alpha Tocopherol, Beta Carotene, and Ascorbic Acid) in Children with Bronchial Asthma." *Turkish Journal of Pediatrics* 42:1 (January-March 2000), 17-21.

9 K.D. Pletsityi et al. "Vitamine E: Immunocorrecting Effect in Bronchial Asthma Patients." *Voprosy Meditsinskoi Khimii* 41:4 (July-August 1995), 33-36.

10 K. Zheng et al. "Effect of Dietary Vitamin E Supplementation on Murine Nasal Allergy." *American Journal of the Medical Sciences* 318:1 (July 1999), 49-54.

11 I. Szorady, E. Hovrath, and E. Toth. "On the Antihistamine Effect of Pantothenic Acid." *Internationale Zeitschrift fur Vitaminforschung* 36:2 (1966), 126-133.

12 A. Mertz-Nielsen et al. "A Natural Flavonoid, IdB 1027, Increases Gastric Luminal Release of Prostaglandin E2 in Healthy Subjects." *Italian Journal of Gastroenterology* 22:5 (October 1990), 288-290.

13 A. Bindoli, M. Valente, and L. Cavallini. "Inhibitory Action of Quercitin on Xanthine Oxidase and Xanthine Dehydrogenase Activity." *Pharmacological Research Communications* 17 (1985), 831-839.

14 K. Johri et al. "Effect of Quercetin and Ablizzia Saponins on Rat Mast Cell." *Indian Journal of Physiology and Pharmacology* 29:1 (January-March 1985), 43-46.

15 J. Galvez. "Application of Natural Products in Experimental Models of Intestinal Inflammation in Rats." *Metabolism* 18:Suppl (1996), B7-B10.

16 I.I. Balaboklin et al. "Use of Vitamins in Allergic Illnesses in Children." *Voprosy Meditsinskoi Khimii* 38:5 (September/October 1992), 36-40.

17 J.P. Tarayre and H. Lauressergues. "Advantages of a Combination of Proteolytic Enzymes, Flavonoids and Ascorbic Acid in Comparison With Non-Steroidal Anti-Inflammatory Agents." *Arzneimittel-Forschung* 27 (1977), 1144-1149.

18 F. Gurkan et al. "Intravenous Magnesium Sulphate in the Management of Moderate to Severe Acute Asthmatic Children Nonresponding to Conventional Therapy." *European Journal of Emergency Medicine* 6:3 (September 1999), 201-205.

19 H. Mangat, G.A. D'Souza, and M.S. Jacob. "Nebulized Magnesium Sulphate Versus Nebulized Salbutamol in Acute Bronchial Asthma: A Clinical Asthma." *European Respiratory Journal* 12:2 (August 1998), 341-344.

20 H. Hill et al. "Investigation of the Effect of

Short-term Change in Dietary Magnesium Intake in Asthma." *European Respiratory Journal* 10:10 (October 1997), 2225-2229.

21 A.V. Emel'ianov and V.I. Trofimov "Effects of Glucocorticoid Therapy on Mineral Metabolism Indicators in Patients with Bronchial Asthma." *Klinicheskaia Meditsina* 73:2 (1995), 23-25.

22 S.E. Wenzel. "Arachidonic Acid Metabolites: Mediators of Inflammation in Asthma." *Pharmacotherapy* 17:1 Part 2 (January/February 1997), 3S-12S.

23 F. Villani et al. "Effect of Dietary Supplementation with Polyunsaturated Fatty Acids on Bronchial Hyperreactivity in Subjects with Seasonal Asthma." *Respiration* 65:4 (1998), 265-269.

24 Ralph Golan, M.D. *Optimal Wellness* (New York: Ballantine Books, 1995), 50.

25 K. Shane Broughton, et al. "Reduced Asthma Symptoms with n-3 Fatty Acid Ingestion are Related to 5-Series Leukotriene Production." *American Journal of Clinical Nutrition* 65 (1997), 1011-1017.

26 Udo Erasmus. *Fats That Heal, Fats That Kill* (Burnaby, BC, Canada: Alive Books, 1993), 264.

27 Vincent Buyck, Sr., Ph.D., National College of Complementary Medicine and Sciences, Washington, D.C.

28 J.A. Dudek and E.R. Elkins, Jr. "Effects of Cooking on the Fatty Acid Profiles of Selected Seafoods." In: A.P. Simopopulos, R.R. Kifer, R.E. Martin, eds. *Health Effects of Polyusaturated Fatty Acids in Seafoods* (New York: Academic Press, 1986), 431-450.

29 W.A. Newman Dorland, M.D. *American Illustrated Medical Dictionary* (Philadelphia: W.B. Saunders, 1946), 1122.

30 Udo Erasmus. *Fats That Heal, Fats That Kill* (Burnaby, BC, Canada: Alive Books, 1993), 112.

31 M. Sugana and I. Ikeda. "Metabolic Interactions Between Essential and Trans-Fatty Acids." *Current Opinion in Lipidology* 7:1 (February 1996), 38-42.

32 Thonnard-Neumann, M.D., and L.M. Neckers,

Ph.D. "Immunity in Migraine: The Effects of Heparin." *Annals of Allergy* 47 (1981), 328-332.

33 P. Mittman. "Randomized, Double-Blind Study of Freeze-Dried Urtica Dioica in the Treatment of Allergic Rhinitis." *Planta Medica* 56 (1990), 44-47.

34 P. Kalix. "The Pharmacology of Psychoactive Alkaloids from Ephedra and Catha." *Journal of Ethnopharmacol-ogy* 32 (1991), 201-208.

35 M. Ling, S. J. Piddlesden, B. P. Morgan. "A Component of the Medicinal Herb Ephedra Blocks Activation in the Classical and Alternative Pathways of Complement." *Clinical Experiments in Immunology* 102:3 (December 1995), 582-588.

36 P. Braquet. *Ginkgolides: Chemistry, Biology, Pharmacology and Clinical Perspectives*, Vol. I (Barcelona, Spain: J. Prous Science Publishers, 1988). See also: P. Braquet, ed. *Ginkolides: Chemistry Biology, Pharmacology and Clinical Perspectives*, Vol. II (Barcelona, Spain: J. Prous Science Publishers, 1989). E. W. Fungfeld, ed. *Rokan: Ginkgo Biloba* (New York: Springer Verlag, 1988).

37 A.C. Markey et al. "Platelet Activating Factor–Induced Clinical and Histopathologic Responses in Atopic Skin and Their Modification by the Platelet Activating Factor Antagonist BN 52063." *Journal of the American Academy of Dermatology* 23:2 (1990), 263-268.; P. Guinot et al. "Inhibition of PAF-Acether Induced Wheal and Flare Reduction in Man by a Specific PAF Antagonist." *Prostaglandins* 32 (1986): 1, 160-163.

38 Simon Y. Mills, M.A. *The Dictionary of Modern Herbalism* (Rochester, VT: Healing Arts Press, 1988), 138.

39 M.F. Chen et al. "Effect of Glycyrrhizin on the Pharmacokinetics of Prednisone Following Low Dosage of Prednisolone Hemisubstinate". *Endocrinologia Japonica* 37:3 (1990), 331-341.

40 S. Teelucksingh, et al. "Potentiation of Hydrocortisone Activity in Skin by Glycyrrhentinic Acid." *The Lancet* 335 (1990), 1060-1063.

41 Kerry Bone. *Phytosynergistic Prescribing: A*

*Professional Prescribers Reference Guide to Herbal Formulas* (Lake Oswego, OR: Communications Medicus), 17, Formula 5.

42 Eugene Zampieron, N.D., A.H.G., and Ellen Kamhi, Ph.D., R.N. *The Natural Medicine Chest* (New York: M. Evans, 1999), 79-81.

43 E.S. Johnson et al. "Efficacy of Feverfew as Prophylactic Treatment of Migraine." *British Medical Journal* 291 (1985), 569-573.

44 David Hoffmann. *The Herb User's Guide* (Northamptonshire, England: Thorsens Publishers, 1987), 55.

45 John Lust. *The Herb Book* (New York: Bantam Books, 1974), 270.

46 J.B. Wu et al. "Biologically Active Constituents of Centipeda minima: Sesquiterpenes of Potential anti-Allergy Activity." *Chemical and Pharmaceutical Bulletin* 39:12 (December 1991), 3272-3275.

47 Hong-Yen Hus, Ph.D., et al. *Oriental Materia Medica: A Concise Guide* (New Canaan, CT: Keats Publishing, 1986), 449.

48 M. Okamoto et al. "Effects of Dietary Supplementation with n-3 Fatty Acids Compared with n-6 Fatty Acids on Bronchial Asthma." *Internal Medicine* 39:2 (February 2000), 107-111.

49 M. Homma et al. "A Novel Inhibitor Contained in Saiboku-To, a Herbal Remedy for Steroid-Dependent Bronchial Asthma." *Journal of Pharmacy and Pharmacology* 46:4 (April 1994), 305-309.

50 Y. Latchman et al. "Association of Immunological Changes in Clinical Efficacy in Atopic Eczema Patients Treated with Traditional Chinese Herbal Therapy (Zemaphyte)." *International Archives of Allergy and Immunology* 109:3 (March 1996), 243-249.

51 "Allergy Medications May Affect Driving More Than Alcohol." *San Francisco Chronicle* (March 7, 2000).

52 E. Vuurman et al. "Seasonal Allergic Rhinitis and Antihistamine Effects on Children's Learning." *Annals of Allergy* 71 (1993), 121.

53 John W. Georgitis, M.D. "Asthma Therapy: What's New and Is it Necessarily Better?" *Chest* 112 (July 1997), 3-5.

54 Suzanne Crowley et al. "Collagen Metabolism and Growth in Prepubertal Children with Asthma Treated with Inhaled Steroids." *Journal of Pediatrics* 132 (March 1998), 409-413.

55 Barry Zimmerman, M.D., et al. "Adrenal Suppression in Two Patients with Asthma Treated with Low Doses of the Inhaled Steriod Fluticasone Porpionate." *Journal of Allergy and Clinical Immunology* 101:3 (March 1998), 425-526.

56 Richard N. Firshein, D.O. *Reversing Asthma* (New York: Warner Books, 1996), 103-108.

57 Samy Suissa, Ph.D., and Pierre Ernst, M.D. "Albuterol in Mild Asthma." *New England Journal of Medicine* 336:10 (March 6, 1997), 729.

58 John W. Georgitis, M.D. "Asthma Therapy: What's New and Is it Necessarily Better?" *Chest* 112 (July l997), 3-5.

## Chapter 12

### Homeopathic and Physical Therapies

1 Ryszard Matusiewicz, M.D. "The Effect of a Homeopathic Preparation on the Clinical Condition of Patients with Corticosteriod-Dependent Bronchial Asthma." *Biomedical Therapy* 15:3 (1997), 70-74.

2 Ryszard Matusiewicz, M.D. "The Homeopathic Treatment of Corticosteroid-Dependent Asthma: A Double-Blind, Placebo-Controlled Study." *Biomedical Therapy* 15:4 (1997), 117-112.

3 R. Ludtke and M. Wiesenauer. "A Meta-Analysis of Homeopathic Treatment of Pollinosis with Galphimia glauca." *Wiener Medizinische Wochenschrift* 147:14 (1997), 323-327. See also: M. Wiesenauer and W. Gaus. "Double-Blind Trial Comparing the Effectiveness of the Homeopathic Preparation Galphimia Potentiation D6, Galphimia Dilution 10(-6) and Placebo on Pollinosis." *Arzneimittle-Forschung* 35:11 (1985), 1745-1747.

4 M. Wiesenauer et al. "Treatment of Pollinosis with Homeopathic Preparation Galphimia glauca." *Allergologie* 10 (1990), S359-S363.

5 K.H. Friese et al. "The Homeopathic Treatment

of Otitis Media in Children—Comparisons with Conventional Therapy." *International Journal of Clinical Pharmacology and Therapeutics* 35:7 (July 1997), 296-301.

6 M. Weiser, L.H. Gegenheimer, and P. Klein. "A Randomized Equivalence Trial Comparing the Efficacy and Safety of *Luffa comp.*-Heel Nasal Spray with Cromolyn Sodium Spray in the Treatment of Seasonal Allergic Rhinitis." *Fortschritte der Komplementarmed* 6:3 (June 1999), 142-148.

7 J.W. Georgitis. "Nasal Hyperthermia and Simple Irrigation for Perennial Rhinitis: Changes in Inflammatory Mediators." *Chest* 106:5 (1994), 1487-1492.

8 Excerpted from "Buffered Hypertonic Saline Nasal Irrigation." Advance/PA (March 1995), 13.

9 J.W. Georgitis. "Nasal Hyperthermia and Simple Irrigation for Perennial Rhinitis: Changes in Inflammatory Mediators." *Chest* 106:5 (1994), 1487-1492.

10 S. Andersson and T. Lundeberg. "Acupuncture—From Empiricism to Science: Functional Background to Acupuncture Effects in Pain and Disease." *Medical Hypotheses* 45:3 (September 1995), 271-281.

11 X. Lai. "Observation on the Curative Effect of Acupuncture on Type 1 Allergic Diseases." *Journal of Traditional Chinese Medicine* 13:4 (December 1993), 243-248.

12 W. Zwolfer et al. "Beneficial Effect of Acupuncture on Adult Patients with Asthma Bronchiale." *American Journal of Chinese Medicine* 21:2 (1993), 113-117.

13 R.A. Aleksandrova et al. "Bronchial Nonspecific Reactivity in Patients with Bronchial Asthma and the Preasthmatic State and Its Alteration Under the Influence of Acupuncture." *Terapevticheskii Arkhiv* 67:8 (1995), 42-45.

14 Y. Yang et al. "Studies on Regulatory Effects of Acupuncture on Mucosal Secretory IgA in Patients with Allergic Asthma." *Chen Tzu Yen Chiu Acupuncture Research* 20:2 (1995), 68-70.

15 E. Wolkenstein and F. Horak. "Protective Effect of Acupuncture on Allergen Provoked Rhinitis." *Wiener Medizinische Wochenschrift* 148:19 (1998), 450-453.

16 R.L Zhou and J.C. Zhang. "Desensitive Treatment with Positive Allergens in Acupoints of the Head for Allergic Rhinitis and Its Mechanism." *Chung Hsi I Chieh Ho Tsa Chih Chinese Journal of Modern Developments in Traditional Medicine* 11:12 (December 1991), 721-723.

17 C.J. Chen and H.S. Yu. "Acupuncture Treatment of Urticaria." *Archives of Dermatology* 134:11 (November 1998), 1397-1399.

18 B.B. Arnetz et al. "A Nonconventional Approach to the Treatment of 'Environmental Illness.'" *Journal of Occupational and Environmental Medicine* 37:3 (July 1995), 838-844.

19 *What Doctors Don't Tell You* 7:2 (May 1996), 11.

## Chapter 13

### Desensitizing the Immune System

1 L. Klimek, A.B. Reske-Kunz, and J. Saloga. "Theories on the Mode of Action of Desensitization." *Wiener Medizinische Wochenschrift* 149:14-15 (1999), 415-420.

2 F. Erel et al. "Effects of Allergen Immunotherapy on the Nasal Mucosa in Patients with Allergic Rhinitis." *Journal of Investigational Allergology and Clinical Immunology* 10:1 (January/February 2000), 14-19.

3 R.M. Naclerio et al. "A Double-Blind Study of the Discontinuation of Ragweed Immunotherapy." *Journal of Allergy and Clinical Immunology* 100:3 (September 1997), 293-300.

4 S.R. Durham et al. "Long-Term Clinical Efficacy of Grass-Pollen Immunotherapy." *New England Journal of Medicine* 341:7 (August 12, 1999), 468-475.

5 H. Yuksel et al. "Sublingual Immunotherapy and Influence on Urinary Leukotrienes in Seasonal Pediatric Allergy." *Journal of Investigational Allergology and Clinical Immunology* 9:5 (September/October 1999), 305-313. See also: D. Mungan, Misirligil, and

L. Gurbuz. "Comparison of the Efficacy of Subcutaneous and Sublingual Immunotherapy in Mite-Sensitive Patients with Rhinitis and Asthma—A Placebo Controlled Study." *Annals of Allergy, Asthma, and Immunology* 82:5 (May 1999), 485-490.

6 R.L. Zhou and J.C. Zhang. "Desensitive Treatment with Positive Allergens in Acupoints of the Head for Allergic Rhinitis and Its Mechanism." *Chung His I Chieh Ho Tsa Chih* 11:12 (December 1991), 721-723.

7 Martha M. Christy. *Your Own Perfect Medicine* (Scottsdale, AZ: Future Medicine, 1994), 28.

8 C.W.M. Wilson, M.D., and A. Lewis, M.D. "Autoimmune Bucal Urine Therapy (AIBUT) Against Human Allergic Disease: A Physiologic Self-Defense Mechanism." Law Hospital in Scotland (1983).

## Chapter 14

### Mind/Body Approaches to Allergy

1 M. Scofield. *Work Site Health Promotion* (Philadelphia: Hanley & Belfus, 1990), 459.

2 Timothy D. Schellhardt. "Company Memo to Stressed-Out Employees: 'Deal With It'." *The Wall Street Journal* (October 2, 1996).

3 J.L. Marx. "The Immune System 'Belongs to the Body'." *Science* 277 (1985), 1190-1192.

4 M. Lekander. "The Immune System is Affected by Psychological Factors. High Stress Levels Can Changes Susceptibility to Infection and Allergy." *Lakartidningen* 3:96 (November 1996), 4807-4811.

5 Hans Selye, M.D. *Stress Without Distress* (New York: New American Library, 1975). J.D. Beasley and J. Swift. *Kellogg Report: The Impact of Nutrition, Environment, and Lifestyle on the Health of Americans* (Annandale-on-Hudson, NY: Institute of Health Policy and Practice, The Bard College Center, 1989).

6 Devi S. Nambudripad, D.C., L.Ac., R.N., Ph.D. *Say Goodbye To Illness* (Buena Park, CA: Delta Publishing, 1993), 8.

7 Arthur Guyton, M.D. *Textbook of Medical Physiology 7th Edition* (Philadelphia: W.B. Saunders, 1986), 910.

8 S. Schmidt-Traub and K.J. Bamler. "Psychoimmunologic Correlation Between Allergies, Panic and Agoraphobia." *Zeitschrift fur Klinische Psychologie, Psychopathologie und Psychotherapie* 40:4 (1992), 325-345.

9 H.R. Wong and J.R. Wispe. "The Stress Response and the Lung." *American Journal of Physiology* 273:1 Part 1 (July 1997), L1-L9.

10 S. Rietveld, I. Van Beest, and W. Everaerd. "Stress-Induced Breathlessness in Asthma." *Psychological Medicine* 29:6 (November 1999), 1359-1366.

11 Stress Management Strategies Benefit Some Asthmatics." *Modern Medicine* 65 (December, 1997), 42-43.

12 J. Chihara. "Stress and Immunoallergy." *Rinsho Byori Japanese Journal of Clinical Pathology* 46:6 (June 1998), 587-592.

13 David A. Mrazek. "Psychological Aspects in Children and Adolescents." *Asthma* 148 (1997), 2177-2183.

14 R. Bussing, R.C. Burket, and E.T. Kelleher. "Prevalence of Anxiety Disorders in Clinic-Based Sample of Pediatric Asthma Patients." *Psychosomatics* 37:2 (March 1996), 108-115.

15 A. Kodama. "Effect of Stress on Atopic Dermatitis: Investigation in Patients after the Great Hanshin Earthquake." *Journal of Allergy and Clinical Immunology* 104:1 (July 1999), 173-176.

16 L.K. Singh et al. "Acute Immobilization Stress Triggers Skin Mast Cell Degranulation Via Corticotropin Releasing Hormone, Neurotensin, and Substance P: A Link to Neurogenic Skin Disorders." *Brain, Behavior, and Immunity* 13:3 (September 1999), 225-239.

17 A. Buske-Kirschbaum et al. "Attenuated Free Cortisol Response to Psychosocial Stress in Children with Atopic Dermatitis." *Psychosomatic Medicine* 59:4 (July/August 1997), 419-426.

18 F.S. Dhabhar. "Stress-Induced Enhancement of Cell-Mediated Immunity." *Annals of the New York Academy of Sciences* 840 (May 1, 1998), 359-372.

19 I.R. Bell et al. "Early Life Stress, Negative Paternal Relationships, and Chemical Intolerance in Middle-Aged Women: Support for Neural Sensitization Models." *Journal of Women's Health* 7:9 (November 1998), 1135-1147.

20 P.L. Ooi and K.T. Goh. "Sick Building Syndrome: An Emerging Stress-Related Disorder?" *International Journal of Epidemiology* 26:6 (December 1997), 1243-1249.

21 Brian Tracy. *The Psychology of Achievement* (Niles, IL: Nightingale-Conant Corporation, 1987), 4.

22 B.B. Arnetz et al. "Endocrine and Dermatological Concomitants of Mental Stress." *Acta Dermato-Venereologica Supplementum* 156 (1991), 9-12.

23 "Stress Management Strategies Benefit Some Asthmatics." *Modern Medicine* 65 (December 1997), 42-43.

24 J.M. Smyth et al. "Effects of Writing About Stressful Experiences on Symptom Reduction in Patients with Asthma or Rheumatoid Arthritis: A Randomized Trial." *Journal of the American Medical Association* 281:14 (April 14, 1999), 1304-1309.

25 R. A. Chalmers et al., eds. *Scientific Research on Maharishi's Transcendental Meditation and TM-Sidih Program: Collected Papers*, Vol. 2-4 (Vlodrop, Netherlands: Maharishi Vedic University Press, 1989).

26 R.K. Wallace et al. "Physiological Effects of Transcendental Meditation." *Science* 167 (1970), 1751-1754. M.C. Dillbeck et al. "Physiological Differences between TM and Rest." *American Physiologist* 42 (1987), 879-881.

27 R. W. Cranson et al. "Transcendental Meditation and Improved Performance on Intelligence-Related Measures: A Longitudinal Study." *Personality and Individual Differences* 12 (1991), 1105-1116.

28 D.H. Shapiro and R.N. Walsh. *Meditation: Classic and Contemporary Perspectives* (New York: Aldine, 1984).

29 Shad Helmsetter, Ph.D. *What to Say When You Talk To Yourself* (Scottsdale, AZ: Grindle Press/Audio, 1986).

30 R. Dilts and T. Hallbom. *Beliefs: Pathways to Health and Well-Being* (Portland, OR: Metamorphous Press, 1990), 1-2.

31 The Burton Goldberg Group. *Alternative Medicine: The Definitive Guide* (Tiburon, CA: Future Medicine Publishing, 1995), 77.

32 Leon Chaitow, N.D., D.O. *Amino Acids in Therapy: A Guide to the Therapeutic Application of Protein Constituents* (Wellingborough, Northhamptonshire, England: Thorsens, 1985), 50-61.

33 T.M. Laidlaw, R.J. Booth, and R.G. Large. "Reduction in Skin Reactions to Histamine after a Hypnotic Procedure." *Psychosomatic Medicine* 58:3 (May/June 1996), 242-248.

34 N. Miller. "Learning of Visceral and Glandular Responses." *Science* 163:866 (January 1969), 434-445, 627.

35 A. Madrid et al. "Subjective Assessment of Allergy Relief Following Group Hypnosis and Self-Hypnosis: A Preliminary Study." *American Journal of Clinical Hypnosis* 38:2 (October 1995), 80-86.

36 The Burton Goldberg Group. *Alternative Medicine: The Definitive Guide* (Tiburon, CA: Future Medicine Publishing, 1995), 245.

37 Patrick Fanning. *Visualization for Change* (Oakland, CA: New Harbinger Publications, 1994), 271-273.

38 Steven Foster. *101 Medicinal Herbs* (Loveland, CO: Interweave Press, 1998).

39 R. McCraty et al. "The Impact of a New Emotional Self-Management Program on Stress, Emotions, Heart Rate Variability, DHEA, and Cortisol." *Integrative Physiological and Behavioral Science* 33:2 (April-June 1998), 151-170.

40 R. McCraty et al. "The Impact of an Emotional Self-Management Skills Course on Psychosocial Functioning and Autonomic Recovery to Stress in Middle School Children." *Integrative Physiological and Behavioral Science* 34:4 (October-December 1999), 246-268.

41 R. McCraty et al. "The Effects of Emotions on Short-term Power Spectrum of Heart Rate Variability." *American Journal of Cardiology* 76:14 (November 15, 1995), 1089-093.

42 Doc Childre and Howard Martin with Donna
   Beech. *The HeartMath Solution* (San
   Francisco: Harper San Francisco, 1999), 67.

43 J.W. Turner, Ph.D., and T.H. Fine, Ph.D.
   "Flotation/REST Used in the Treatment of
   Arthritis Pain." A paper presented at the
   Fourth Annual International Conference on
   REST, Washington, D.C. (1990). Roderick A.
   Borrie, Ph.D., et al. "Flotation/REST for the
   Management of Rheumatoid Arthritis."
   *Proceedings of the Ninth Annual Conference
   on Interdisciplinary Health Care* (Stony
   Brook, NY: SAHP/SUNY, 1988), 277-282.
   T.H. Fine and J.W. Turner, Jr. "Flotation REST
   and Chronic Pain." Presented at the
   International Congress of Psychology,
   Acapulco, Mexico (1984).

44 Peter Suedfeld, Ph.D., et al. "Water
   Immersion and Flotation: From Stress
   Experiment to Stress Treatment." *Journal of
   Environmental Psychology* 3 (1983), 147-
   155.

45 T.H. Fine, Ph.D., and J. W. Turner, Jr., Ph.D.
   "The Effect of Flotation/REST on EMG
   Biofeedback and Plasma Cortisol." In: T.S.
   Fine and J.W. Turner, Jr., eds. *Proceedings of
   the First International Conference on REST
   and Self Regulation* (Toledo, OH: IRIS,
   1985), 148-155.

46 Based on clinical observations of Eugene R.
   Zampieron, N.D., A.H.G., Naturopathic
   Medical Center, Middlebury, CT (1993-
   1998).

47 R.B. Tisserand. *The Art of Aromatherapy*
   (Rochester, VT: Healing Arts Press, 1977).

48 Ibid.

49 G.H. Dodd. "Receptor Events in Perfumery."
   In: S. van Toller and G. H. Dodd, eds.
   *Perfumery: The Psychology and Biology of
   Fragrance* (London: Chapman and Hall,
   1988).

50 J. Steele. "Brain Research and Essential Oils."
   *Aromatherapy Quarterly* 3 (Spring 1984), 5.

51 "Aromatherapy on the Wards: Lavender Beats
   Benzodiazepines." *International Journal of
   Aromatherapy* 1:2 (1988), 1.

52 Hoon Ryu et al. "Effect of Qigong Training on
   Proportions of T Lymphocyte Subsets in
   Human Peripheral Blood." *American Journal

of Chinese Medicine* 23:1 (1995), 27-36.

53 Eugene Zampieron, N.D., A.H.G. Interview
   with Ameni Harris on WPKN, 89.5 FM's "The
   Natural House Call" (May 1998).

54 W. Gruber et al. "Alternative Medicine and
   Bronchial Asthma—A Review from a Pediatric
   Perspective." *Monatsschrift Kinderheilkunde*
   145 (1997), 786-796.

55 P.K. Vendanthan et al. "Clinical Study of Yoga
   Techniques in University Students with
   Asthma: A Controlled Study." *Allergy &
   Asthma Proceedings* 19:1
   (January/February 1998), 3-9.

# Index

impaired, 88, 220, 264
intestinal, 67, 212–19
liver, 88, 219–23
mercury, 154, 155–56
organs for, 49, 56, 212
overload. *See* Toxic overload
respiratory system, 276–77
skin, 257–58
strategies, 65
Detoxification Profile, 88
DHEA (dehydroepiandrosterone), 101, 104, 248
Diagnosis, 65, 279. *See also* Tests and testing
Diet, 38. *See also* Foods; Nutrition
for allergy testing, 82–83, 158
anti-asthma, 268
anti-fungal, 182–83, 281
anti-parasitic, 233
children's, 110, 118
for detoxification, 156
EFAs in, 289
elimination, 158, 174–76
healthful, 64, 106, 122–26
for leaky gut, 188–90
for liver support, 221–22
poor, 57
rotation, 174, 177–78
standard American (SAD), 50, 168, 172
Stone Age, 177–78
sugar in, 63–64
for thyroid support, 196
variety in, 168, 174
vegetarian, 123
Digestion
barrier function of, 45, 184
incomplete. *See* Maldigestion
in infants, 47–48
optimal, 180, 198
process, 214
Digestive dysfunction, 46–52, 89–96. *See also* Maldigestion
Digestive tract, 46, 47, 214–15
function tests, 89–96
healing, 67
tonifying, 200
Disaccharidase, 202–3
Disease. *See* Illness
DMPS Challenge test, 87
Donovan, Patrick, 180
Drugs. *See* Medicines
Dust, 147
Dust mites, 121, 137–38, 147
Dysbiosis, 172
internal, 46, 48–49, 172
intestinal, 89, 90, 216

Ear infections (otitis media), 27, 41, 118, 159–60
homeopathic remedies for, 309–10, 315–17
treatments, 279
Eck, Paul C., 62
Eczema, 16, 17, 30–31

bacteria and, 244
case studies, 239–42, 345–46
causes of, 41, 107
foods and, 238
inhalant allergies and, 239
tendency toward, 15
treatments, 251
triggers, 31
Edelson, Stephen B., 257, 258, 331, 333–34
Edema (swelling), 21
EDP (enzyme-potentiated desensitization), 68, 331–34
EDS. *See* Electrodermal screening
EDTA Lead Versonate 24-Hour Urine Collection test, 87
EFAs. *See* Essential fatty acids
Egger, Joseph, 162
Electrodermal screening (EDS), 77–80, 83
information gathering via, 342, 343
for parasite testing, 99
for reaction prevention, 117–18
ELISA (enzyme-linked immunoserological assay) test, 75–76
Endocrine glands, 45, 61, 63
Endocrine system, 60
Endotoxins, 62
Enemas, 216, 217, 219
for parasite removal, 226, 227–28, 229
Energy. *See also* Prana; Qi
adrenal glands and, 63
balancing, 328, 342, 344
as field, 343
flow, 80, 339
Enuresis, 165–66
Environment
detoxifying, 146–52
internal, 93–94, 152–56
outside, 146–47
Environmental illness, 17, 37, 138. *See also* Multiple chemical sensitivity
Environmental medicine, 17, 35, 139
Enzyme deficiencies, 36, 51–52, 200
testing for, 101–4
Enzyme-potentiated desensitization (EPD), 68, 331–34
Enzymes, 51, 101
digestive, 47, 200–203
functions of, 201
sources of, 51, 201
supplementing, 210
Eosinophils, 25
EPD (enzyme-potentiated desensitization), 68, 331–34
Ephedra, 292
Epidermis, 54, 236
Epilepsy, 21
Epinephrine (adrenaline), 32, 101, 280, 351
Essential fatty acids (EFAs), 53
deficiencies, 287
defined, 100, 127, 243, 287
in diet, 286–91
metabolism of, 64

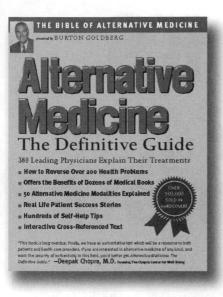

**THE BIBLE OF ALTERNATIVE MEDICINE**

presented by BURTON GOLDBERG

# Alternative Medicine
## The Definitive Guide

380 Leading Physicians Explain Their Treatments

- How to Reverse Over 200 Health Problems
- Offers the Benefits of Dozens of Medical Books
- 50 Alternative Medicine Modalities Explained
- Real Life Patient Success Stories
- Hundreds of Self-Help Tips
- Interactive Cross-Referenced Text

OVER 500,000 SOLD IN HARDCOVER!

"This book is long overdue. Finally, we have an authoritative text which will be a resource to both patients and health-care providers. If you are interested in alternative medicine of any kind, and want the security of authenticity in this field, you'd better get *Alternative Medicine: The Definitive Guide*." —Deepak Chopra, M.D. Founder, The Chopra Center For Well Being

Millions of people are searching for a better way to health—this is the book they're reaching for. *Alternative Medicine: The Definitive Guide* is an absolute must for anyone interested in the latest information on how to get healthy and stay that way.

At 1,100 pages, this encyclopedia puts all the schools of alternative medicine—50 different therapies—under one roof.

The *Guide* is packed with lifesaving information and alternative treatments from 380 of the world's leading alternative physicians. Our contributors give you the safest, most affordable, and most effective remedies for over 200 serious health conditions.

From cancer to obesity, heart disease to PMS, the *Guide* gives you dozens of actual patient stories and physician treatments to show you how this medicine really works.

The *Guide* does something no other health book has ever done. It combines the best clinical information from doctors with the most practical self-help remedies all in a format that is easy-to-read, practical, and completely user-friendly.

The *Guide* gives you the knowledge you need today so you can make intelligent choices about the future of your health.

# TO ORDER, CALL 800-841-BOOK

# BOOKS *your* *health* depends on

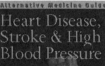

### Alternative Medicine Guide

## Heart Disease, Stroke & High Blood Pressure

**Heart Problems Can Be Prevented and Reversed Using Clinically Proven Alternative Therapies**

» Hold the Angioplasty
...Cancel the Bypass
» Avoid Heart Attack
» Reverse Stroke Damage
» Lower Your Blood Pressure
» Overcome Cholesterol's
Deadly Effects

*BURTON GOLDBERG*

---

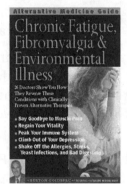

### Alternative Medicine Guide

## Chronic Fatigue, Fibromyalgia & Environmental Illness

26 Doctors Show You How They Reverse These Conditions with Clinically Proven Alternative Therapies

» Say Goodbye to Muscle Pain
» Regain Your Vitality
» Peak Your Immune System
» Climb Out of Your Depression
» Shake Off the Allergies, Stress,
Yeast Infections, and Bad Digestion

*BURTON GOLDBERG*

---

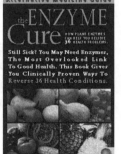

### Alternative Medicine Guide

## the ENZYME Cure

HOW PLANT ENZYMES CAN HELP YOU RELIEVE 36 HEALTH PROBLEMS.

**Still Sick? You May Need Enzymes, The Most Overlooked Link To Good Health. This Book Gives You Clinically Proven Ways To Reverse 36 Health Conditions.**

---

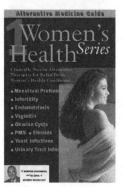

### Alternative Medicine Guide

## 1 Women's Health *Series*

Clinically Proven Alternative Therapies for Relief From Women's Health Conditions

» Menstrual Problems
» Infertility
» Endometriosis
» Vaginitis
» Ovarian Cysts
» PMS » Fibroids
» Yeast Infections
» Urinary Tract Infections

---

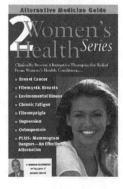

### Alternative Medicine Guide

## 2 Women's Health *Series*

Clinically Proven Alternative Therapies for Relief From Women's Health Conditions...

» Breast Cancer
» Fibrocystic Breasts
» Environmental Illness
» Chronic Fatigue
» Fibromyalgia
» Depression
» Osteoporosis
» PLUS: Mammogram
Dangers—An Effective
Alternative

---

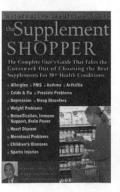

### Alternative Medicine Guide

## the Supplement SHOPPER

The Complete User's Guide That Takes the Guesswork Out of Choosing the Best Supplements For 50+ Health Conditions.

» Allergies » PMS » Asthma » Arthritis
» Colds & Flu » Prostate Problems
» Depression » Sleep Disorders
» Weight Problems
» Detoxification, Immune
Support, Brain Power
» Heart Disease
» Menstrual Problems
» Children's Illnesses
» Sports Injuries

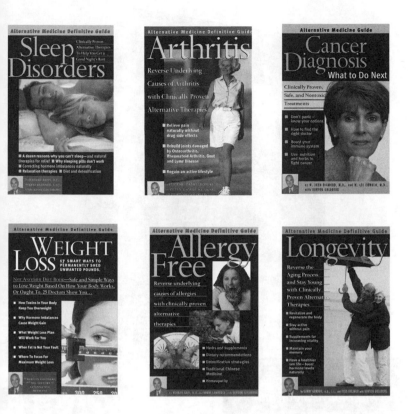

These titles are part of our *Alternative Medicine Guide* paperback series—healing-edge advice that may mean the difference between sickness and robust health. We distill the advice of hundreds of leading alternative physicians from all disciplines and put it into a consumer-helpful format—medical knowledge without the jargon. Essential reading before—or instead of—your next doctor's visit. Because you need to know your medical alternatives.

## To order, call 800-841-BOOK or visit www.alternativemedicine.com. You can also find our books at your local health food store or bookstore.

MAINTAINING MALE SEXUAL VITALITY ■ ANTI-AGING SKIN REPAIR

# Alternative Medicine

The Voice of Alternative Medicine®

Detect Breast Cancer Years Earlier

Bach Flower Essences
Easing Life's Difficulties

Everything You
Wanted to Know About
PROGESTERONE
CREAMS

Metabolic Typing—
The Latest Skinny on LOSING WEIGHT

Your Thyroid Might Be
Low, After All

How Mammography
Causes Cancer

ISSUE 31
1999

TIPS TO BEAT INSOMNIA ■ HEALTHY HAUTE CUISINE

# Alternative Medicine

Saving Sight
Beating the Macular
Degeneration Epidemic

The Voice of Alternative Medicine

WHAT IS
Naturopathy?
And What Is Not

The Threat
of Meat
Irradiation

BioPulse
An Extraordinary Clinic for
Degenerative Diseases

Heart Health Breakthrough
The End of Bypass Surgery Is in Sight

Anti-Cancer Foods
What's New in Medicine
Don't Poison Your Pet

We digest it for you—
*Alternative Medicine
Magazine* tracks the entire
field—all the doctor's jour-
nals, research, confer-
ences, and newsletters.
Then we summarize what
is essential for you to
know to get better and
stay healthy. We're your
one-stop read for what's
new and effective in
alternative medicine.

# TO ORDER,
# CALL 800-841-BOOK

# THE BOOK
# THAT EVERYONE WITH
# CANCER NEEDS

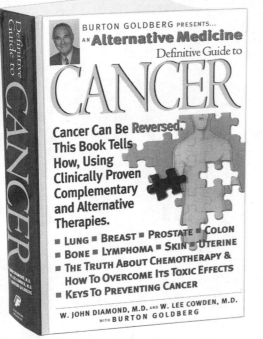

There has never been a book like this about cancer. The message is simple, direct, and lifesaving: cancer can be successfully reversed using alternative medicine. This book shows how.

The clinical proof is in the words and recommendations of 37 leading physicians who treat and restore life to thousands of cancer patients. Read 55 documented patient case histories and see how alternative approaches to cancer can make the difference between life and death. Learn about the 33 contributing causes to cancer.

These doctors bring to alternative cancer care decades of careful study and practice. They know that there is no magic bullet cure for cancer. They also know that many factors contribute to the development of cancer and many modalities and substances must be used to reverse it.

Hardcover ■ ISBN 1-887299-01-7 ■ 6" x 9" ■ 1,200 pages

# TO ORDER, CALL 800-841-BOOK